"Interesting, well written, and totally reliable. Warmly recommended as a comprehensive guide to what is currently known about the effects of lifestyle and diet on women's health. The Nurses' Health Study demonstrates how sound, sustained epidemiological investigation can lead to important new medical information and better health."
—Marcia Angell, M.D., and Arnold S. Relman, M.D., former editors in chief, *New England Journal of Medicine*

"We all make choices every day that affect our health and well-being. Of all the source books available to guide women in making sound choices, this is the one to trust. It's comprehensive, readable, consistent, and grounded in years of careful and sophisticated research. It is the definitive text on how we can maximize our chances of living healthy and full lives."
—Diana Chapman Walsh, Ph.D., president of Wellesley College

"The contributions of the Nurses' Health Study to our understanding of women's health issues and the development of chronic diseases like heart disease, cancer, and diabetes are unsurpassed. This outstanding book brings together these seminal research results, providing understandable descriptions about the meaning of these research findings and clear messages about the implications for all women. This book accomplishes its purpose stunningly, by making sense of the research results and providing guidance for women on which aspects of a healthy lifestyle will lead to a healthier life."
—Leslie Bernstein, Ph.D., Keck School of Medicine, University of Southern California

# Healthy Women, Healthy Lives

*A Guide to Preventing Disease
from the Landmark Nurses' Health Study*

A HARVARD MEDICAL SCHOOL BOOK

SENIOR EDITORS

Susan E. Hankinson, R.N., Sc.D.

Graham A. Colditz, M.D., Dr.P.H.

JoAnn E. Manson, M.D., Dr.P.H.

Frank E. Speizer, M.D.

WRITERS

Hank Dart, M.S.

Catherine Tomeo Ryan, M.P.H.

FIRESIDE

NEW YORK • LONDON • TORONTO • SYDNEY • SINGAPORE

*This book is dedicated to the women in the Nurses' Health Study*

*and the Nurses' Health Study II*

FIRESIDE
Rockefeller Center
1230 Avenue of the Americas
New York, NY 10020

FIRESIDE and colophon are registered trademarks
of Simon & Schuster, Inc.

For information regarding special discounts for bulk purchases, please contact Simon & Schuster
Special Sales at 1-800-456-6798 or business@simonandschuster.com

DESIGNED BY KEVIN HANEK

Manufactured in the United States of America

10  9  8  7  6  5  4  3  2  1

The Library of Congress has cataloged the Simon & Schuster Source edition as follows:
Healthy women, healthy lives: a guide to preventing disease from the landmark Nurses'
Health Study / senior editors, Susan E. Hankinson . . . [et al.].
    p.  cm.
"A Harvard Medical School book."
Includes bibliographical references and index.
    1. Women—Diseases—Prevention.   2. Women—Health and hygiene.   I. Hankinson,
Susan E.
RG121 .H435     2001
613'.04244—dc21        2001034154

ISBN 0-684-85519-4
    0-7432-1774-8 (Pbk)

# Acknowledgments

THE NURSES' HEALTH STUDY had its origins in 1967 when Drs. Martin Vessey and Frank Speizer shared an office in the Statistical Research Unit of the Medical Research Council of Great Britain in London. They were receiving reports about healthy young women who were using birth control pills and having episodes of blood clots in their legs. The doctors became concerned that there was no mechanism in place to study the long-term consequences of what was potentially a powerful drug being given to healthy women. Together they devised several schemes to identify cohorts of women that could be followed prospectively. Dr. Speizer returned to the United States and began the study we summarize in this book.

This undertaking would not have been possible without the support and efforts of many very talented co-investigators. From the beginning, the project needed leaders who both learned on the job and provided their own expertise to improve the effort. Under Dr. Speizer's direction, the first of these was Charles Hennekens, who became involved in 1975 and helped launch the first mailings to the nurses. He continued for many years, focusing mainly on cardiovascular outcomes and eventually rising to the rank of professor at Harvard Medical School. He was followed by Christopher Bain, a talented Australian who is now professor of epidemiology in the Department of Social and Preventive Medicine at the University of Queensland. Walter Willett became the next project director, and it was during his period of involvement that the diet portion of the questionnaires was developed, tested, and validated. He has remained actively involved in the study despite taking on more administrative duties as professor and chairman of the Department of Nutrition at the Harvard School of Public Health. Under his leadership, we expanded the effort in 1989 to include a second cohort of over 116,000 nurses who are now participants in the Nurses' Health Study II. We concurrently expanded both studies to include a wide variety of lifestyle issues that might affect the health of middle-aged women. Finally, and for the longest period, Graham Colditz assumed the directorship; he continues as project director and has recently assumed the role of principal investigator of the Nurses' Health Study. From the beginning of the study, we have had the active involvement of Bernard Rosner, a most able statistician, who in the early days helped devise the analytical tools needed to deal with the large volume of data being collected.

Many other investigators have been involved with the study, some staying for only a few years. They have helped by taking on specific research tasks and have learned by being part of the team effort. Over forty-five individuals have received graduate degrees from Harvard University for the intellectual contributions they made while working with the Nurses' Heath Study. In addition, visiting scientists from other institutions have joined us for periods of up to two years to work on some of the data. Others have identified specific research components in which they have assumed senior leadership roles in developing the intellectual structure that has made the Nurses' Health Study a successful scientific enterprise.

In bringing together this summary of the data from the Nurses' Health Study, we have benefited greatly from the outstanding talents of the current group of investigators involved in the study. Each participated by helping to collect the background data for a particular chapter and by reviewing the initial drafts of that chapter. We have identified them as contributing editors. The authors are indebted to these individuals for their superb work. However, we must take full responsibility for the way in which the final versions of the summaries are presented in this book.

We have been fortunate to have an exceptional staff working on the study, a few members for as many as twenty-five years. Barbara Egan, who coordinates documentation of newly reported illnesses among the nurses, has been with the study since its inception. Gary Chase has been responsible for the development of the questionnaire formatting, mailing, and processing, and for keeping track of the many thousands of address changes that have occurred over the last twenty-five years. And the management of all of these data would have been much more difficult without the able talents of Karen Corsano and her group of well-trained data managers and programmers.

Several other institutions and individuals must be mentioned. First and foremost has been the public financial support supplied through the offices of the National Institutes of Health (NIH), mostly from the National Cancer Institute. We have had the good fortune to work most directly with two project officers over all these years, Drs. Genrose Copley and Joe Patel. We have also had federal support from other institutes in NIH that have funded our efforts to study diseases other than cancer. Over the years, we have received funds from private and other nonprofit agencies, both to aid in the testing of specific hypotheses unrelated to our NIH support and to generally support the Nurses'

Health Study effort. Some of this financial assistance has actually come from the nurses themselves. At the suggestion of the nurses who attended the Twentieth Anniversary Symposium of the Nurses' Health Study, we established the Friends of the Nurses' Health Study Fund at Harvard University to support educational and research activities related to the study.

This book would not have been possible without the able direction and support of Dr. Tony Komaroff and his talented assistants, particularly Matthew Brim, at Harvard Health Publications and, through his office, the support of Simon & Schuster. Not only did Dr. Komaroff handle the administrative issues related to this project, but he was also an invaluable editor of each chapter and regularly attended the editorial review meetings.

We must also thank our respective families who sacrificed time with us so that we could complete the many reviews and meetings that went well beyond our usual work days.

Finally, none of this would have been possible without the sustained and outstanding contributions and commitment of the women who make up the Nurses' Health Study. It has been their devotion and trust that has made this study possible, and it is with this in mind that we dedicate *Healthy Women, Healthy Lives* to them.

Susan E. Hankinson, R.N., Sc.D.
Graham A. Colditz, M.D., Dr.P.H.
JoAnn E. Manson, M.D., Dr.P.H.
Frank E. Speizer, M.D.
June 2001

# Contents

# Introduction

I T IS WITH GREAT PLEASURE that I introduce the Nurses' Health Study, which I consider to be one of the most significant studies ever conducted on the health of women. *Healthy Women, Healthy Lives* summarizes in easy-to-understand language what has been learned about how women can reduce the risk of developing diseases that cause great suffering and premature death.

There is no better time to reflect on what we have learned about women's health than now. Just a hundred years ago, an American woman was lucky to live beyond her forty-eighth birthday. She was often considered too physically fragile to get a higher education, let alone enter the workforce. Public health interventions, including better sanitation practices, immunizations, and improved childbirth techniques, have helped give women an extra thirty years of life.

But while women's health has moved ahead, our understanding of it has too often lagged behind. Twenty-five years ago, medical researchers became painfully aware of the dearth of information on the disease process in woman. With remarkable vision, scientists at Harvard Medical School recognized that the answers could only be found with meticulous research spanning not years but decades. Knowing that nursing professionals were among those likely to be most conscientious in their participation, these scientists launched the Nurses' Health Study in 1976.

The Nurses' Health Study has since become the longest-running and the largest prospective observational study of women's health ever conducted. Even more, it has laid the foundation for subsequent clinical trials on a variety of women's health questions. It currently includes more than 120,000 women who have been participants for more than two decades.

This volume presents information on a woman's probability of developing specific diseases and suggests how that probability may change with certain alterations in diet, weight control, physical activity, and other lifestyle changes. It tackles some of the most difficult and confusing health questions, including postmenopausal hormones, the risk of Alzheimer's disease, the risk of breast and ovarian cancers, and obstacles to exercise. The authors also offer specific lifestyle programs that can help encourage and empower women to make positive health choices.

The U.S. Department of Health and Human Services, through the National Institutes of Health, is proud to have been instrumental in supporting the Nurses' Health Study. This research is now being complemented by the NIH Women's Health Initiative (WHI), a fifteen-year clinical study of the effects of postmenopausal hormones, a low fat diet, and calcium and other dietary supplements on postmenopausal women's health. The WHI also encompasses an observational study and a community prevention study.

These and other research initiatives may yield results exceeding the greatest hopes of the first researchers at Harvard a quarter century ago. Today, at the dawn of the most technologically advanced era the world has ever known, the possibilities for women are endless. Women today are likely to live forty years after their reproductive time has passed. And as we learn more about the prevention and treatment of many diseases, women will live even longer and healthier lives.

This new era has also produced a deluge of information about women's health, not all of it accurate. That is why it is critical, when we have come so far in improving women's health care, that we also work to ensure that all women get the accurate, scientifically based health information they need. Fulfilling that mission is made far easier thanks to the research presented here.

Elizabeth Blackwell, the first woman physician in the United States, once said: "It is not easy to be a pioneer . . . but I would not trade it for the world." I would like to commend the leadership and vision of the fine team of scientists who have worked over the years to bring life and meaning to volumes of health data—and to the thousands of women who have participated in the Nurses' Health Study. Their legacy will lay a foundation of better health for generations of American women.

Donna Shalala
President, University of Miami
Former Secretary of U.S. Department of Health and Human Services

# Preface

O VER TWENTY-FIVE YEARS AGO, we started the landmark Nurses' Health Study. Still ongoing, it is one of the largest and longest-running studies of women ever conducted. Thanks to the participation of over 120,000 registered nurses from across the United States, we have been able to gather invaluable information on a wide range of health issues, from the risk factors for cancer and heart disease to the benefits of a diet rich in fruits and vegetables. And the resulting twenty-five plus years' worth of data have been influential in identifying lifestyle choices that women can make to lower their risk of illness and improve their overall health.

In this book, we have used this rich source of data to provide you with a resource for achieving and maintaining good health throughout life. With the Nurses' Health Study as an anchoring point, but also presenting results from other large studies of women, we explore the major diseases and risk factors responsible for the greatest disability and premature death among women in the United States. Throughout, we try to help you make sense of this vast amount of scientific information.

Designed to help you easily find the information you are looking for, *Healthy Women, Healthy Lives* is divided into four distinct sections:

*PART I. GETTING STARTED.* The three chapters in Part I provide important information for getting the most out of *Healthy Women, Healthy Lives.* Chapter 1 offers background information on the history and current state of women's health and discusses the issues women should consider when making their own personal health choices. Chapter 2 discusses the history of the Nurses' Health Study and its contribution to health research, and explains its place among other health studies. Chapter 3 introduces important concepts and provides a key to understanding the levels of risk outlined in Parts II and III.

*PART II. LOWERING THE RISK OF DISEASES.* This section describes in depth the diseases that have the greatest impact on women's health. Each chapter identifies those factors that affect the risk of the disease and then outlines the steps you can take to help lower your risk. Each chapter concludes with recommendations and tips from some of our colleagues at Harvard Medical School who are primary care providers. Drawing on their experiences counseling thousands of patients, they provide their perspectives on making healthy choices and trying to lower the risk of disease.

Beginning with those diseases that have the greatest overall impact on women, we discuss in detail: coronary heart disease, breast cancer, lung cancer, stroke, diabetes, colon cancer, osteoporosis, endometrial cancer, ovarian cancer, and skin cancer. A selection of other diseases—arthritis, eye diseases related to aging (such as cataracts and macular degeneration), Alzheimer's, and asthma—are also included, though in less detail and in a single chapter that concludes this section. Although we have yet to study these latter conditions thoroughly in the Nurses' Health Study, each is very important, and we feel strongly that they should be included in this book, even if only briefly. One obvious absence is a chapter on depression, a serious and relatively common condition in women. Unfortunately we have only very limited data in the study on depression and its risk factors. We are, however, actively collecting such information from our participants and hope to make important contributions to this field in the near future.

PART III. CHANGING BEHAVIORS. This section discusses the major behaviors linked to health and disease in women. Generally ordered by overall importance, these chapters cover: exercise, weight control, smoking, diet, drinking, postmenopausal hormones, birth control pills, and aspirin. Each chapter reviews the major diseases linked to a specific behavior and—as in Part II—includes recommendations and tips for changing behavior from primary care providers.

PART IV. APPENDICES AND GLOSSARY. These provide materials to supplement Parts I through III. The Appendices include three sections. The first discusses in detail the different types of research studies mentioned throughout the book. The second provides tips for becoming an informed consumer of health information, whether from the classic mass media of television, books, magazines, and newspapers, or the new mass media of the Internet and World Wide Web. The third section includes the formulas for calculating body mass index, the glycemic index of selected foods, and a listing of Dietary Reference Intakes. Finally, the glossary defines many of the health and medical terms used throughout *Healthy Women, Healthy Lives.*

We recommend that most women begin by reading the three introductory chapters in Part I before moving on to the rest of the book. The background information they provide will help you get the most out of Parts II and III. If you are already familiar with the Nurses' Health Study and have some knowledge about the workings of health research, you may not need to begin with Part I; however, you may find it to be a valuable refresher if you do. Whatever level of knowledge you bring to *Healthy Women, Healthy Lives*, we have organized the book so that the information is valuable, understandable, and easy to locate. How you use the book will be up to you, but we believe that the information provided can help change the way women behave, and that these behavioral changes can have an impact on healthy lives.

# Contributors

## Senior Editors

**Susan E. Hankinson, R.N., Sc.D.**
Associate Professor of Medicine
Harvard Medical School
Channing Laboratory, Department of Medicine,
Brigham and Women's Hospital
Associate Professor of Epidemiology
Harvard School of Public Health

**Graham A. Colditz, M.D., Dr.P.H.**
Professor of Medicine
Harvard Medical School
Channing Laboratory, Department of Medicine,
Brigham and Women's Hospital

**JoAnn E. Manson, M.D., Dr.P.H.**
Professor of Medicine
Harvard Medical School
Preventive Medicine, Department of Medicine,
Brigham and Women's Hospital

**Frank E. Speizer, M.D.**
Edward H. Kass Professor of Medicine
Harvard Medical School
Channing Laboratory, Department of Medicine,
Brigham and Women's Hospital

# Primary Care Physicians

### Carol Bates, M.D.
Assistant Professor of Medicine
Harvard Medical School
Director of Primary Care Education
Beth Israel Deaconess Medical Center

### Nancy Rigotti, M.D.
Associate Professor of Medicine and Ambulatory Care and Prevention
Harvard Medical School
Director, Tobacco Research and Treatment Center
Massachusetts General Hospital

### Celeste Robb-Nicholson, M.D.
Assistant Professor of Medicine
Harvard Medical School
Associate Physician
Massachusetts General Hospital

# Contributing Editors from the Channing Laboratory

**Robin Blum, S.M.**
Department of Nutrition
Harvard School of Public Health

**Celia Byrne, Ph.D.**
Instructor in Medicine
Harvard Medical School
Associate Epidemiologist,
    Department of Medicine,
    Brigham and Women's Hospital

**Carlos Camargo, Jr., M.D., Dr.P.H.**
Assistant Professor of Medicine
Harvard Medical School
Associate Physician, Department of
    Medicine, Brigham and Women's
    Hospital

**Wendy Chen, M.D., M.P.H.**
Instructor in Medicine
Harvard Medical School
Associate Physician, Department of
    Medicine, Brigham and Women's
    Hospital

**Gary Curhan, M.D., Sc.D.**
Assistant Professor of Medicine
Harvard Medical School
Associate Physician, Department of
  Medicine, Brigham and Women's
  Hospital

**Kathleen Fairfield, M.D., Dr.P.H.**
Instructor in Medicine
Harvard Medical School
Associate Physician, Beth Israel
  Deaconess Medical Center

**Diane Feskanich, Sc.D.**
Instructor in Medicine
Harvard Medical School
Research Fellow, Department of
  Medicine, Brigham and Women's
  Hospital

**Alison Field, Sc.D.**
Assistant Professor of Medicine
Harvard Medical School
Associate Epidemiologist,
  Department of Medicine, Brigham
  and Women's Hospital

**Laurie Fisher, S.M.**
Brigham and Women's Hospital

**Edward Giovannucci, M.D., Sc.D.**
Associate Professor of Medicine
Harvard Medical School
Associate Epidemiologist,
  Department of Medicine, Brigham
  and Women's Hospital

**Francine Grodstein, Sc.D.**
Assistant Professor of Medicine
Harvard Medical School
Associate Epidemiologist,
  Department of Medicine, Brigham
  and Women's Hospital

**Michelle Holmes, M.D., Dr.P.H.**
Assistant Professor of Medicine
Harvard Medical School
Associate Physician, Department of
  Medicine, Brigham and Women's
  Hospital

**Frank Hu, M.D., Ph.D.**
Assistant Professor of Nutrition,
Harvard School of Public Health

**David Hunter, MB.B.S., M.P.H., Sc.D.**
Professor of Epidemiology and
  Nutrition
Harvard School of Public Health
Associate Epidemiologist,
  Department of Medicine, Brigham
  and Women's Hospital

**Ichiro Kawachi, M.D., Ph.D.**
Associate Professor of Health and
  Social Behavior
Harvard School of Public Health
Associate Epidemiologist,
  Department of Medicine, Brigham
  and Women's Hospital

**Laura Kubzansky, Ph.D., M.P.H.**
Assistant Professor of Health and
  Social Behavior
Harvard School of Public Health

**Jing Ma, M.D., Ph.D.**
Assistant Professor of Medicine
Harvard Medical School
Associate Epidemiologist,
    Department of Medicine, Brigham
    and Women's Hospital

**Kathryn Rexrode, M.D., M.P.H.**
Instructor in Medicine
Harvard Medical School
Associate Physician, Department of
    Medicine, Brigham and Women's
    Hospital

**Janet Rich-Edwards, Sc.D., M.P.H.**
Instructor in Medicine
Harvard Medical School

**Beverly Rockhill, Ph.D.**
Instructor in Medicine
Harvard Medical School
Epidemiologist, Department of
    Medicine, Brigham and Women's
    Hospital

**Bernard Rosner, Ph.D.**
Professor of Medicine (Biostatistics)
Harvard Medical School
Senior Biostatistician, Department
    of Medicine, Brigham and
    Women's Hospital

**P. J. Skerrett**
Brigham and Women's Hospital

**Caren Solomon, M.D., M.P.H.**
Assistant Professor of Medicine
Harvard Medical School
Associate Physician, Department of
    Medicine, Brigham and Women's
    Hospital

**Meir Stampfer, M.D., Dr.P.H.**
Professor of Epidemiology and
    Nutrition
Harvard School of Public Health
Physician, Department of Medicine,
    Brigham and Women's Hospital

**Walter Willett, M.D., Dr.P.H.**
Professor of Epidemiology and
    Nutrition
Harvard School of Public Health
Associate Physician, Department of
    Medicine, Brigham and Women's
    Hospital

# PART ONE

# Getting Started

# CHAPTER ONE

# An Exciting Time
# for Women's Health

IT IS AN EXCITING TIME for women's health. Women are living longer lives today than ever before, and research on the treatment and prevention of disease in women is finally catching up with that of men. Even more notable, women are increasingly making health a top priority in their own lives. Traditionally women, as the primary caregivers in the family, have looked after the health of others before their own, but now they are realizing how important their own health is to leading productive, fulfilling, and happy lives.

The average life span of American women has increased from around fifty years in 1900 to close to eighty years today. Yet there is more to good health than a long life. Quality of life throughout the years is also important. Chronic conditions (such as heart disease and osteoporosis) that can make doing the things you enjoy more difficult are much more common as people age. And, with the aging of the U.S. population as a whole—by 2030, one out of every four women will be over the age of sixty-five—taking steps to avoid such disorders is even more important.

While most chronic diseases occur fairly late in a woman's life, they often stem, in part, from much earlier behavior. Coronary heart disease, the leading killer of women, begins to develop as early as adolescence, and the risk of diabetes and breast cancer also seems to have roots in youth and young adulthood. Establishing healthy habits early on and maintaining them throughout life is essential to enhancing overall health—at every stage of life.

Until fairly recently, much of the research on ways to lower the risk of chronic diseases was conducted mainly on men. One reason for this was convenience. Because men tend to develop chronic diseases earlier in their lives than women do, data on the risk factors for such diseases could be collected over a shorter period of time. This was not the only reason, however. Unwitting bias also served to exclude women from research studies, and for years, women had to follow health recommendations based primarily on data in men. Today, however, the situation has improved. Equal participation in research studies is now a national priority, and there is an increasing body of data solely on women's health issues. Not surprisingly, men and women are very similar when it comes to the steps they need to take to optimize their health and lower their risk of chronic diseases, but we now know that there are also some important differences.

Over the past twenty-five years, the Nurses' Health Study has made many important contributions to the field of women's health, leading the way in numerous areas. Most important, the study has helped identify many of the behaviors that contribute to good health in women. Based on these data, we have found that a huge proportion of the leading diseases in the United States could be avoided by healthy lifestyle choices. Fully 80 percent of the cases of heart disease and diabetes and 70 percent of the cases of stroke and colon cancer could be significantly delayed or prevented by women's leading healthier lives. Of course, 90 percent of lung cancers could be prevented by not smoking. And for smokers, there are huge benefits to stopping, even as an older adult. Quitting at age sixty can cut the lifetime risk of lung cancer in about half.

Of course, not everything that determines health is under a person's control. Genes also play a role in many disorders. But contrary to what many people think, your genes are not your destiny. Even women with a mutation in the BRCA 1 gene—the "breast cancer gene" mutation—are not destined to get breast cancer. Up to half of women with a BRCA 1 mutation do *not* go on to develop the disease. Clearly, there is more to good health than the hereditary hand you were dealt by your mother and father. For most illnesses, a combination of heredity, lifestyle, and other factors (both known and unknown) cause disease to develop. For some diseases, such as coronary heart disease, diabetes, colon cancer, and melanoma, lifestyle factors play quite a large role in making up risk. For others, the contribution of lifestyle to risk is smaller.

## PERSONAL HEALTH CHOICES

With an almost overwhelming amount of health information available to women today, what is the best way for you to approach making personal health choices and getting answers to such important questions as: "What diseases should I be most concerned about, and what are the most important changes I should make to try to lower my risk of illness?" Although each woman has a unique set of goals and concerns when it comes to her own health, all women can use some universal strategies to make the best health choices possible.

First—as we discuss in detail throughout the book—certain key lifestyle choices have such large health benefits that it pays for everyone to make them. An overall healthy lifestyle—avoiding smoking, eating a healthy diet, being physically active, and maintaining a healthy weight—can not only lower the risk of many serious diseases but also enhance the overall quality of life. Regular physical activity alone lowers the risk of coronary heart disease, stroke, diabetes, high blood pressure (hypertension), osteoporosis, and colon cancer as well as improves energy levels, helps combat stress, and enhances mood.

Not everything, though, has such wide-ranging benefits and so few risks as the key lifestyle choices. Many factors lower the risk of some disorders while increasing the risk of others. Deciding whether or not to concern yourself with these is a bit more complicated. A good example is regular aspirin use. Studies show that using aspirin regularly can lower the risk of colon cancer as well as of heart attack and ischemic stroke in people with cardiovascular disease. But aspirin can also have some serious side effects, increasing the risk of bleeding in the stomach, intestines, and brain. Weighing such potential risks and benefits is essential to the health decision-making process. If you have cardiovascular disease or are at high risk of colon cancer, it likely makes sense for you to use aspirin regularly. However, if you are not at high risk of cardiovascular disease or colon cancer, it may not make sense, given aspirin's potentially serious side effects.

## The Key Healthy Lifestyle Messages

Following some basic lifestyle rules can greatly lower your risk of disease and enhance your overall health. By simply going for a walk at lunch time or adding an extra serving of vegetables to your meals, you are taking an important step toward lowering your risk of coronary heart disease, stroke, diabetes, hypertension, osteoporosis, and many cancers. These five key lifestyle choices have a huge number of health benefits and virtually no risks:

- Do not smoke (see Chapter 17)
- Be more physically active (see Chapter 15)
- Eat a diet rich in fruits, vegetables, whole grains, and fiber, and low in saturated and trans fats (see Chapters 18 and 19).
- Maintain a healthy weight and do not gain excessive weight as an adult (see Chapter 16).
- Take a multivitamin every day (see Chapter 21).

In addition to the risks and benefits of a specific health choice, the number and type of diseases affected by that choice also go into the decision-making process. The biggest potential payoff comes from health choices that lower the risk of a number of serious diseases. Focusing your efforts on a single risk factor that is linked to only one or two uncommon diseases is probably not the best use of your energy. That energy is best spent on health choices that may protect you from a number of diseases and improve your overall health.

Of course, there are always exceptions. If you happen to be at high risk for a certain disease (because of a family history, for example), you may want to take all the steps possible to lower your risk of that disease, even if it means making choices that may protect you against only that disease and no other. For

## Beyond the Individual—Promoting Health in Your Community

While most of this book is focused on helping women make the best individual health choices they can, there are many other avenues they can explore that will have a broad impact on health. As you know, there is often more to making positive lifestyle changes than personal motivation. Many external factors—such as the flexibility of work hours, availability of healthy food choices, and access to safe recreational areas—also play a role in whether we are able to make healthy behaviors part of our daily lives. By working toward making changes on the community level (on the job, at school, and in city hall) that help support healthy behaviors, women can go a long way toward improving the health and well being of the broader community. And such opportunities for change are available in every woman's community. Some can be as simple as talking to a school principal about adding more fresh fruit to your child's school cafeteria menu. Others can be more involved, such as lobbying for legislation that bans smoking in any indoor public place in your county. Examples of community-focused actions women can work toward include:

- Flexible hours in the workplace so that employees can have time to exercise during the day or attend periodic health screenings
- Healthier food choices in workplace and school cafeterias
- Support for more, and better, physical education in schools
- Better access to safe places to exercise, such as parks, bike paths, and walking trails
- Bans on smoking in *any* indoor public place
- Stiff penalties for businesses selling tobacco to minors

most people, though, making healthy choices is like making most other choices in life: it is usually best to choose the options with the most advantages and the fewest disadvantages.

## HEALTH CHOICES IN THE REAL WORLD

In a perfect world, we would all have the time and energy to weigh these factors and to make (and put into practice!) an in-depth plan for improving our health. But as we know, reality is quite different. The time we have to devote to our health can be limited. It competes with all the other important parts of our lives—family, friends, jobs, the home, and good old-fashioned free time. So what is the best way to approach making healthy choices?

To begin, it is important not to become overwhelmed. As you go through this book, you will read about a large number of risk factors for a wide variety of diseases. But relax. This book is not meant to be a lengthy checklist of every single healthy choice you should make, nor is it intended to make you feel guilty for past choices. Rather, it is a resource that can help you explore the details of women's health and decide where your efforts are best placed.

Throughout, you will be pointed toward the key lifestyle choices. Beyond these, the healthy choices you decide to make depend very much on your level of concern about a certain disease and the benefits and risks of certain choices. Essential to making any good decision, though, is being well informed. Often this means gathering information on your own, such as reading this book. Sometimes, when the issues are more serious or complicated (as with aspirin or postmenopausal hormone use), it means meeting with a health care provider.

Everyone is unique, and when it comes to strategies for successfully making healthy choices in your life, what works for somebody else may not necessarily work for you. Overall, however, people tend to have the greatest success when they begin with only one or two changes and slowly add on others. You can pick the one thing you think will be the easiest to change—such as taking a multivitamin every day—or the one thing you think will have the biggest benefit for your health—such as stopping smoking—and then build from there. Changing too many things at once can be overwhelming and set you up for failure. Beginning slowly allows time for new behaviors to become ingrained in your daily routine. This way, when you tackle the next behaviors, the first ones are already part of your lifestyle. And it is never too late to make these changes; there are still many benefits to be gained by making healthy choices later in life.

Of course, despite any amount of planning, some factors that influence our health decisions may be hard to control. Although running may be your favorite form of exercise, it can be difficult to run as often as you would like during the early evenings of winter. Similarly, it may be a challenge for you to get more fruits and vegetables if the office cafeteria favors pizza and hamburgers. Like most things in life, health decisions often require compromise, but with a little creativity and forethought, you can usually find your way around these types of obstacles.

Whether you are able to make one healthy change in your life or ten, the important thing is that you play an active role in your own health. There is a lot you can do—as we detail throughout this book—to try to lower your risk of disease and improve your overall health. Any positive steps you take, no matter how small, are positive ones in the right direction.

Women's health has come a long way from the time its primary focus was on issues of childbearing and family health. Now, thankfully, a woman's health is much more broadly defined, including her well-being across her entire lifetime. By sharing our experiences and the knowledge we have gained over the last twenty-five years of the Nurses' Health Study, we hope that *Healthy Women, Healthy Lives* will become one of your indispensable resources for learning about women's health and making healthy choices throughout your life.

# What Is the Nurses' Health Study?

## The Nurses' Health Study

### THE QUESTION THAT GOT US STARTED: "DO BIRTH CONTROL PILLS HAVE LONG-TERM HEALTH EFFECTS?"

More than twenty-five years ago, this question sparked the beginning of what has since become one of the largest and most comprehensive studies of women's health. From birth control pills to exercise, from alcohol to zinc, the Nurses' Health Study has helped to identify many of the factors that protect health, as well as those that contribute to disease.

The study began in the mid-1970s, when birth control pills had been in widespread use for about a decade. Pleased with their effectiveness and convenience, many women were intending to use the pills for decades to come. Yet there was considerable uncertainty about whether this practice was safe. Taking the pill had already been shown to increase the risk of blood clots, heart attacks, and stroke. And as other side effects of the pill began to emerge, researchers also suspected a link with breast cancer. It was the possibility of this last link that led us to propose a bold new study: we would survey thousands of women about their method of birth control and then track their health status over time.

Because birth control pills were quickly emerging as a public health issue, the National Institutes of Health (the federal agency primarily responsible for prioritizing and funding medical research in the United States) was willing to consider funding our study. However, they first required that we submit a grant proposal so that our scientific peers could review what we had done so far—and what we planned to do if our study was funded. We submitted a grant proposal in 1973 and received the funding to start the study in 1974. After two years of pilot-testing the methods for the study, we began recruiting participants in 1976.

## FINDING THE NURSES

Our first major challenge was to identify a large group of women—ideally tens of thousands—who would be willing to complete a questionnaire about their method of birth control and their health status. In addition, the information they provided had to be accurate, and we had to be able to follow the women over time to determine if the pill had any long-term effects.

We realized that nurses would be the ideal study participants—and in fact they have been. As health professionals, they are extremely aware of the value of medical research and have thus been willing to make a long-term commitment to the study. In addition, they have been relatively easy to follow over the past twenty-five years, largely because they are prompt in notifying us of address changes. Finally, and perhaps most important, because of their knowledge and training, the nurses have been able to provide us with health information that is both accurate and reliable. This accuracy has been documented repeatedly. For example, whenever a study participant reports that she has been diagnosed with a serious illness, we ask permission to review her medical records to both confirm the diagnosis and gather additional details about the disease. The vast majority of the time we find that the nurse has provided us with accurate information.

## BEGINNING THE STUDY

Having chosen nurses as our study participants, we contacted the boards of nursing in eleven U.S. states and obtained the names and addresses of 170,000 female nurses. They were all married and between the ages of thirty and fifty-five to ensure that a large number would have used birth control pills. They were also primarily white due to the makeup of the nursing population at the time.

We sent our first questionnaire to these nurses in 1976. Though fairly straightforward, this questionnaire was actually the product of much deliberation and debate. The questions were designed so that they could be answered relatively easily, while still providing us with enough information to establish scientific relationships. For example, we asked the women if they had ever used birth control pills, and if so, for how long. We also asked about various medical conditions: had they ever had breast disease or a heart condition, and if so, when were they diagnosed? Because we already knew some of the factors that were linked to these conditions, we asked about those as well: how many children did they have, had they ever smoked, and had their parents developed breast cancer or heart disease?

Despite the depth of these questions, the entire survey was only two pages. This helped minimize the amount of time and effort needed to complete the survey and also helped maximize the number of responses we received. More than 120,000 nurses responded to our first questionnaire, and in doing so, became part of one of the largest and longest-running studies of women's health in the world.

## TWENTY-FIVE YEARS OF LOYALTY

For the past twenty-five years, the nurses in the study have completed a questionnaire every other year. Not surprisingly, given the duration and scope of the study, the questions included in our biennial survey have changed substantially over time (see Figure 2-1). While there are certain questions that we have asked on every survey (such as current weight and smoking status), many different questions have been added or dropped throughout the years. This is for several reasons.

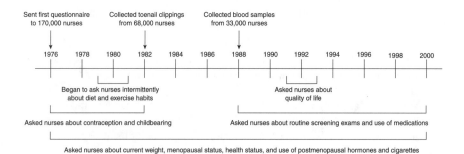

FIG. 2-1. In the past twenty-four years, the questionnaires used in the Nurses' Health Study have changed immensely. While this figure could not possibly encompass all of those changes, it does give an idea of how our questionnaires have changed over time. For example, while we have repeatedly asked the nurses about their current weight throughout the course of the study, we have only intermittently asked about their diet and physical activity.

First, the nurses have obviously grown older during the course of the study, and certain behaviors are no longer relevant to them. For example, during the first decade, we routinely asked women to update us about their contraceptive methods and childbearing. However, as the majority of the women reached menopause, these questions became less relevant and were replaced with others.

Second, the questionnaires have changed over time to reflect the emergence of new and potentially important issues in women's health. For example, in recent years scientists have suggested that a woman's health in middle age might be determined in part by how much she weighed as a baby. To address this possibility, we added to our 1992 survey a question about birth weight.

Finally, our questionnaires have evolved as a function not only of our own interests but also those of the nurses. Study participants repeatedly told us that they were concerned about their quality of life and how it was affecting their health. In response, we added a series of questions about caregiving, work stress, and social relationships. Although our questionnaires are much longer and more detailed than they were originally, more than 90 percent of the women continue to complete them.

---

### In the Nurses' Own Words . . .

I am glad to comment on my participation in the Nurses' Health Study. First of all, I am proud to be a participant. I read the newsletter with interest, and when articles appear in the media about women and cholesterol, the effects of supplemental vitamins on health—anything that comes out of the study—I read it with interest and am glad that I have contributed to a better understanding of women's health. In the midst of all the diet fads that swirl around us constantly, I do try to just eat sensibly, conscious of the fact that I filled out my form for the study in a certain pattern. I guess I am trying to be the best I can be, not only for myself and family, but also conscious of the fact that the statistics are part of a much bigger picture. I would gladly fill out more forms and donate anything asked for (blood, hair, etc.) to further understanding of women's health. I think you were brilliant to pick nurses—we're compulsive about forms and willing to give of ourselves. Thank you for using those traits for the common good.

—From ADN

---

## ADDING BIOLOGICAL SAMPLES TO THE STUDY

Over the years, many of the women in the study have provided more than questionnaire responses; they have literally given a piece of themselves. On a number of occasions, when questionnaires could not provide the information we needed, we asked the nurses to send us biological samples.

The first such request was prompted by scientific evidence that the mineral selenium might help prevent certain cancers. Though we typically do not need biological samples to study the effects of dietary components, selenium is somewhat different. For most minerals, the amount found in one vegetable is equivalent to the amount found in another vegetable of the same type. However, the same is not true for selenium. The amount of selenium in one carrot may be vastly different from that of another carrot, depending on how much selenium was in the soil where the carrot grew. Thus, even if we know how many carrots (and other selenium-rich foods) a woman eats, we still will not know how much selenium she consumes. To learn this, we needed to ask for a piece of each nurse in the study: her toenail clippings.

Toenail clippings can provide an accurate indication of how much selenium, as well as other trace materials, a woman has consumed in the past sev-

## Substudies of the Nurses' Health Study

Over the past twenty-five years, many of the women in the study have gone beyond their call of duty as participants. On multiple occasions, we have asked some of them to participate in small studies we were conducting on specific topics. These substudies, some of which are described below, have contributed greatly to our understanding of women's health.

- To determine whether the dietary component of our questionnaire could be answered reliably, we asked about 200 women in the greater Boston area to participate in a small study. Each woman completed two questionnaires about her usual diet and also kept detailed diaries of what she ate and drank for four one-week periods. By comparing the questionnaire responses with the information in the diaries, we were able to determine that women could accurately report their diet using a simple questionnaire.

- Recognizing that a woman's choice of contraception might affect not only her own health but also her partner's, we asked 28,000 women to provide detailed information about their partner's health. Using this information, we found a modest increased risk of prostate cancer among men who had previously had a vasectomy.

- Since 1986, more than 1,700 women with benign breast disease have granted us permission to obtain tissue samples from their breast biopsies. By classifying these samples based on their cell type, we have been able to determine that certain types of benign breast disease raise the risk of breast cancer. More recently, these same women have allowed us to review their mammograms to determine whether the density of the breast is also related to the risk of breast cancer.

- To study age-related changes in the eye, we asked about 600 women in the Boston area to have an extensive eye exam, performed by our ophthalmology colleagues. The results of these exams will allow us to better understand how lifestyle factors like diet contribute to the development of eye disease.

eral months. In 1982 we asked 92,000 participants to mail nail clippings from each toe to our research center in Boston; more than 68,000 women did so.

In 1988, we made our second request for a biological sample. This time we asked the nurses to send us several tubes of their blood. Again, the response was overwhelming: we received about 33,000 samples of blood, some of which have been analyzed for cholesterol, hormone levels, environmental chemicals, and even genetic markers.

We have since made other requests for biological samples, including cheek cells and additional blood. All of these samples have allowed us to study scientific relationships that we would otherwise never have been able to study. For this, we are incredibly grateful to the thousands of nurses who provided their samples.

## LEARNING FROM THE NURSES WHILE PROTECTING THEIR PRIVACY

Despite having amassed huge amounts of information about the women in our study, we take great care to ensure that no one but researchers can ever link that information back to the individuals who provided it. Even the researchers have limited access, with the information available only on a need-to-know basis. Each woman in the Nurses' Health Study was assigned an identification number in 1976, and her information is identifiable by that number only. Her questionnaire data are stored in one secure computer system, and her name and address in another. This helps ensure that the privacy and confidentiality of study participants are protected at all times. We also have a certificate of confidentiality from the Department of Health and Human Services to further ensure that the data provided are kept confidential.

## Other Research Studies

In the last two decades, the Nurses' Health Study has made many advances in identifying the factors that contribute to the development and prevention of major illnesses affecting women. However, we have not been alone in our efforts. There are many other important research studies on women's health, and together with the Nurses' Health Study, they have created the body of scientific evidence that guides health recommendations.

Three studies in particular have provided a great deal of evidence to support the topics covered in this book: the Framingham Heart Study, the American Cancer Society Cancer Prevention Study II, and the Iowa Women's Health Study. These ongoing studies have contributed substantially to the vast advances made in women's health in the past fifty years and will continue to do so for years to come. Two additional studies, the Nurses' Health Study II and the Women's Health Initiative, will also be contributing tremendously in the near future.

## THE FRAMINGHAM HEART STUDY

In the 1930s, cardiovascular disease reached epidemic proportions in the United States, and by the late 1940s, it had become the leading cause of death among American men and women. In the hope of learning how to prevent this deadly disease, researchers at the U.S. Public Health Service started a series of studies, including the Framingham Heart Study in 1948. This study has tracked participants' health for the past fifty years and has contributed greatly to our understanding of cardiovascular disease, as well as a variety of other diseases and conditions. As its name indicates, the study is made up of men and women who lived in Framingham, Massachusetts, at the time the study began. This town had a very stable population, and most residents obtained their health care from one major hospital in the area; both of these factors made it easier for researchers to follow the participants over time.

When the study began, the 5,200 participants were between the ages of thirty and sixty and were free from heart disease. Since then, surviving participants have undergone extensive medical exams every two years consisting of detailed medical histories, laboratory tests, and interviews about lifestyle. The Framingham Heart Study is notable not only for its duration and the extended commitment of its participants, but also because it was one of the first major cardiovascular studies to recruit women.

## THE AMERICAN CANCER SOCIETY CANCER PREVENTION STUDY II

In September of 1982, volunteers from the American Cancer Society invited their friends, neighbors, and relatives to join the Cancer Prevention Study II, which was similar to another study conducted by the American Cancer Society in the 1960s. Within a month and a half, over a million men and women had joined the second study and completed a four-page questionnaire about their health habits and personal and family medical history. Although most participants have not provided information on their lifestyles since then, researchers have continued to track their health status over the years. They have done this by having volunteers make personal inquiries about the friends and family members they recruited and by checking national death records. This study is notable particularly for its size (it includes over 675,000 women) and for its nineteen-year duration.

## THE IOWA WOMEN'S HEALTH STUDY

Hoping to determine which lifestyle factors might be related to the development of cancer in older women, researchers at the University of Minnesota in 1986 sent a sixteen-page questionnaire to 100,000 Iowan women between the ages of fifty-five and sixty-nine. About 41,000 women responded and completed subsequent questionnaires.

The questionnaires used in this study were similar to those used in the Nurses' Health Study, with one notable exception: they did not ask women whether they had been diagnosed with cancer. Without this pertinent information, how can researchers possibly determine a link between lifestyle factors and cancer risk? The answer is relatively simple and explains why researchers chose Iowa as their study site: whenever someone in Iowa is diagnosed with any type of cancer, it is immediately reported to the State Health Registry. Each year, the Registry provides the study's researchers with a list of participants who have been diagnosed with cancer. For the past fifteen years, researchers have successfully tracked women's health in this manner and produced dozens of reports about what leads to cancer and what lowers the risk of cancer.

## THE NURSES' HEALTH STUDY II

This study, which has grown out of the ongoing Nurses' Health Study, began in 1989, thirteen years after the start of the original study. The purpose was to examine reproductive health issues that had arisen in recent years and could not be addressed by the original study. For example, birth control pills contained substantially lower doses of hormones in 1989 than they did when the women in the Nurses' Health Study were taking them. In addition, most of the women in the Nurses' Health Study had already been pregnant by the time birth control pills became available. To study the health effects of the low dose pills, particularly before a first pregnancy, we decided to start a study with younger women.

In 1989, we mailed a four-page questionnaire to tens of thousands of nurses between the ages of twenty-five and forty-two and received responses from more than 116,000. These nurses have continued to complete questionnaires every two years not only about their reproductive history but also about their health status, diet, physical activity, and medication use. For any given questionnaire, about 90 percent of the nurses respond, which is a reflection of their commitment and dedication to this study. Overall, the Nurses' Health

## Studying the Nurses' Children: The Growing Up Today Study

In 1995, we sent a letter to the Nurses' Health Study II participants who had children between the ages of nine and fourteen. We asked the women if they would allow their children to participate in a new observational study called the Growing Up Today study. Its goal was to examine the impact of diet and exercise on adolescent weight gain.

More than 18,000 mothers agreed to let their children participate, and in 1996, we sent our first questionnaire to 27,000 children. More than 9,000 girls and 8,000 boys responded, providing us with much-needed information about the lives of adolescents today. The children continue to complete questionnaires on an annual basis, and as a result have become part of one of the largest ongoing studies of adolescent health in the world.

Study II promises to provide a better understanding of how women's lifestyle choices in early childhood affect their health both then and in later years.

### THE WOMEN'S HEALTH INITIATIVE

The Women's Health Initiative is a research effort that began in 1992 and eventually included forty different clinical centers across the United States. At each center, researchers invited postmenopausal women between the ages of fifty and seventy-nine to take part in a nine-year randomized controlled trial.

*The Randomized Controlled Trial.* This type of study is quite different from the other studies in this chapter (including the Nurses' Health Study), which are called observational studies. In observational studies, the participants live as most women do—they choose their own diets, exercise when they want to, and take the medications their health care providers prescribe. They regularly report their activities to researchers, who then use this information to determine how lifestyle choices affect health. In a randomized controlled trial, participants are more like subjects in a traditional scientific experiment. They are asked to adhere to a certain diet or take a particular medication so that researchers can study the health effects of the assigned diet or medication. Appendix A explains the different types of epidemiologic studies further.

In the Women's Health Initiative (WHI), researchers are conducting three separate trials to determine the health effects of three specific factors: low fat diets, postmenopausal hormones, and calcium and vitamin D supplements. In the first study, which includes nearly 50,000 women, researchers have asked about half the women to adhere to a special low fat diet (which was taught through several nutritional counseling sessions) and have allowed the other half to consume their usual diet. After the women have been on their respective diets for nine years, researchers will look to see which group has lower rates of breast cancer, colon cancer, and heart disease. In this way, they can determine whether the low fat diet carries a greater health benefit than the usual diet.

In the second trial, researchers assigned a daily dose of postmenopausal hormones to one group of women and a daily placebo (or sugar pill) to the other group. Again, researchers will track the health status of the women in each group and eventually determine which group has lower rates of heart disease and fractures. In the third and final trial, researchers assigned half of the women to take daily supplements of calcium and vitamin D, and the other half to take daily placebos. From this trial, researchers hope to determine whether the supplements protect against hip fractures and colon cancer, as suggested by several smaller studies.

*The Observational Study.* In addition to the three randomized controlled trials in the Women's Health Initiative, there is also an observational study, which includes nearly 94,000 women who volunteered for the study but were unable or unwilling to participate in the trials described above. These women have completed annual questionnaires about their lifestyle practices and have undergone routine medical exams. With this observational study, researchers have a much broader aim than with the intervention studies: to examine the multitude of lifestyle factors that contribute to heart disease, stroke, cancer, fracture, diabetes, and other major illnesses in women.

Overall, the Women's Health Initiative promises to provide some of the most conclusive evidence yet about women's health. It is distinct from other studies in this chapter not only because of its interventional approach, but also because of its study population: nearly 20 percent of the women—about 30,000—are African American, Latino, Asian American, or American Indian. This is in contrast to most other research studies, where more than 95 percent of all participants are white.

## Conclusions

Although this book focuses on the Nurses' Health Study and other long-term observational studies, there are many additional studies that have also contributed to our understanding of women's health. We must rely on all of these if we are to reach firm conclusions about how women can lower their risk of chronic diseases. The most substantiated and well-accepted health information is that which has been supported by a number of different studies.

In this book, we balance findings from our own study within the context of other studies' results. For example, there are now over thirty studies on birth control pills and ovarian cancer. Taken collectively, these studies suggest that taking the pill does lower the risk of ovarian cancer. We use findings from the Nurses' Health Study to explain this relationship, while making clear that ours is just one of the many studies to have shown this. When our results contradict the larger body of evidence, we note that, too. By providing a balanced summary of what is currently known about women's health, we hope to guide women toward healthier lifestyle choices.

# CHAPTER THREE

# Making Sense of Health Research

BEFORE EXPLORING THE EPIDEMIOLOGIC EVIDENCE on women's health, it would be helpful to understand more about the science of epidemiology. The roots of the word are in *epidemic,* which means prevalent among the people. Epidemics occur when there is an unusually high incidence of a particular disease in a population. Though epidemics were once thought of only as infectious diseases, the term has since been broadened to include chronic diseases like cancer and heart disease. For example, lung cancer reached epidemic proportions in the United States during the twentieth century: in 1983, it was three times as common as it had been in 1950.

In epidemiology, we study how and why these epidemics occur. We do this by comparing how often a disease occurs in one group versus another and then trying to determine why the rates are different between the groups. For example, the Nurses' Health Study began with the goal of comparing breast cancer rates among women who used birth control pills and women who did not. Based on comparisons like these, we can tell whether or not the characteristic of interest (in this case, pill use) influences a woman's risk of disease. We do this by examining both absolute risk and relative risk.

## Absolute Risk

Absolute risk is the chance or probability that a woman will develop a specific disease during a specified period of time. It is estimated by looking at a large group of women who are similar in some respect (in terms of age, for example) and counting the number of women in the group who develop the disease over the specified time period. For example, to estimate the chance that a fifty-year-old woman will develop breast cancer in the next ten years, researchers would follow a group of fifty-year-old women for ten years to see what percent of them developed breast cancer. Because this group would be diverse in every respect except age, the absolute risk estimated would be for the "average" fifty-year-old woman.

Throughout this book, when we present an absolute risk, we generally present the chance that a woman who is fifty will develop a given disease by the time she is eighty. Thus, we present thirty-year absolute risks. We do this with the following graphic, which depicts a group of a hundred women (see Figure 3-1). Each figure in the graphic represents a woman who is fifty years old, and each highlighted figure represents a woman who will develop the disease before she turns eighty. The graphic represents the absolute risk of breast cancer for a woman who is fifty years old. Of the one hundred figures shown, nine are highlighted. This means that in a group of a hundred women who are fifty years old, nine will develop breast cancer by age eighty. The average fifty-year-old woman thus has a 9 in 100 chance of developing breast cancer by the age of eighty. For diseases that occur less frequently (that is, they affect fewer than 1 in 100 women), the graphic will show a thousand figures. Thus nine highlighted figures in such a graphic would indicate a 9 in 1,000 chance, or less than 1 in 100.

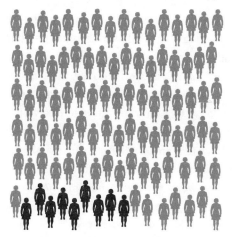

FIG. 3-1. In a group of 100 women who are fifty years old, 9 will develop breast cancer before reaching age eighty. (Source: National Cancer Institute)

## Relative Risk

A relative risk is the ratio of two absolute risks. The numerator (or top half of the ratio) is the absolute risk of disease in women who have a particular characteristic (often called a risk factor). The denominator (or bottom half of the ratio) is the absolute risk in women who do not have that characteristic. The group in the denominator is usually called the reference group. For example, to calculate the relative risk of breast cancer among women who have a family history of breast cancer compared to women who do not, we use the following ratio:

$$\frac{\text{Absolute risk of breast cancer among women with a family history}}{\text{Absolute risk of breast cancer among women without a family history}}$$

If the numerator is the *same* as the denominator, then the relative risk is 1.0. This means that the same percent of disease occurs in those with the characteristic as those without. Thus, the characteristic is not linked to the risk of disease.

If the numerator is *greater* than the denominator, then the relative risk is greater than 1.0. A relative risk greater than 1.0 means that women with the characteristic of interest (in this example, family history) have a higher absolute risk of disease than women in the reference group. In other words, women who have the characteristic are more likely to develop the disease than women who do not. We could also say that the characteristic increases a woman's risk of developing the disease.

If the numerator is *smaller* than the denominator, then the relative risk is less than 1.0. A relative risk less than 1.0 means that women who have the characteristic being studied have a lower absolute risk of disease than the reference group. In other words, women who have the characteristic are less likely to develop the disease than women who do not. We could also say that the characteristic reduces or lowers a woman's risk of the disease.

The size of a relative risk indicates the extent to which a particular characteristic increases or decreases the risk of the disease being studied (see table on page 23). Relative risks that are less than 1.0 are usually expressed as a percent decrease. For example, the relative risk of breast cancer in women who have children compared to women who do not is 0.90. We would say then that women with children are 10 percent less likely to develop breast cancer than women without children. Here's the math: $1.0 - 0.9 = 0.10$; $0.10 \times 100\% = 10\%$.

Relative risks that are between 1.0 and 1.99 are usually expressed as a percent increase. For example, the relative risk of breast cancer for women who drink one alcoholic beverage daily compared to those who do not is 1.40. Based on this, we would say that women who drink daily are 40 percent more likely to develop breast cancer than women who do not drink. Here's the math: $1.0 - 1.0 = 0.4$; $0.4 \times 100\% = 40\%$.

Relative risks that are greater than 2.0 are expressed somewhat differently. They are usually stated as the number of times that the risk is increased in the group with the characteristic compared to the group without. For example, the relative risk of breast cancer for women with a family history of breast cancer is 2.0, so we would say that women with a family history are two times as likely

| Relative risk | How does having this characteristic or risk factor affect a woman's risk of disease? | Percent change in risk |
|---|---|---|
| ≥5.00 | Increases the risk enormously | 400% or more |
| 2.00–4.99 | Increases the risk greatly | 100–399% |
| 1.35–1.99 | Increases the risk moderately | 35–99% |
| 1.10–1.34 | Increases the risk slightly | 10–34% |
| 1.01–1.09 | Increases the risk minimally | 1–9% |
| 1.0 | No effect | No change |
| 0.91–0.99 | Decreases the risk minimally | 1–9% |
| 0.76–0.90 | Decreases the risk slightly | 10–24% |
| 0.51–0.75 | Decreases the risk moderately | 25–49% |
| 0.21–0.50 | Decreases the risk greatly | 50–79% |
| ≤0.20 | Decreases the risk enormously | 80% or more |

to develop breast cancer as women without a family history. We might also say that there is a twofold increase in the risk of breast cancer among women with a family history.

As demonstrated in the table above, a characteristic that has a relative risk of 1.50 has only a moderate effect on a woman's risk of disease, while a characteristic that has a relative risk of 0.50 has a large effect. This means that a 50 percent increase in risk is not equivalent to a 50 percent decrease. The reason for this is somewhat complex and is best illustrated by an example. Say that the relative risk of a disease for those who exercise compared to those who do not is 0.50. This would mean that active women are 50 percent less likely to get the disease than sedentary women. If active women are less likely to get the disease, then the reciprocal of this relationship must also hold true: that sedentary women are more likely to get the disease. We can calculate how much more likely by taking the reciprocal of the relative risk for active women. (A reciprocal of a number is calculated by dividing 1.0 by that number.) In this example, the reciprocal would be 1.0 / 0.5, which is 2.0 (see Figure 3-2). Thus, we could say that sedentary women are two times more likely to develop the disease than active women. This would mean the same thing as saying that active women are half as likely to develop the disease as sedentary women.

Throughout this book, we present relative risks using graphics like Figure

Half

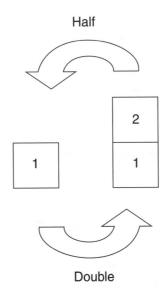

Double

FIG. 3-2. Cutting your risk of a disease in half, or by 50 percent, is the opposite of doubling your risk. Thus, if active women have half the risk of disease as sedentary women, then sedentary women have double the risk of active women.

3-3. Each vertical bar on the figure represents a group of women with a certain characteristic. The characteristic (or risk factor) is described on the horizontal axis (the bottom of the figure). The height of the bar indicates the relative risk of disease for that group. The scale for the relative risk is on the vertical axis (or left-hand side of the figure), with a horizontal line crossing a relative risk of 1.0. If a vertical bar is above that line, then the relative risk for the group represented by that bar is greater than 1.0. This means that the group has an *increased* risk of disease. If the bar is below that line, then the relative risk for that group is less than 1.0. This means that the group has a *decreased* risk of disease. In the graph, the vertical bar on the left represents the reference group (that is, women without a family history), and the bar on the right represents women with a family history. The relative risk for the reference group is set at 1.0, as demonstrated by the left-hand bar being even with the line at 1.0. The relative risk for women with a family history is 2.0, as demonstrated by the right-hand bar being twice as high as the left-hand bar. This means that women with a family history are twice as likely to develop breast cancer as women without a family history.

Notably, some figures in this book have a scale on the left that goes as high as 25, and some have a scale that goes only to 2.0. Why the difference? Relative

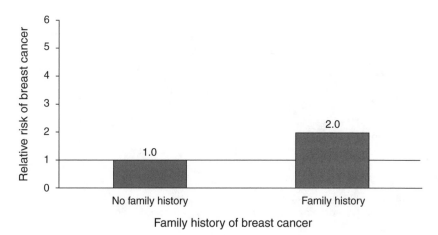

FIG. 3-3. The risk of breast cancer is twice as high among women with a family history of breast cancer as among women without a family history. (Source: Nurses' Health Study)

risks can be infinitely large, but there is a limit to how small they can be. The largest relative risks observed in epidemiology exceed 30, while the smallest have to be somewhere between 0 and 1.0. As a result, relative risks that fall below 1.0 cannot be compared on the same scale as relative risks that are above 1.0. For example, as we noted earlier, a 50 percent decrease in risk (as demonstrated by a relative risk of 0.5) is much more significant than a 50 percent increase in risk (as demonstrated by a relative risk of 1.5). Why? Because the most a factor could possibly decrease the risk of disease by is 100 percent; a 50 percent decrease in risk is half of what is achievable. A 50 percent increase in risk, however, is only a moderate increase, given that other factors might increase risk by 200 percent or even 900 percent.

It is critical to recognize that the importance of a relative risk depends largely on the underlying absolute risks. When a disease is less common, a relative risk that sounds high will still mean that the disease is uncommon, even among those with the characteristic of interest. For example, the chance that a fifty-year-old woman will develop ovarian cancer before the age of eighty is about 1 in 100. Even if a woman has a characteristic that doubles her risk of ovarian cancer, her chances of developing it are still only 2 in 100. When a disease is common, however, a relative risk that is high is of greater concern. For example, the chance that a fifty-year-old woman will develop coronary heart disease before the age of 80 is 20 in 100. Thus, if a woman has a characteristic that doubles her risk of heart disease, her chances of getting it rise to 40 in 100, which is clearly a concern.

## Relative Risks: Making Comparisons

You see the headline "Taking hormones raises the risk of breast cancer by 5 percent." If you're a postmenopausal woman on hormones, you might be concerned with this finding but feel that a 5 percent increase in risk is pretty minimal. However, as is often the case, such headlines may not include important additional information that you need to correctly assess your risk. In reality, the risk of breast cancer goes up by about 5 percent for every year that you take hormones. What does this mean? In the first year or two, you are just slightly more likely to develop breast cancer than if you had never taken hormones. Fifteen years later, though, if you're still on hormones, you are much more likely to develop the disease than if you'd never taken them. This is because those small per-year increases in risk slowly accumulate, resulting over time in a substantially increased risk, which may change the way you balance the overall risks and benefits of long-term hormone use.

The same thing can happen with reductions in risk. For every hour and a half a week that you walk briskly, your risk of heart disease goes down by 20 percent. On first glance at this statistic, you might wonder why you should even bother getting off the couch. After all, 20 percent is a pretty modest benefit. But again, the gradient is what is important: the more you walk, the greater the benefit. Sure, an hour and a half a week is only a 20 percent reduction in risk, but if you can squeeze in three hours a week, you'll cut your risk by 40 percent.

These examples illustrate an important point: the size of a relative risk depends on the comparison that is being made. Most health risks do occur on a gradient: the more you do something, the more or less likely you are to develop a given disease. Thus, the relative risk depends largely on what two points on the gradient are being compared. The change in risk could be very small if two points close together are being compared (for example, one hour of walking a week compared to two hours of walking a week). Or it could be quite large if two distant points are being compared (one hour of walking a week compared to one hour of walking a day). Throughout this book, we make clear what comparisons are being made, so that you can better understand how certain factors affect your risk of disease.

### Drawing Conclusions

The results of single epidemiologic studies are now widely touted in the media, but it is important to remember that the results of a single study are rarely conclusive. Conclusions cannot be drawn about a relationship, or health recommendations made, without understanding how the findings of one study fit with the findings of other studies. For example, if a new study shows that alcohol protects against breast cancer, we cannot simply conclude that this is true.

Some studies are more persuasive than others because of how they are conducted or designed, and this must be considered when weighing results. In addition, study findings can occasionally occur by chance. Thus, in this example, we would need to consider that more than forty other studies have shown alcohol to increase the risk of breast cancer. This accumulated evidence would lead us to conclude that alcohol probably does raise the risk of breast cancer—a conclusion very different from the one we might have reached had we simply accepted the new study's findings. One way that researchers often examine the weight of evidence for a particular relationship is to combine the results of all of the studies that have been done on that relationship.

## Differences in Study Results

Why might the results of one study differ from the results of so many others? There are several possible explanations.

First, although it is not very common, study results sometimes occur simply by chance. For example, suppose all of the pregnant women in your neighborhood gave birth to boys. Some people might wonder if something special in your neighborhood made these women more likely to have sons. However, this is probably just due to chance. In health research, we try to eliminate the possibility of chance findings by using certain statistical methods.

An alternative explanation for differences in study results is related to the way studies are conducted. As discussed in Appendix A, some studies are designed and carried out in a way that makes them less likely to give accurate results than other studies. For example, the results of one type of observational study will not be accurate if a large number of women refuse to participate, and their reasons for refusing are related to the topic being studied.

Finally, factors that influence the risk of disease often cluster together, and sometimes studies do not do a good job of disentangling the effects of one factor from the effects of another. For example, in the United States, people who exercise tend also to take a multivitamin. If researchers do not take this into account when looking at how multivitamins affect the risk of disease, they could easily mistake the benefits of the exercise as a benefit of multivitamins. In most high quality studies, statistical methods are used to help sort out the effects of different risk factors.

Throughout this book, we try always to give a sense of how findings from the Nurses' Health Study fit into the larger body of scientific evidence. Each relationship that we explore between a factor and a disease is identified either as established, probable, or possible, depending on how much evidence there is to support it. To determine this, we consider four things: how many studies support the relationship, the strength of the relationship, whether the studies that support it are of high quality, and whether there is a sound biological reason for the relationship. An *established* relationship is one that has been demonstrated consistently in a large number of high quality studies, generally increases or decreases risk at least moderately, and has been shown to be biologically plausible. An example is the relationship between smoking and lung cancer, which has been confirmed in hundreds of studies over the past fifty years. A relationship that has been demonstrated in most studies but not all would be considered *probable*. For example, though some studies have found no link between physical activity and breast cancer, the majority suggest that activity probably does offer some protection. In addition, the relationship makes sense biologically. Finally, a *possible* relationship is one that is supported by a few good studies, but still needs to be confirmed by additional research. A possible relationship also exists when a few studies support the relationship, but it is either not very strong or not consistently observed. An example of this is the relationship between the consumption of green leafy vegetables and the decreased risk of ovarian cancer, which has been demonstrated in a few studies but not in others.

Overall, epidemiologic studies provide a framework for understanding how women can take charge of their health by making simple lifestyle changes. In the next section, we will take what we have learned about epidemiologic studies one step further—by explaining what findings from large research studies mean to the individual woman.

## The Boundaries of Research

Medical research was responsible for some of the most amazing accomplishments of the twentieth century, including the eradication of polio, the discovery of penicillin, and the use of radiation for diagnosing and treating disease—to name just three. With such a distinguished pedigree, however, we are likely to forget that research also has its limitations. And you need to understand the boundaries of research—what it can and can't do—as you make important choices about your health.

In epidemiologic research, we analyze what has happened to one group of people and then use that information to predict what might happen to a similar group in the future. Because our research is based on probabilities, we can make fairly accurate predictions about large groups of people. Thus, moving many people toward a healthy lifestyle will have a large impact on decreasing risk in the population overall. However, we can never determine with certainty what will happen to a specific individual.

For example, we can look at a group of a thousand women, five hundred of whom are physically active and five hundred of whom are not, and compare how many women in each group go on to develop heart disease. If during a five-year period, ten active women develop heart disease, as do twenty sedentary women, we would say that physically active women are half as likely to develop heart disease as those who are sedentary. We would then use this information to predict that, in a similar group of women, regular physical activity might cut the risk of heart disease by 50 percent. We could not, however, determine which particular women in the group will be the ones to develop the disease.

Using probabilities to estimate an individual woman's risk is a lot like forecasting the weather. A meteorologist uses past data to make a prediction about an individual day. She gathers all the information she can, compares the current weather pattern with previous weather patterns, and then makes a best guess, telling viewers to carry their umbrellas that day because the probability of showers is 60 percent.

As you well know, however, a weather forecast is either right or wrong on a particular day. It either rained, and you needed your umbrella, or it did not rain. The same goes for physical activity and heart disease in the example above (although a 60 percent chance of rain on one day is astronomically high compared to the risk of developing heart disease from a sedentary lifestyle). Even though being active lowers the risk of heart disease by 50 percent in women, when it comes to your own personal risk, either you will develop the disease or you will not. Making changes in your lifestyle for the sake of your health is not a guarantee that you will avoid disease. We all know people who lead healthy lifestyles and still develop heart disease, and we also know those who smoke, drink excessively, and never exercise—and still live to be ninety years old. Overall, there are no guarantees when it comes to your health, only important opportunities to better your chances of leading a long and healthy life.

With *Healthy Women, Healthy Lives,* we hope to lead you toward those opportunities by giving you the information you need to make the best possible choices for your health.

# PART TWO

# Lowering the Risk
# of Diseases

# CHAPTER FOUR

# Lowering the Risk of Coronary Heart Disease

## BACKGROUND

Coronary heart disease is a leading killer of women in the United States—a fact often overshadowed by the media attention given to other diseases, such as breast cancer. While approximately 180,000 women will develop breast cancer during the course of a year, nearly a million women will develop coronary heart disease. Often perceived as a man's disease, it is clearly not. Nearly equal numbers of men and women die of coronary heart disease each year, and though men tend to develop the disease earlier than women—the average woman has the same risk as the average man ten years her junior—women tend to live longer, giving them a longer period of time in which to develop the disease.

Even though it is such a large health burden, the good news is that the risk

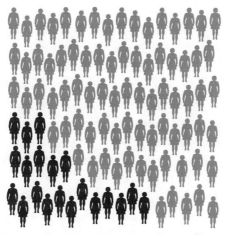

FIG. 4-1. In a group of 100 women who are fifty years old, 20 will develop coronary heart disease before they reach the age of eighty. (Source: Lloyd-Jones et al.)

of heart disease is largely modifiable. Only a few of the risk factors for the disease are completely out of your control, and the rest—such as smoking, high blood pressure (also called hypertension), high blood cholesterol, and diet—you can control. Taking steps to control these factors and reduce the risk of the disease may be particularly important for women. The Framingham Heart Study found that nearly two-thirds of the women in their study who had died suddenly from coronary heart disease had no previous symptoms—highlighting the need to keep the disease from developing initially.

## The Heart and Coronary Heart Disease

The heart is a muscle that pumps blood throughout the body. Like all muscles, it needs a constant supply of oxygen and nutrients to work properly, which it receives through the coronary arteries. When these arteries become narrowed by a disease called atherosclerosis, the condition is called coronary heart disease (CHD).

In atherosclerosis, cholesterol and fat build up inside the artery walls. The process most likely begins when the artery wall is injured—by factors such as hypertension, high blood cholesterol, smoking, and diabetes—and the body overreacts in repairing the damage. White blood cells (cells that respond to injury in the body) enter the artery wall and bring with them, through a complex process, fat and cholesterol, which get deposited. Over time, enough fat and cholesterol can accumulate that the wall bulges inward, and the artery begins to narrow. In advanced stages, the site of the buildup (plaque) develops a hard, fibrous cap.

When the artery is significantly narrowed by the buildup, a person can experience chest pain (angina), caused by the heart muscle's not getting all the blood it needs to work properly. The condition becomes dangerous when an artery becomes completely blocked. This occurs most often when the hard cap over a buildup suddenly ruptures, and a blood clot forms that cuts off all blood flow. A portion of the heart then starves for oxygen and nutrients. If this continues for even a relatively short period of time (about 5 to 10 minutes), part of the heart muscle dies, an episode called a heart attack (myocardial infarction) (see Figure 4-2).

In some instances, blood flow to the heart may be blocked by a spasm in a coronary artery that constricts the vessel. Spasms can occur in arteries with or without atherosclerosis and often result in chest pain. If a spasm occurs at the site of atherosclerosis, it can rupture the hard cap, which can lead to blood clots and then a heart attack.

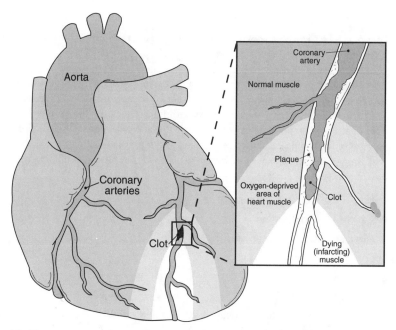

Aorta

Coronary
arteries

Clot

Coronary
artery

Normal muscle

Plaque

Oxygen-deprived
area of
heart muscle

Clot

Dying
(infarcting)
muscle

FIG. 4-2. The coronary arteries supply oxygen and nutrients to the heart. When they become narrowed and obstruct the blood supply, the condition is called coronary heart disease. A heart attack occurs when an artery becomes completely blocked, most often due to a blood clot forming at the narrowing, and part of the heart muscle fed by the artery dies.

A potentially dangerous, immediate result of coronary heart disease, particularly a heart attack, is an irregular heartbeat (arrhythmia) called ventricular fibrillation, in which the main pumping chambers of the heart (ventricles) start quivering (fibrillating) and lose their ability to pump blood throughout the body. Ventricular fibrillation is the main cause of sudden death in women with coronary heart disease.

Although heart disease most often develops in women over sixty, many studies have shown that atherosclerosis may actually begin very early in life. Children as young as ten to fourteen years of age have been found to have the earliest form of the buildup, called a fatty streak. Not all fatty streaks develop into atherosclerosis, but over time, some do.

## Don't Hesitate! Recognize the Symptoms of a Heart Attack and Get Care Immediately

Women are more likely than men to die after a heart attack. Why? One reason is that women are less likely than men to seek immediate medical care for a heart attack in progress, denying their symptoms because they mistakenly think that coronary heart disease is a man's disease. All women, especially as they get older, should be able to recognize the symptoms of a heart attack and seek immediate care—as well as take an aspirin—if they have a combination of the following symptoms:

- Chest pain, discomfort, or pressure
- Left arm pain or discomfort
- Pain radiating to the neck or jaw
- Shortness of breath
- Sweating
- Upset stomach or nausea
- Discomfort in the area between the breastbone and navel
- Unexplained anxiety or fatigue

### REVERSING THE PROCESS—REGRESSION

Fortunately, the development of atherosclerosis and, subsequently, CHD is not a one-way street. Many studies have shown that the process can be reversed to a certain degree or at least stopped from progressing. By choosing a healthy lifestyle and bringing under control those factors responsible for injuring artery walls and depositing fat and cholesterol—hypertension, high blood cholesterol, smoking, and diabetes, for example—you can actually reverse the process of atherosclerosis, and have the same white blood cells that originally deposited fat and cholesterol within the artery walls taking the substances away.

## LESSONS FROM THE NURSES' HEALTH STUDY AND OTHER STUDIES

Despite the fact that much of the heart disease research in the past was conducted on men (in part because the disease develops at an earlier age in men), there now exists a substantial amount of evidence on the causes of coronary heart disease in women. While many of the factors linked to heart disease are

## Coronary Heart Disease: The Larger Picture

- Coronary heart disease (CHD) is a leading killer of women in the United States, killing 1 in 4 women.
- Nearly a million women will be diagnosed with CHD in the course of a year.
- The risk of CHD for women begins to increase dramatically between the ages of forty-five and fifty-four.
- Whether due to similar genes or similar lifestyles, CHD tends to run in families.
- The large majority of CHD cases could be prevented or significantly delayed if women follow some simple rules of lifestyle, including not smoking, eating a healthy diet, and being physically active.

the same for both men and women, there are some factors that are unique to women—such as postmenopausal hormones and birth control pills—and some that affect risk differently in women than in men—such as diabetes and blood cholesterol.

## Factors You Cannot Control

Some factors you cannot control put you at higher risk for developing coronary heart disease (CHD). The reason that you should know about these is simple: if you have them, and they put you at extra risk, it is even more important for you to work on the factors that you can control.

### AGE

For both men and women, the risk of CHD increases with age. In general, though, women have a risk of heart disease similar to men ten years their junior. For men, the risk of heart disease begins to increase dramatically between the ages of thirty-five and forty-four. For women, this increase does not occur until between the ages of forty-five and fifty-four.

### FAMILY HISTORY

Coronary heart disease runs in families. Having a parent or sibling who has been diagnosed with heart disease greatly increases a woman's risk of developing it herself, especially if the relative developed it at a young age. In the Nurses' Health Study, we found that women who had a parent who had developed CHD before age sixty had an increased risk of the disease compared to women whose parents had not had the disease (see Figure 4-3). For women

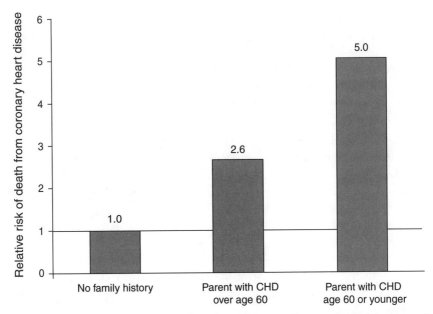

FIG. 4-3. The relative risk of fatal coronary heart disease increases if a parent has had the disease. It is greatest in those whose parent developed CHD at age sixty or younger. (Source: Nurses' Health Study)

who had a parent who developed the disease after age sixty, risk was still increased, but to a lesser degree.

One reason family history increases the risk of CHD is biological: family members share genes that make them vulnerable. Another reason is social: family members often have similar lifestyles that influence modifiable CHD risk factors such as smoking, diet, and physical activity level. Controlling these factors provides the best opportunity to lower the chances of developing the disease.

## RACE AND ETHNICITY

There are significant racial and ethnic differences in the rates of CHD (see Figure 4-4). Most notably, the rate of death from the disease is nearly 35 percent higher in African American women than in white women. In males, the difference in death rates between African Americans and whites is much lower, with the rate in white males slightly higher than that in African American males. It is unclear why the disparity exits between white women and African American women, although there are a number of possibilities. Compared to white women, African American women have about twice the rate of diabetes and obesity, two major risk factors for CHD. African American women may

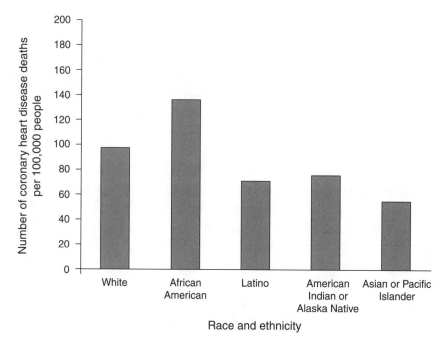

FIG. 4-4. The risk of heart disease varies with race and ethnicity. African Americans tend to have higher rates than whites, while Latinos, American Indians, and Asian/Pacific Islanders tend to have lower rates than whites. (Source: National Center for Health Statistics)

also be less likely to seek or receive proper care for their disease, and therefore may be more likely to die from the condition.

In contrast, Asian American women tend to have the lowest rates of CHD in the United States, though their rates have been increasing slightly. Not entirely clear is how the disease affects Latina women compared to other ethnic groups. There is some evidence that Latina women have lower rates than white women, but other evidence suggests that Latina women are more likely to be hospitalized and to die from CHD. Further study should produce a clearer picture of how CHD affects the various ethnic groups in the United States.

## Factors You Can Control

You can modify many of the risk factors for coronary heart disease (CHD)—an encouraging fact given that the disease kills one in four women in the United States. In combination, these modifiable factors have a powerful influence on your risk of the disease. So powerful, in fact, that studies of migrating populations show that in as little as one generation, a population's risk for the disease can significantly increase when they move from a country with a low rate of

CHD (such as Japan) to a country with a high rate of CHD (such as the United States)—due largely to individuals' adopting the lifestyle of the new country. The Nurses' Health Study suggests that at least 80 percent of heart attacks in women may be prevented or delayed by modifications of lifestyle. Of particular importance are the same lifestyle choices that can also lower your risk of many other diseases: not smoking, maintaining a healthy weight, eating a healthy diet, and being active.

## SMOKING

For over thirty-five years, since the release of the first U.S. Surgeon General's Report on Smoking and Health in 1964, smoking has been linked to an increased risk of CHD. Tobacco smoke not only promotes the dangerous buildup of fat and cholesterol in artery walls, it can also promote the formation of the blood clots that can be the ultimate cause of a heart attack.

As with many other studies, we found in the Nurses' Health Study that women who currently smoke have a greatly increased risk of CHD compared to women who have never smoked, and the more a woman smokes, the greater her risk. Women who smoke more than two packs of cigarettes a day have a risk of CHD that is nearly eleven times greater than the risk in those who have never smoked. Even light smokers—those who smoked only one to four cigarettes a day—have double the risk of the disease.

Despite the implications of cigarette advertisements, smoking lower tar or lower nicotine cigarettes increases the risk of CHD just as much as smoking regular cigarettes does. Women who smoke such "lite" cigarettes often smoke more or inhale more deeply to compensate for the lower nicotine levels.

Most of the increased risk from smoking, however, is not permanent. After quitting, the risk begins to drop. We found that two years after a smoker had quit, her risk was cut in half, and ten or more years after she quit, it nearly equaled that of women who had never smoked.

In addition to its direct effect on the risk of CHD, there is also a great deal of evidence that smoking increases the effect of other risk factors for the disease—for example, hypertension, diabetes, and high blood cholesterol. We found that smokers with hypertension had 22 times the risk of CHD compared to nonsmokers with normal blood pressure. Similarly large increases in risk were also seen in smokers with diabetes or high blood cholesterol.

*Passive Smoking.* Breathing the smoke from other people's cigarettes, called passive smoking, also increases the risk of CHD. Based on the results of numerous studies, passive smoking appears to increase the risk of CHD in nonsmokers by about 20 to 30 percent. In the Nurses' Health Study, we found that those nonsmoking women who were regularly exposed to passive smoke had nearly double the risk of CHD compared to those not exposed to passive smoke. Moreover, a woman's risk increased as the amount of smoke to which she was exposed increased.

## Stopping Smoking—Difficult but Well Worth It

Stopping smoking is a difficult prospect, but it is something most smokers want to do. And while it isn't easy, it can be done. Every day, a thousand people in the United States quit for good. In addition to lowering the risk of stroke, osteoporosis, diabetes, and many types of cancer, stopping smoking also significantly lowers the risk of coronary heart disease. And the benefits begin almost immediately after stopping. After a few hours, the body begins to carry oxygen more efficiently, and after a week, circulation improves. See page 339 for tips on how to quit and more details on the immediate and long-term benefits of quitting.

## BLOOD CHOLESTEROL

Blood cholesterol level (the amount of cholesterol circulating in the blood) is a well-established risk factor for CHD. There are two main types of cholesterol that relate to the risk of CHD: low-density lipoprotein (LDL) cholesterol, often referred to as "bad" cholesterol, and high density lipoprotein (HDL) cholesterol, often referred to as "good" cholesterol. LDL cholesterol can promote atherosclerosis by contributing to the buildup of cholesterol in the coronary arteries, which is why it is bad. HDL cholesterol has the opposite effect, removing cholesterol from the blood and helping to eliminate it from the body, which is why it is good. One analysis that combined the results from over twenty studies found a doubling of heart disease risk among middle-aged women who had either a high total cholesterol level, a high LDL cholesterol level, or a low HDL cholesterol level (see Figure 4-5).

For women, HDL level seems to be especially important. Not only is a low HDL level a stronger predictor of CHD risk in women than in men, but it may even be more important than a high LDL level, traditionally thought of as the most important marker of CHD risk.

The following table shows cholesterol levels that are desirable, borderline high, and high according to a federal report by a panel of experts. Such categorizations are somewhat arbitrary, however. It is true that a desirable cholesterol

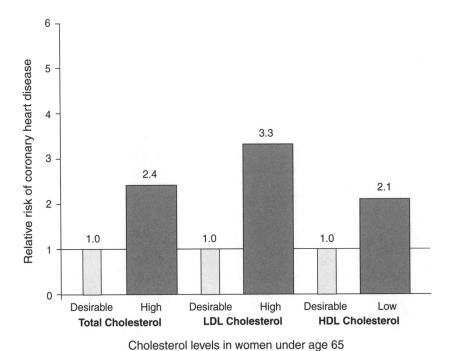

Cholesterol levels in women under age 65

FIG. 4-5. The relative risk of coronary heart disease increases with high total cholesterol, high LDL cholesterol, and low HDL cholesterol levels, compared to women with desirable levels for each of these. (Source: National Heart, Lung, and Blood Institute)

level is better than a borderline high level and that a borderline high level is better than a high level. But the risk of CHD does not just increase when someone crosses from one category into the next; it actually increases steadily with cholesterol levels. For example, an LDL level at the upper end of the borderline

## Recommended Blood Cholesterol Levels (milligrams per deciliter)

| | DESIRABLE | BORDERLINE HIGH | HIGH |
|---|---|---|---|
| Total cholesterol | Less than 200 mg/dL | 200–239 mg/dL | 240 mg/dL and above |
| LDL cholesterol | Less than 130 mg/dL | 130–159 mg/dL | 160 mg/dL and above |

An **HDL cholesterol** level of less than 35 mg/dL is a major risk factor for coronary heart disease. An HDL level of 60 mg/dL or higher is protective.

Source: National Heart, Lung, and Blood Institute

## Treating Blood Cholesterol with Drugs

Lifestyle changes are the first choice for improving blood cholesterol levels, but in many cases drugs are needed as well. Total blood cholesterol level and the levels of LDL and HDL are not the only factors that go into the decision to start a person on drug therapy. A person's overall risk of heart disease is also taken into account. Together with their health care providers, women can plan the best approach to bringing poor blood cholesterol levels under control.

## The Life Span and Blood Cholesterol

Cholesterol levels tend to naturally change over the course of a woman's lifetime. Between adolescence and middle age, women tend to have better cholesterol profiles than men. Their HDL levels are higher and their LDL levels are lower. Around the age of fifty, however, as women enter the menopausal years, they lose some of this advantage. HDL levels fall slightly and LDL levels start to rise, eventually becoming higher than men's. Several lifestyle factors can help lower LDL levels and increase HDL levels. Postmenopausal hormones may also improve blood cholesterol, although the decision to take hormones after menopause is not a simple one. Because postmenopausal hormones have both risks and benefits, women should talk to their health care providers about whether hormones are right for them.

high category will increase the risk of CHD more than an LDL level at the lower end of the borderline high category, even though both levels are in the same category. The same goes for the high as well as the desirable categories.

Improving blood cholesterol levels can lower the risk of CHD. Studies show that for every 1 percent drop in total blood cholesterol level, there is an approximately 2 to 3 percent drop in the risk of CHD. Though the subjects in these studies were primarily men, it is likely that women would show similar benefits. Even more important than lowering total cholesterol, however, is trying to decrease LDL levels. The results of numerous studies show that lowering LDL cholesterol can significantly lower the risk of CHD. Though not as extensively studied, there is good evidence that increasing HDL levels can also lower the risk of CHD and may be of particular importance in women.

A number of factors influence blood cholesterol levels—diet, physical activity, weight, and smoking (see table on page 44). Substituting polyunsaturated fat and monounsaturated fat for the saturated fat and trans-unsaturated fat in the diet (see below) can lower LDL levels and increase HDL levels. Stopping smoking, being physically active, and drinking moderate amounts of alcohol can increase HDL levels. For those who are overweight, losing weight can also increase HDL levels and decrease LDL levels. Making such changes can help maintain optimal cholesterol levels or at least bring cholesterol levels into the desirable ranges.

Only after these approaches fail to improve cholesterol levels would a physician generally recommend drug treatment. Though a few blood cholesterol drugs specifically target HDL levels, most people are prescribed drugs that lower LDL levels, which tend to be easier to change—through drugs or lifestyle—than HDL levels.

## Behaviors and Cholesterol Levels

| BEHAVIOR | EFFECT ON HDL LEVELS— "GOOD" CHOLESTEROL | EFFECT ON LDL LEVELS— "BAD" CHOLESTEROL |
|---|---|---|
| Changing diet | | |
| Cutting back on saturated fat | ↓ | ↓ |
| *Sources: animal fat (dairy, meat)* | | |
| Cutting back on trans-unsaturated fat | ↑ | ↓ |
| *Sources: shortening, hydrogenated oils* | | |
| Eating more polyunsaturated fat | ↑ | ↓ |
| *Sources: liquid vegetable oil, fatty fish* | | |
| Eating more monounsaturated fat | ↑ | ↓ |
| *Sources: olive oil, canola oil* | | |
| Being physically active | ↑ | ↓ |
| Drinking moderate amounts of alcohol | ↑ | – |
| Stopping smoking | ↑ | – |
| Losing weight (if overweight) | ↑ | ↓ |

## Triglycerides

Triglycerides are the main chemical form of the fats that circulate in the bloodstream. Although we have not studied triglycerides in the Nurses' Health Study, high blood triglyceride levels (hypertriglyceridemia) have been shown in numerous studies to increase the risk of coronary heart disease, especially in women. In addition to being associated with low HDL levels, high blood triglycerides may change the structure of the LDL cholesterol in blood, making it even more likely to contribute to the buildup of fat and cholesterol inside artery walls. Maintaining a healthy weight, increasing physical activity, and cutting back on alcohol can help lower triglyceride levels. Women with very high levels (see table below) may be prescribed drugs that lower either triglycerides or LDL cholesterol.

## Blood Triglyceride Levels

| | |
|---|---|
| Normal | Less than 200 mg/dL |
| Borderline high | 200–400 mg/dL |
| High | 400–1,000 mg/dL |
| Very high | Greater than 1,000 mg/dL |

Source: National Heart, Lung, and Blood Institute

### BLOOD PRESSURE

"Blood pressure" refers to the force in the arteries created when the heart pumps blood throughout the body. Hypertension, the term for high blood pressure, is a major risk factor for CHD and is also exceptionally common in the United States. More than 30 million Americans suffer from the disorder, including half of all women over the age of forty-five. When blood pressure rises, the heart must pump with more force and the walls of the arteries are put under greater pressure. This increased pressure can injure the inner lining of the artery walls, starting the process of atherosclerosis.

Blood pressure is reported as two numbers—systolic blood pressure and diastolic blood pressure. Systolic blood pressure—the higher of the two numbers—measures the force of the blood in millimeters of mercury (mm Hg) as the heart is contracting and pumping blood. Diastolic blood pressure—the lower of the two numbers—measures the force of the blood as the heart rests in between beats. Although blood pressure varies with age, the optimal blood pressure is 120/80 mm Hg or lower (see Figure 4-6). Blood pressures over 140 mm Hg for systolic or 90 mm Hg for diastolic are considered high. Below age fifty-five more men than women have hypertension. At age fifty-five or over, this reverses, with the rate in women exceeding that in men.

**Figure 4-6. Classification of Blood Pressure for Adults Age 18 and Older\***

| Category | Systolic  (mm Hg) | | Diastolic (mm Hg) |
|---|---|---|---|
| Optimal† | Less than 120 | and | Less than 80 |
| Normal | Less than 130 | and | Less than 85 |
| High-normal | 130–139 | or | 85–89 |
| High | | | |
| Stage 1 | 140–159 | or | 90–99 |
| Stage 2 | 160–179 | or | 100–109 |
| Stage 3 | 180 or greater | or | 110 or greater |

\* Not taking blood pressure drugs and not acutely ill. Blood pressure varies with age.
†Optimal blood pressure with respect to cardiovascular risk is below 120/80 mm Hg.
  However, unusually low readings should be evaluated for clinical significance.
(Source: National Heart, Lung, and Blood Institute)

The link between hypertension and CHD in women has been well established in many studies. In the Nurses' Health Study, we found that women who reported that they had hypertension had 3.5 times the risk of the disease as women reporting normal blood pressure. When we specifically assessed fatal heart attacks, the risk linked to hypertension was even greater—more than 6 times the risk of women with normal blood pressure.

One specific type of hypertension—isolated systolic hypertension—is very common in women, especially as they age. Isolated systolic hyptertension affects only systolic blood pressure, while diastolic blood pressure remains normal. It was once thought that systolic hypertension alone was of little consequence to CHD and that diastolic blood pressure was the component that increased risk. A number of studies, however, including the Framingham Heart Study, have found that isolated systolic hypertension greatly increases the risk of coronary heart disease and stroke—perhaps even more so than diastolic hypertension.

As with blood cholesterol, numerous studies show that lowering blood pressure can reduce the risk of CHD. Studies of drug treatment show that treating isolated systolic hypertension—for example, reducing blood pressure from 165/90 to 154/90—can lower the risk of CHD in women by 25 percent. And a drop of 6 mm Hg in diastolic blood pressure—for example, from 130/100 to 130/94—can lower the risk of the disease by approximately 16 percent.

But medicines aren't always needed to treat hypertension. Lifestyle changes can also lower blood pressure and are sometimes all that is required (see the box). Losing weight (if necessary), limiting alcohol intake, being physically active, and eating a healthy diet that is low in salt and provides nutrients that help control blood pressure (e.g., potassium, magnesium, and calcium) are approaches that can help lower blood pressure or maintain a normal blood pressure. A recent study sponsored by the National Heart, Lung, and Blood Institute that enrolled approximately half women found that a diet rich in fruits, vegetables, and low fat dairy products (called the DASH diet) could significantly lower blood pressure. When combined with a low salt diet, the benefits of the DASH diet were even greater, and both people with and without hypertension experienced lowered blood pressure.

Change in lifestyle is the preferred first approach to treating hypertension. Only if someone has very high blood pressure (160/100 mm Hg or greater) or a number of other risk factors for CHD should drugs be used as a first approach to treatment. If lifestyle changes cannot bring blood pressure under control after six to twelve months, most doctors will likely recommend drug treatment.

## Behaviors That Help Prevent Hypertension

- Stopping smoking
- Maintaining a healthy weight or losing weight if necessary
- Limiting alcohol intake—*no more than one drink per day for women*
- Being physically active—*30 to 45 minutes of aerobic activity on most days*
- Eating a diet rich in fruits, vegetables, and low fat dairy products
- Limiting salt intake—*no more than 6 grams (approximately one teaspoon) of salt per day*

Source: National Heart, Lung, and Blood Institute, 1997.

## DIABETES

Diabetes is a very powerful risk factor for CHD, especially in women. Of the two main types of diabetes, the most common by far is adult-onset diabetes, also referred to as type 2 or non-insulin-dependent diabetes mellitus. Adult-onset diabetes develops most often in adults and especially in people who are overweight. A person with adult-onset diabetes can often control blood sugar with lifestyle changes and/or oral medicine. The other type of diabetes is juvenile-onset diabetes, also referred to as type 1 or insulin-dependent diabetes, and it most often develops before the age of thirty. A person with juvenile-onset diabetes requires insulin to control blood sugar. Both types increase the risk of coronary heart disease.

Women with diabetes essentially lose the overall age advantage they have over men when it comes to developing CHD. The results of numerous studies show that while men with diabetes have 2 to 4 times the risk of CHD compared to men without diabetes, women with diabetes have 3 to 7 times the risk compared to women without the disorder, making their risk of the disease about equal to that of men of the same age. In the Nurses' Health Study, we found a very large risk of CHD in women with adult-onset diabetes compared to women without.

Diabetes increases the risk of CHD in part by increasing the risk of high blood cholesterol and hypertension. Diabetes may also promote injury to the artery wall, formation of blood clots, and changes to nerves in the heart that can increase the risk of a deadly arrhythmia after a heart attack.

We have also found that the increased risk of CHD linked to diabetes is heightened still further by other heart disease risk factors. A woman with both diabetes and high blood cholesterol has a risk of developing CHD that is 2 times higher than that of a woman with diabetes and normal cholesterol. If a woman has diabetes and also smokes or is very overweight or has hypertension, her risk of developing CHD is 3 times higher than if she had diabetes but none of these other risk factors. Thus, for a woman with diabetes, the best way to lower the risk of CHD is to control other risk factors for the disease. Women with diabetes who have one or more of these other risk factors for heart disease may also benefit from taking an aspirin regularly, but only on the recommendation of their health care provider. Of course, controlling blood sugar levels, whether a woman has juvenile-onset or adult-onset diabetes, is critically important as well.

## PHYSICAL ACTIVITY

Physical activity lowers the risk of CHD. Despite the fact that only a quarter of the more than forty studies assessing physical activity and CHD have included women, these few studies have been extremely consistent in demonstrating that physical activity helps protect women from CHD, reducing the risk of the disease by 30 to 50 percent. In addition to helping prevent hypertension, high blood cholesterol, obesity, and diabetes, physical activity may also help prevent CHD by lowering the chances of blood clots forming at a site of atherosclerosis.

In the Nurses' Health Study, we have drawn some important conclusions about the link between physical activity and the risk of CHD. First, we have shown that women do not need to train for marathons or spend hours at a health club to lower their risk of coronary heart disease. Women who walked briskly for at least three hours a week received the same protection against CHD as women who exercised vigorously for at least an hour and a half a week. Both groups of women were 30 to 40 percent less likely to develop heart disease than women who were sedentary. Second, we found that the more time women spend being physically active each week, the lower their risk of heart disease (see Figure 4-7). Finally, it is never too late to reap the protective benefits of physical activity. Women who have been sedentary for many years but then start a program of regular exercise, have a lower risk of heart disease than those who remain sedentary. We also showed that the more active women become, the lower their risk of heart disease.

Although nearly anyone can safely begin a walking program, women who have not been active for a while should check with their health care providers before embarking on a more active lifestyle. Begin slowly, with just enough ex-

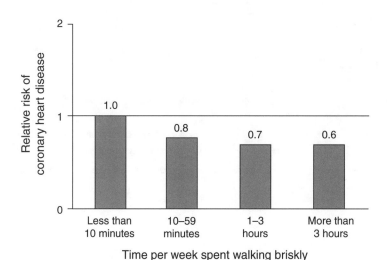

FIG. 4-7. Women who walk at a brisk pace (more than 3 miles per hour) for at least one hour a week receive moderate protection against coronary heart disease. (Source: Nurses' Health Study)

ercise to get the muscles and joints accustomed to the increased activity level. Then slowly increase the length and intensity of the activity over time.

## Coronary Heart Disease: Weighing the Risks

### INCREASED RISK

- Women who smoke more than two packs of cigarettes a day have an exceptionally high risk of coronary heart disease (CHD) compared to women who have never smoked. Even women who smoke only one to four cigarettes a day have a high risk.
- Women with hypertension have a large risk of CHD compared to women reporting normal blood pressure.
- Women with diabetes have a very large risk of CHD compared to women without the disorder, making their risk about equal to that of men of the same age.
- Women who are overweight or gain a lot of weight as adults have a large risk of CHD compared to women of normal weight or women whose weight has remained steady throughout adulthood.
- Women who eat high amounts of saturated fat and trans-unsaturated fat have an increased risk of CHD.
- Women who are sedentary have a large risk of CHD compared to women who are regularly active.

### LOWERED RISK

- Women who eat high amounts of polyunsaturated fat and monounsaturated fat have a lower risk of CHD.
- Women who eat five or more ounces of nuts per week—about five airline packets' worth or more—have a moderately lower risk of CHD than women who rarely or never eat nuts.
- Women who eat more servings of fruits and vegetables a day are less likely to develop CHD than women who rarely eat fruits and vegetables.
- Women who have about one drink of alcohol a day have a moderately lower risk of CHD than nondrinkers.

## WEIGHT

A number of large cohort studies—including the Nurses' Health Study, the Iowa Women's Health Study, and the Framingham Heart Study—have found that the risk of CHD increases as weight increases. In the Nurses' Health Study, we specifically found that the risk of CHD was slightly elevated among women whose weight fell within the upper reaches of the normal range, and it rose to be very large in obese women (see Figure 4-8). Where a woman carried her weight influenced her risk of CHD as well. Those women carrying the most weight around their middles—often referred to as apple-shaped—had a large risk of the disease compared to those women carrying the least. A waist size of more than 35 inches is considered high and is easy for women to monitor themselves.

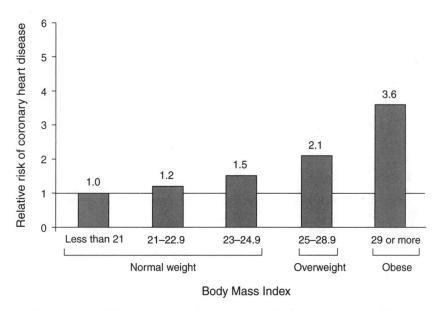

FIG. 4-8. The relative risk of coronary heart disease increases the heavier you are, even if you are in the upper end of the normal range. See Appendix C for information on calculating body mass index. (Source: Nurses' Health Study)

We also found that gaining substantial amounts of weight after age eighteen increased the risk of CHD, even for women whose weight stayed in the normal range. Women who gained 12 to 18 pounds after age eighteen had a slightly greater chance of developing CHD than women whose weight remained nearly the same throughout adulthood. The more weight gained, the greater the risk. Women who gained 44 pounds or more had more than double the risk of CHD.

Although many studies have found that being overweight seems to increase the risk of CHD on its own, the main reason that being overweight increases risk of the disease is that it increases the risk of hypertension, diabetes, and high blood cholesterol—all intermediate factors that also increase the risk for CHD.

## DIET

Diet has long been recognized as a risk factor for CHD. However, much of the public is confused—and rightfully so—about which specific types of food increase the risk and which types of food decrease the risk of the disease. Recommendations from national experts appear to change every few months. While such changes are inevitable as science advances, the results can be confusing. Here we present what is currently known about diet and the risk of CHD, and we try to do it in as clear and straightforward a manner as possible.

Along with the results from other studies, we have found in the Nurses' Health Study that dietary fat, nuts, fiber, whole grains, fruits and vegetables, alcohol, and foods that are quickly converted to glucose all have significant effects—some positive and some negative—on the risk of CHD.

## DIETARY FAT

A low fat diet has long been recommended as a way to lower the risk of CHD. However, this now seems to be an oversimplification of the relationship. In the Nurses' Health Study, we have found that it is not the total intake of fat that affects the risk of CHD but rather the level of intake of the different kinds of fats—saturated, trans-unsaturated, polyunsaturated, and monounsaturated. Both saturated fat and trans-unsaturated fat increase the risk of CHD, while polyunsaturated fat and monounsaturated fat lower the risk.

Fats are thought to influence the risk of CHD primarily by affecting HDL and LDL cholesterol levels, but they may also affect other factors linked to CHD, such as blood clotting, sensitivity to insulin, and the chances of having a fatal arrhythmia following a heart attack.

*Saturated Fat.* Saturated fats come primarily from animal sources and are solid at room temperature in their pure form, such as butter and lard. Other sources of saturated fat are red meat, cheese, nonskim milk, and tropical vegetable oils, such as palm kernel oil and coconut oil. Studies looking at the influence of saturated fat on cholesterol level have found that saturated fat raises both LDL ("bad") cholesterol levels and HDL ("good") cholesterol levels. Possibly due to the fact that it raises both levels, we found in the Nurses' Health Study that increases in saturated fat consumption only slightly increase the risk of CHD.

*Trans-unsaturated Fat.* Trans-unsaturated fats are vegetable fats that have been altered during a heating process and, like saturated fats, are solid at room temperature. Stick margarine and vegetable shortening are examples, and they are widely used in commercially baked products—cookies, cupcakes, pies—often appearing on food labels as "partially hydrogenated vegetable oil." Commercially fried foods, such as the french fries and onion rings from fast food restaurants, are also major sources. Studies of trans-unsaturated fats have found that they have a particularly adverse effect on blood cholesterol levels, lowering HDL while also raising LDL. We found that increased consumption of trans-unsaturated fat led to a large increase in the risk of CHD. Replacing only about 30 calories a day of carbohydrates with about 30 calories of trans-unsaturated fats nearly doubled the risk of CHD.

*Polyunsaturated Fat.* Polyunsaturated fats come primarily from plant and fish sources—though there are some animal sources as well—and are liquid at room temperature. Common sources are liquid vegetable oils, oil-based salad dressing, and fatty fish (like salmon). Studies have consistently found that polyunsaturated fats lower LDL cholesterol while they either slightly lower or have no effect on HDL cholesterol. In the Nurses' Health Study, we found that replacing about 80 calories a day of carbohydrates with about 80 calories of polyunsaturated fats lowered the risk of CHD by about 40 percent. We also found that one specific type of polyunsaturated fat, alpha-linolenic acid (see box for sources), was particularly effective at preventing death from coronary heart disease. Women who consumed the most alpha-linolenic acid had a 45 percent lower risk of dying from CHD than women consuming the least. In addition to improving cholesterol levels, alpha-linolenic acid may also help protect against the deadly arrhythmias that can follow a heart attack.

Some studies have also shown that the polyunsaturated fat found primarily in fatty fish (omega-3) may help lower the risk of CHD. Although studies to date have not consistently found a benefit, in the Nurses' Health Study we found a 20 percent reduction in the risk of heart disease among women who ate fish at least once a month. Those who ate fish more frequently received even greater protection.

## Good Sources of Alpha-Linolenic Acid

Alpha-linolenic acid, a polyunsaturated fat, may lower the risk of sudden death caused by a heart attack. Good sources include:

- Salad dressings with a vegetable oil base
- Canola oil
- Soybean oil
- Flaxseed oil
- Wheat germ oil
- Walnuts

*Monounsaturated Fat.* Monounsaturated fats are usually liquid at room temperature. Major sources include olive oil, canola oil, and, in the American diet, red meat. Not only have monounsaturated fats been found to lower LDL levels, they have also been found to increase HDL levels. In the Nurses' Health Study, we have seen that monounsaturated fats help protect against coronary heart disease. We found that replacing about 80 calories a day of carbohydrates with about 80 calories of monounsaturated fats lowered the risk of CHD by about 30 percent. Even though red meat is a major source of monounsaturated fat in the United States, it is not recommended that those wanting to increase their monounsaturated fat consumption do so by eating more red meat. In addition to containing a good deal of saturated fat, a high red meat intake may also increase the risk of colon cancer. Olive oil and canola oil are much healthier choices, as they contain very little saturated fat.

## NUTS

A number of large cohort studies, including the Iowa Women's Health Study and our Nurses' Health Study, have found that regularly eating nuts in moderation can lower the risk of CHD. In the Nurses' Health Study, women who ate five or more ounces of nuts per week had a 35 percent lower risk of CHD than women who rarely or never ate nuts. Nuts may lower the risk of CHD because they are naturally high in polyunsaturated fats and can therefore help lower LDL levels. In addition to their effect on blood cholesterol, nuts may also lower the risk of CHD by preventing blood clots and arrhythmias as well as providing nutrients that may help prevent atherosclerosis and hypertension (for example, vitamin E, potassium, magnesium, and folate).

## Cereal Fiber

Eating a moderate to high amount of cereal fiber appears to lower the risk of CHD. Cereal fiber is found in whole grain products, such as whole wheat bread, wild rice, oatmeal, and many cold breakfast cereals. In the Nurses' Health Study, we found that, compared to women who ate the least amount of cereal fiber, those who ate average to high amounts had a fairly large reduction in their risk of heart disease. Results from the Iowa Women's Health Study found similar results.

In addition to lowering LDL cholesterol, increasing the amount of cereal fiber in the diet may also reduce the risk of CHD by lowering the risk of diabetes, high blood triglycerides, and blood clots.

## Whole Grains

Several large studies have shown that whole grain foods can reduce the risk of CHD. These foods tend to be packed with heart-healthy vitamins and nutrients, including fiber, folate, and vitamin E. In the Nurses' Health Study, we found that the more frequently women ate whole grains, the less likely they were to develop heart disease. Women eating the most whole grains had an approximately 30 percent lower risk of CHD than women eating the least. When we looked at specific whole grain foods, we found that brown rice, whole grain breakfast cereal, bran, and popcorn offered the most protection.

## Glycemic Index

Glycemic index measures how quickly a food is converted to the simple sugar glucose during digestion. A food with a high glycemic index (such as white rice or white bread) is converted quickly to glucose; one with a low glycemic index (such as broccoli or dried beans) is converted slowly to glucose. A quick conversion causes spikes in blood glucose levels, which in turn cause spikes in levels of insulin, the hormone that helps cells take up glucose so they can use it for energy. Spikes in insulin levels can be bad for the heart. Not only do they increase the risk of diabetes (a major heart disease risk factor), they also adversely affect blood cholesterol levels, triglyceride levels, and blood pressure, each of which can increase the risk of CHD.

In the Nurses' Health Study, when we assessed how the glycemic index of foods related to the risk of CHD, we found that overweight women who ate the most servings of high glycemic index foods were twice as likely to develop heart disease than overweight women who ate the fewest servings of high glycemic index foods. For women of normal weight, glycemic index seemed to have no apparent effect on risk. This may be because the effect of high glycemic index foods on insulin levels may be more pronounced if a woman is experiencing problems using insulin efficiently (called insulin resistance), something strongly linked to being overweight. For a list of the glycemic index of selected foods, see Appendix C.

## FRUITS AND VEGETABLES

Fruits and vegetables are rich in vitamins and nutrients that offer cardiovascular benefits. For example, potassium helps lower blood pressure, folate helps lower the level of the atherosclerosis-promoting protein homocysteine, and fiber helps lower the risk of diabetes, high blood cholesterol, and the formation of blood clots. And although not all studies are consistent, eating fruits and vegetables does seem to offer modest protection against heart disease. We found in the Nurses' Health Study that women who ate three servings of fruits and vegetables a day were about 20 percent less likely to develop CHD than women who rarely ate fruits and vegetables, and the more women ate, the lower their risk. Green leafy vegetables (such as spinach and kale), cruciferous vegetables (such as broccoli and cauliflower), and foods rich in vitamin C (such as oranges and green peppers) seemed particularly beneficial.

## ALCOHOL

Given its coverage in the media, most people are aware that moderate alcohol consumption can lower the risk of CHD. Initial reports said that it was red wine in particular that lowered CHD risk. However, numerous studies have now shown that moderate consumption of any type of alcohol helps protect against the disease, possibly by increasing the level of HDL cholesterol or decreasing the risk of blood clots. In the Nurses' Health Study, we found that women who drank about one drink a day (for example, a 12-ounce glass of beer, a glass of wine, or a shot of hard alcohol) had a 40 percent lower risk of CHD than nondrinkers.

Despite its overall heart health benefit, moderate alcohol consumption can increase blood triglyceride levels. High blood triglycerides can increase the risk of heart disease, especially in women, and cutting back on alcohol intake is one way to bring high triglyceride levels down to normal.

Although there are clear health benefits to moderate drinking, there are also some health risks. For a detailed discussion on alcohol consumption, see Chapter 20.

## Vitamins

The link between vitamins and CHD is an active area of research, and there is substantial evidence that consuming certain vitamins can lower the risk of CHD.

*Vitamin E.* Vitamin E is an antioxidant that helps protect cells and tissue from damage by a certain form of oxygen, called oxygen free radicals. These free radicals can oxidize LDL cholesterol, a chemical change that makes the LDL cholesterol more likely to injure artery walls and to be deposited at a site of atherosclerosis. Vitamin E is carried in LDL and can help prevent its oxidation.

Although the results from some recent randomized trials—performed primarily in high risk men—have found no link between vitamin E and CHD, we have had encouraging results in the Nurses' Health Study. We found that women with the highest intake of vitamin E (an average of about 200 IU a day) had a nearly 35 percent lower risk of CHD than women with the lowest intake. Vitamin E from food alone was not enough to see any benefit, however; it was necessary to supplement the food they ate with vitamin E capsules. Even those women with the highest vitamin E in their diet averaged only 7.7 IU a day and did not show any decrease in their risk of CHD. More studies—including randomized clinical trials in women—on the benefits of vitamin E need to be performed before conclusive recommendations can be made about its intake.

*Vitamin $B_6$ and Folate.* A number of studies, including the Nurses' Health Study, have linked a high intake of vitamins $B_6$ and folate with a lower risk of CHD. In our study, it appeared that women needed to supplement their diets with $B_6$ tablets in order to get enough of the vitamin to lower their risk. With folate, however, women were able to benefit from either the amount they got through either food alone or supplements alone (see Figure 4-9).

Vitamin $B_6$ and folate are thought to decrease the risk of CHD by lowering blood levels of the protein homocysteine. Animal and human studies have demonstrated that very high levels of homocysteine greatly increase the risk of developing CHD, and more recent studies have shown that even less drastic elevations in homocysteine can also raise the risk of the disease. Homocysteine may contribute to CHD risk by injuring artery walls and increasing the risk of blood clots.

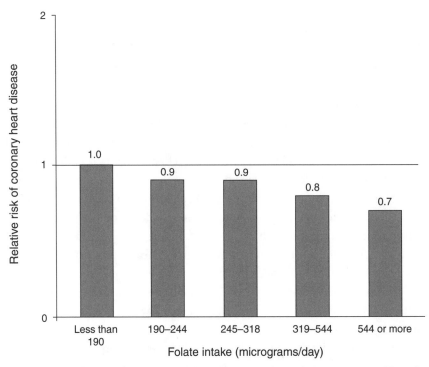

FIG. 4-9. The risk of heart disease drops as folate intake increases. (Source: Nurses' Health Study)

## The Good News

- Quitting smoking has large health benefits, some of which start almost immediately. Over the long term—ten or more years after quitting—a former smoker's risk of coronary heart disease (CHD) nearly equals that of women who have never smoked.

- Not all types of blood cholesterol are "bad." In fact, HDL cholesterol—often called "good" cholesterol—actually helps to remove cholesterol from the blood and eliminate it from the body.

- Women don't need to run marathons to benefit from exercise. Women who walk briskly for at least three hours a week receive the same protection against CHD as women who exercise vigorously for at least an hour and a half a week.

## ASPIRIN

Aspirin has been proven to reduce heart damage when taken during a heart attack, and to help prevent a second heart attack. Aspirin may also lower the risk of initially developing CHD. While regularly taking a low-dose aspirin (three to four times a week) has been shown to reduce the risk of initially developing CHD in men, there have been fewer studies in women, and the results of these have been mixed. In the Nurses' Health Study, we found that women who took one to six aspirins a week had a moderately lower risk of initially developing CHD than women who did not take any aspirin. Women over fifty years of age seemed to benefit the most, showing a slightly greater drop in risk than younger women. Taking more than six aspirins per week did not affect the risk of CHD.

Aspirin is an anticoagulant that reduces the risk of CHD primarily by hampering the ability of blood to clot. While lack of clotting is beneficial for heart disease, it can also raise the risk of hemorrhagic stroke and bleeding in the stomach and intestines. More studies are needed before clear recommendations can be made to women about the risks and benefits of aspirin use to lower the risk of initially developing CHD. However, we encourage women with risk factors for heart disease to discuss the potential benefits of regularly taking aspirin with their health care providers.

## POSTMENOPAUSAL HORMONES

A large number of U.S. women take postmenopausal hormones to alleviate the short-term symptoms and longer-term health effects of menopause. While such hormone therapy has some risks associated with it, such as an increased risk of breast cancer and clots in the large veins of the legs, it also appears to be beneficial in many ways—lowering the risk of osteoporosis and possibly colon cancer.

Postmenopausal hormones have also long been recommended for the prevention of CHD. However, there is now uncertainty about this recommendation. Emerging evidence suggests that postmenopausal hormones may raise the risk of heart disease during the first one to two years that women are using them. This new evidence raises concerns about who should take postmenopausal hormones and makes it doubly important for women to talk to their health care providers about this issue.

The prior recommendation that women take hormones for the prevention of heart disease is based on evidence from a large number of observational studies. Most of these studies examined the risk of heart disease among women who had never used postmenopausal hormones compared to those who had already been using them for at least five years. We combined the results of more than forty of these studies and found that while women were taking estrogen, they were about half as likely to develop heart disease as women who had never taken estrogen. This was true whether estrogen was taken alone or in combination with progestin.

Although the evidence from observational studies does suggest that hormones protect against heart disease, the relationship is not that simple. Randomized controlled trials recently have been begun to examine this. In these trials, postmenopausal women take either a daily placebo or a daily dose of hormones for an extended period of time. Researchers then determine which group is less likely to develop heart disease. In the earliest trial of this nature, researchers studied the effects of estrogen on women who already had heart disease. During the first year of the trial, women on hormones were more likely to have a heart attack than women on placebo pills. As the trial progressed, however, the women on hormones became less likely to have a heart attack. When we looked at short-term hormone use among women with heart disease in the Nurses' Health Study, we found similar results.

Whether healthy women also experience an increase in risk during the first years of hormone use is not yet known. Preliminary results from the on-going Women's Health Initiative suggest that they do. In that trial, researchers are studying the effects of hormones on healthy women—that is, women with no prior history of heart disease. During the first one to two years of the trial, women on hormones were slightly more likely than women on placebo pills to experience a heart attack, stroke, or blood clot. As the trial progresses, the rate of cardiovascular events seems to be equaling out between the two groups of women, much like it did in the previous trial. Since the Women's Health Initiative is ongoing, more conclusive evidence will not be available from this trial until 2005.

In the meantime, how should postmenopausal women proceed with making decisions about the use of hormones? Unfortunately, there is no clear answer right now. The available evidence suggests an *increase* in the risk of CHD during the first one to two years of hormone use and a *decrease* in risk during subsequent years of use. Because this is an ongoing area of research, with new evidence constantly emerging, women should periodically discuss the issue with their health care providers.

## BIRTH CONTROL PILLS

Older, high dose birth control pills—used most often by women in the United States from the early 1960s through the mid-1970s—have been linked to a moderate to high increase in the risk of CHD, especially among women who smoked. But this was only in women who were currently using the pill, and the risk of CHD in this generally young group of women was so small that the increase in risk resulted in only a relatively few extra cases of the disease. Once women stopped taking the pill, their risk returned to that of women who had never used the pill, regardless of how long they had used it initially.

For women using the newer, low dose formulations, there appears to be little or no increase in the risk of CHD, except if they are smokers, who experience large increases in the risk of heart attack compared to nonsmokers (especially after the age of thirty-five). Smoking, in combination with using the pill, greatly increases the risk of blood clots that can lead to a heart attack.

## Other Risk Factors

Though not as well established, a number of other factors may affect the risk of developing coronary heart disease (CHD).

### EMOTIONAL AND PSYCHOSOCIAL FACTORS

A number of emotional and psychosocial factors have been linked to CHD, including anger, anxiety, lack of social support, and depression. While such factors are often associated with behaviors that increase the risk of CHD—for example, hostile people may be more likely to smoke and to have poor diets—they likely have a direct effect on the heart as well. High levels of anxiety and hostility and low levels of social support can stimulate the autonomic nervous system and the production of certain hormones that promote hypertension, high blood cholesterol, and atherosclerosis.

*Social Support.* Social support describes a person's social networks. If you are married, have a large number of friends, and participate in group activities, you have a high level of social support. A number of studies have linked low levels of social support with CHD. One study found that women with a medium or low level of social support had 2 to 2.5 times the risk of atherosclerosis of women with high levels.

*Caregiving.* Women are often the primary caregivers of the family, and there is some evidence that this role can take a toll on health, increasing the risk of heart disease, high blood pressure, and even premature death. In preliminary results from our study, we found that women who spent nine or more hours a week caring for an ill spouse had an 80 percent greater risk of CHD than women who did no caregiving at all. Possibly surprisingly, even women spending nine or more hours a week caring for healthy grandchildren experienced a 55 percent higher risk of the disease.

*Severe Anxiety.* Severe anxiety, or extreme worry, has been linked to CHD in a number of studies of both men and women. In the Framingham Heart Study, female homemakers who showed signs of severe anxiety had nearly 8 times the risk of CHD compared to women showing the least signs of anxiety. In a study of male health professionals, we found that the most anxious men had more than double the risk of coronary heart disease compared to the least anxious.

*Anger.* Like anxiety, anger and hostility have been linked to CHD in numerous studies. One of these—the National Heart, Lung, and Blood Institute's Family Heart Study—found that women who were at high risk of CHD and who also showed hostility had a 40 percent greater risk of having a heart attack compared to those high-risk women not showing hostility.

*Depression.* Many studies have shown that depression can be bad for your heart. If you have already had a heart attack, it can increase your risk of having and dying from a second heart attack. Depression may even moderately increase your risk of initially developing CHD. One study found that women who were the most depressed were 70 percent more likely to have a first heart attack than those who were the least depressed. Depression may increase the risk of CHD in many ways, including raising hormone levels that can cause hypertension and arrhythmias as well as making it less likely that someone will adhere to a healthy lifestyle.

*Shift Work.* Approximately 22 million people in the United States do shift work, which means they work outside of the standard eight-hour workday. Some people work nights, others work unscheduled hours, and still others continually rotate work around different eight-hour shifts of the twenty-four-hour day. Only a small number of studies—almost all of men—have looked at the link between shift work and coronary heart disease, with some showing an effect and some not. In the Nurses' Health Study, we found that women who worked a rotating shift schedule for six or more years had a 50 percent greater risk of CHD compared to women who had worked only a standard eight-hour day.

Shift work may increase the risk of CHD in a number of ways. Shift workers may be more likely than people working regular hours to smoke, not get enough exercise, or eat an unhealthy diet. Shift work itself, though, may also affect the body directly by disrupting its normal rhythms. One study found that workers new to shift work showed increases in blood cholesterol and blood sugar. Additional studies are needed before it is known exactly why and how shift work affects the risk of CHD.

*Snoring.* Snoring, for both men and women, may increase the risk of coronary heart disease. If you snore, you are more likely to experience sleep apnea, a condition in which you stop breathing temporarily while asleep. The lack of oxygen caused by these breathless periods can possibly increase blood pressure and blood clotting and promote atherosclerosis. We found in the Nurses' Health Study that the risk of CHD was increased in women who snored compared to women who never snored, and the more frequently women snored, the greater their risk. Regular snorers had over twice the risk of CHD as women who never snored.

*Infections That May Cause Atherosclerosis and CHD.* Recent research studies have pointed to the possibility that a long-term infection of the lining of the arteries might be one cause of atherosclerosis. The evidence is strongest for a microorganism called *Chlamydia pneumoniae.* Some studies have also found that people with severe periodontal disease—which is linked to infection—are at increased risk of heart disease. If the link between heart disease and infections proves to be true, it could mean that antibiotic treatment or immunization against such organisms might protect against CHD. However, it will be some time before the evidence is in.

## WHAT IT ALL MEANS

You have great control over your risk of coronary heart disease (CHD). Unlike some disorders where lifestyle factors play a relatively minor role, the risk of CHD is largely made up of factors you can control. Astonishingly—and fortunately—we found in the Nurses' Health Study that over 80 percent of the cases of CHD could be eliminated by some simple rules of lifestyle. Most important: do not smoke or quit if you do, eat a healthy diet, and be physically active. You also should see a health professional regularly to be checked for high blood cholesterol, high blood pressure, and high blood sugar (a sign of diabetes). While you might have symptoms from these conditions that would prompt you to seek care, these conditions sometimes exist for many months or years before symptoms or a serious event occurs.

## Established, Probable, and Possible Factors Associated with the Risk of Coronary Heart Disease

| RISK FACTOR | APPROXIMATE RISK* |
|---|---|
| *Established* | |
| Smoking | ↑↑↑↑ |
| Diabetes | ↑↑↑↑ |
| High blood pressure | ↑↑↑ |
| Poor blood cholesterol levels | ↑↑↑ |
| Age (greater than 65 vs. under 45) | ↑↑↑ |
| Family history of coronary heart disease | ↑↑↑ |
| (parent with coronary heart disease vs. no family history) | |
| Weight | |
| Being overweight | ↑↑↑ |
| Gaining more than 15 pounds in adulthood | ↑↑ |
| Having a large waist (35 inches or larger) | ↑↑↑ |
| Ethnicity (African American vs. white) | ↑↑ |
| High glycemic index foods (high intake vs. low intake) | ↑↑ |
| (overweight women only) | |
| Dietary fat intake | |
| High saturated fat | ↑ |
| High trans fat | ↑↑↑ |
| High polyunsaturated fat | ↓↓ |
| High monounsaturated fat | ↓↓ |
| Cereal fiber intake (high vs. low intake) | ↓↓ |
| Physical activity (regularly active vs. sedentary) | ↓↓↓ |
| Alcohol intake (1 drink per day vs. none) | ↓↓ |
| Low dose aspirin | |
| Lowering the risk of heart attack in women | ↓↓ |
| with coronary heart disease | |
| Lowering the risk of dying from a heart attack in progress | ↓↓ |
| Whole grain foods (high intake vs. low intake) | ↓↓ |
| Fruit and vegetable intake (high intake vs. low intake) | ↓↓ |

*Probable*

    Low dose aspirin—for lowering the risk of initially      ↓↓

       developing heart disease

    Vitamins

       Vitamin E (high intake vs. low intake)      ↓↓

       Folate and vitamin $B_6$ (high intake vs. low intake)      ↓↓

    Nut intake (5 ounces per week vs. none)      ↓↓

*Possible*

    Lack of social support      ↑↑↑

    Severe anxiety      ↑↑↑

    Anger and hostility      ↑↑↑

    Depression      ↑↑

    Having a shift work job      ↑↑

    Snoring      ↑↑

    High level of caregiving      ↑↑

    Birth control pills—new, low dose formulations      ↑

       (current or recent use)

    Postmenopausal hormone use for 5+ years      ↓↓

| *↑Small increase in risk | ↓ Small decrease in risk |
|---|---|
| ↑↑Moderate increase in risk | ↓↓ Moderate decrease in risk |
| ↑↑↑Large increase in risk | ↓↓↓ Large decrease in risk |
| ↑↑↑↑Very large increase in risk | ↓↓↓↓ Very large decrease in risk |

# WHAT I TELL MY PATIENTS ABOUT LOWERING THEIR RISK OF CORONARY HEART DISEASE

DR. CAROL BATES

Coronary heart disease (CHD) is not only the number one cause of death among women. It also is a disease, unlike some others, where a woman really can take charge of her life and protect her health. The Nurses' Health Study demonstrated that many cases of CHD could be eliminated by adopting changes in lifestyle.

I find that many of my patients aren't concerned enough about CHD to ask about risk reduction. They tend to be more concerned about cancer, especially breast cancer. Those who are interested in risk reduction often don't think they can do the three things that offer the most protection: quit smoking, eat a healthy diet, and become physically active.

So when I talk with my patients about reducing their risk of CHD, I try to provide more than just advice. I also share tips on how to take action in spite of all the pressures and demands of day-to-day life.

## Stop Smoking

This may be the single most important step you can take to reduce your risk of developing CHD. If you smoke more than two packs a day, your risk is already II times greater than that of a nonsmoker. Even if you smoke only one to four cigarettes a day, you have double the risk. Strategies for how you can quit smoking successfully are discussed at length in Chapter 17.

## Avoid Secondhand Smoke

Inhaling someone else's cigarette smoke also increases your risk of CHD, by anywhere from 20 to 30 percent. The risk is even greater if you inhale passive smoke on a regular basis for a prolonged period (for instance, if you live with a smoker); in that event, your risk doubles. So what do you do?

- If you live with a smoker, ask him or her to stop smoking. If your partner can't quit, ask that he or she smoke outside the house only.
- Choose the nonsmoking sections of restaurants.
- Avoid bars, which tend to be enclosed and—if they permit it—full of smoke. Meet a friend for drinks at a restaurant or an outdoor café.

## Eat a Healthy Diet

Sure, you've heard the advice before, but it bears repeating: eat a diet with plenty of fruits and vegetables (at least five servings a day), high in fiber (found in whole grains and beans) and low in fat. And when you do consume fat, try to make it polyunsaturated fats and monounsaturated fats rather than saturated and trans-unsaturated fats.

Of course, the key to dietary change is to have practical information on hand when you're in the grocery store after a long day at work and the path of least resistance is microwaving a pizza and drinking a beer. You can start by making small changes to your diet and then to building on those changes. See Chapter 19 for some good ideas.

## Increase Your Physical Activity

Being overweight increases your risk of CHD. It's not just the calories you consume that cause you to gain weight: it's also the calories you don't burn. The Surgeon General recommends that we do moderate physical activity, which includes brisk walking, for at least thirty minutes a day on most days. But if you can remain active for at least ten minutes at a time, three times a day, you will enjoy most of the same health benefits.

I've described strategies for increasing your physical activity in Chapter 15. Briefly, they include:

- Consider exercise part of your normal routine rather than something you add in to an already busy day.
- Start slowly and build gradually.
- Do an activity that you enjoy.
- Reward yourself with flowers, a new exercise outfit, or another nonedible treat.
- Remember to warm up and cool down.

## Get Your Blood Cholesterol Tested

This is usually done every five years. If your cholesterol has been abnormal, it should be checked more frequently. If your total blood cholesterol or LDL cholesterol level is too high, or your HDL cholesterol level is too low, you can take steps to achieve a better profile. Stop smoking, become physically active, drink no more than one alcoholic drink per day, and substitute more polyunsaturated and monounsaturated fat in your diet for saturated and trans-unsaturated fat. If this initial approach is not sufficient to improve your cholesterol levels, then talk with your health care provider about medications that may be appropriate. And remember that blood cholesterol levels fluctuate over the course of your lifetime, so you should monitor this periodically.

## If You Have High Blood Pressure, Reduce It

Typically, your blood pressure is measured as part of a routine physical examination, so make sure that you see your health care provider regularly (once a year). As many as half of all women older than forty-five have high blood pressure, so if yours is high, you are not alone. What can you do? As with blood cholesterol levels, your first step should be to change your diet to a more heart-healthy mix of foods and increase your physical activity. Stop smoking, drink no more than one alcoholic drink per day, and decrease your salt intake.

## Have Your Blood Sugar Levels Checked Regularly

One type of diabetes (adult-onset diabetes) develops during adulthood and can increase your risk of CHD. You can reduce your risk of developing this disease by not smoking, being physically active, eating a healthy diet, and avoiding significant weight gain during adulthood. If you are sedentary, above your ideal body weight, or have a family history of diabetes, ask your health care provider to check your blood sugar periodically.

## Identify and Treat Depression, Anger, and Anxiety

There is growing evidence that women with depression or with unexpressed anger are more likely to develop and to die from CHD. There is no proof yet that proper treatment will reduce the chance of developing heart disease, but treating these emotional conditions obviously can greatly improve the quality of a woman's life in many other ways.

Unfortunately, we still live in a society where many people regard emotional illnesses as a kind of personal weakness or character flaw. They therefore do not seek medical attention, or they reject the diagnosis or refuse treatment. The Surgeon General recently called attention to the importance of emotional disorders in our society, and pointed out that most such disorders have a *physical* basis: emotional disorders are caused by altered brain chemistry, although they are also strongly influenced by life events.

If you think you may have an emotional disorder, you should seek help for it. Meditation, relaxation tapes, and physical activity are potential ways to cope with emotions. You should also discuss your symptoms and treatment options with your health care provider.

## Other Helpful Hints

In addition to the broad strategies detailed above, you can take additional small steps to reduce your risk of developing CHD. These include:

- If you can keep it in moderation, a drink of alcohol every day may lower your risk by about 40 percent. But don't exceed that amount, because drinking more can increase your risk of other diseases, not to mention the risk of developing an addiction.
- Start eating nuts occasionally as a snack. If you eat five ounces of nuts a week (about two handfuls a day), you can reduce your risk of

CHD by about 35 percent (as long as your don't increase your calorie intake).

- Eat fortified cereal in the morning. Not only will this provide many of the vitamins and nutrients you need, but it also supplies fiber, which can help to reduce your risk of coronary heart disease and some types of cancer.
- Foods rich in vitamin E may reduce the risk of CHD. There is some evidence that consuming a vitamin E supplement (400 IU) every day, especially if you are at risk for CHD already, may also reduce your risk, although this is unproven, and several recent studies have not shown a benefit. However, there is virtually no risk from taking this much vitamin E as a supplement. Vitamin E is sometimes listed in milligrams (mg) as well as in IU. For vitamin E supplements, 1 mg of vitamin E equals 1 IU of vitamin E.
- Taking 400 micrograms (the amount found in most multivitamins) of folic acid each day may protect against CHD, and is generally recommended in women of childbearing years, to protect against birth defects in children.
- There is some evidence that taking a vitamin $B_6$ supplement (100 milligrams) each day may also protect against CHD, but this is unproven. Nevertheless, there is no risk from taking this much vitamin $B_6$.
- If you have a history of heart disease or a history of risk factors for heart disease, taking an aspirin a day may offer you protection against CHD. However, since aspirin can also cause bleeding, you should talk with your health care provider about the risks and benefits of aspirin use.

# CHAPTER FIVE

# Lowering the Risk of Breast Cancer

## BACKGROUND

You likely recognize the ratio one in eight as an American woman's lifetime risk of developing breast cancer. In addition to being an alarming reminder to some women of how common breast cancer is, the one in eight ratio can also raise a host of important questions. Why is the lifetime risk so high? What causes the disease? And most important, how can I lower my risk? While the recent attention given to breast cancer by the media and various health organizations has increased general awareness of the disease, many women are still confused about the answers to these questions. And with media reports on scientific studies appearing to contradict each other on a weekly basis, it is easy to understand why. One story says eating too much fat increases the risk of breast cancer; another says the fat found in olive oil actually lowers risk; and the next week a different issue altogether goes through this type of cycle.

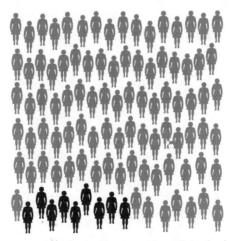

FIG. 5-1. In a group of 100 women who are fifty years old, 9 will develop breast cancer before they reach the age of eighty. (Source: National Cancer Institute)

Despite the confusion that often seems to surround the topic, breast cancer deserves much of the attention it gets. Approximately 180,000 American women are newly diagnosed with the disease each year, and it is the leading killer of women in midlife (ages forty to fifty-five). The only cancer that kills more women overall is lung cancer (see Figure 5-2), but breast cancer is actually responsible for more years of life lost because it generally afflicts younger women. On top of the physical health problems, breast cancer can also exact a large emotional and psychological toll, because it affects a part of the body that

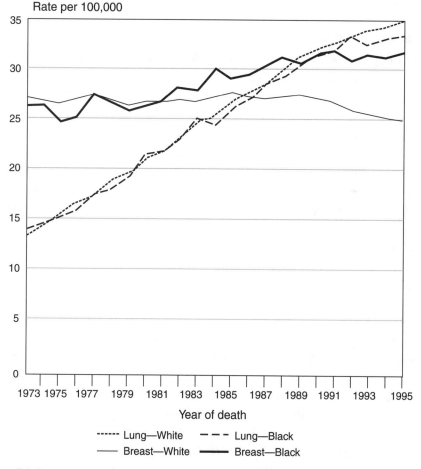

FIG. 5-2. Breast Cancer and Lung Cancer Mortality. Age-adjusted to the 1970 U.S. standard. (Source: National Cancer Institute)

many women associate directly with their femininity. Surveys have consistently found that women perceive breast cancer to be their greatest health threat.

Over the last twenty years, substantial strides have been made in treating breast cancer and in identifying factors that contribute to its development. Today, quality of life is significantly better for women treated for breast cancer than in the past, and the rate of new cases of the disease has leveled off and even started to decline slightly in some groups of women. Much work remains, however, as overall rates of the disease remain high and not all women have benefited equally from the recent decrease in disease rates. The rate of new cases of breast cancer is actually increasing in African American women, and even though white women have higher rates of breast cancer overall, African American women are still more likely to die from the disease.

## The Breast and Breast Cancer

Breasts are made up of several sections called lobes. Each lobe has smaller sections called lobules, which produce milk when a woman is breast-feeding. The lobes and lobules are linked by tubes called ducts. Ducts are the tubes that carry the milk from the lobules to the nipple. The rest of the breast is mostly made up of fat but also consists of veins, arteries, nerves, and other tissue (see Figure 5-3).

In breast cancer, cells in the breast divide and grow at an abnormal rate, clump together, and form a malignant (cancerous) tumor. There are two main types of breast cancer. Most common is breast cancer that begins in the ducts and spreads to nearby tissue, called invasive ductal carcinoma. The other main type is breast cancer that begins in the lobes and spreads to nearby tissue, called invasive lobular carcinoma.

There is also a condition called carcinoma in situ, where there are abnormal cells in the breast, but they are not cancerous and have not spread to other nearby tissue. *In situ* means "in place." Still, carcinoma in situ is a sign that breast cancer may develop at a later time. The two main categories of carcinoma in situ are ductal carcinoma in situ (DCIS)—where the abnormal cells originate in the milk ducts—and lobular carcinoma in situ (LCIS)—where the abnormal cells originate in the lobules.

The most common outward sign of breast cancer is a hard lump in the breast that is usually not movable and may or may not be painful. The skin over the lump may be thickened and dimpled (like the skin of an orange) or indented in areas where the cancer has spread. The nipple may be inverted (turned inward) or leak dark fluid.

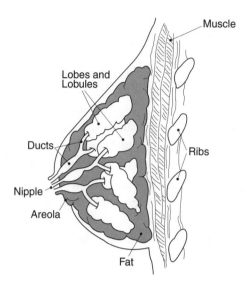

FIG. 5-3. The breast is composed primarily of fat and breast tissues. But the breast also has nerves, arteries, and veins, as well as lymphatic vessels that carry lymph fluid to and from the lymph nodes. The *lobules* are milk-producing glands, and the *ducts* carry the milk to the nipples during lactation. Breast cancer usually starts in the ducts or the lobules but may spread to other parts of the body through the lymph channels or blood vessels.

The best chance of surviving breast cancer comes from the early detection of cancerous tumors through regular clinical breast exams and mammograms. Reducing the risk of the disease ever occurring, however, should be every woman's goal.

## The Importance of Early Life in Breast Cancer Risk

Ideally the prevention of breast cancer would start in youth and young adulthood, as this period has been found to be extremely important in determining a woman's risk of developing breast cancer later in life. Breast tissue during this time (from youth up until a woman gives birth to her first child) appears to be more susceptible to elements that can cause cells to subsequently become cancerous. Exposure to radiation is a good example. The risk for adult breast cancer is very high for a girl under ten exposed to a high dose of radiation (such as exposure to the atomic bomb in 1945 Japan), moderate for a teenager, and small for a young adult.

Unfortunately, by the time an individual woman begins to think concretely about how she can lower her risk of breast cancer, this critical period has likely passed. Parents, however, can help their daughters adopt healthy lifestyles that can impact some of the factors that affect risk during young adulthood, as we discuss later in this chapter. Important factors include age at menarche (the first menstrual period), alcohol consumption, and smoking. Especially important is encouraging daughters to be physically active and to maintain a healthy weight, which, along with many other health benefits, can delay age at menarche.

It has been estimated that breast cancer rates could be reduced by as much as half in the United States by focusing prevention efforts on youth and making certain social changes (for example, so that women who give birth at an early age are not handicapped professionally). While the social changes to support such efforts may be far off, this estimate highlights the fact that rates of breast cancer in the United States can be reduced and that women are far from helpless in the fight against the disease.

## LESSONS FROM THE NURSES' HEALTH STUDY AND OTHER STUDIES

To many women it would seem that just about everything affects the risk of developing breast cancer. While this is not the case, the scientific community has

---

*In the Nurses' Own Words . . .*

I have enjoyed participating in the Nurses' Health Study over the past twenty-four years and consider it a privilege to be part of important research to improve women's health. Completing the biennial survey provides me with an opportunity to take inventory of my lifestyle practices. Specifically, it forces me to take a more thoughtful and detailed look at my dietary choices. Along the way, I have added more fruit and vegetables, reduced fat intake and portion size, and included vitamin supplements in my daily regime. Now, at fifty-three, I am following the research to help guide my efforts to add quality to the post-menopausal years, especially maintaining mobility and flexibility and a positive, healthy outlook toward the aging process.

As a five-year cancer survivor, I know all too well that many things are out of my control. So it has become very important for me to exert control where I am able. The Nurses' Health Study helps to provide direction in the choices I make.

—From CC

come a long way in identifying many factors that increase the risk of the disease. These factors can range from family history to lifestyle factors to reproductive variables.

Although there are a few factors that substantially increase a woman's risk of breast cancer, most individually elevate or lower risk by only a small amount. Some of these factors are those over which a woman has control (such as alcohol consumption and use of postmenopausal hormones) and some are not (such as breast cancer in an immediate family member and age at menarche). By knowing how each of these factors affects her risk, a woman can take appropriate steps to try to protect herself from the disease.

Ultimately, it seems that most cases of breast cancer are caused by a combination of factors, some of which are known and some of which are currently unknown.

## Breast Cancer: The Larger Picture

- Approximately 180,000 American women are newly diagnosed with breast cancer each year, and it is the leading killer of women between the ages of forty and fifty-five.
- The lifetime risk of breast cancer is approximately 12 percent, which means that for all adult women, one in eight is at risk of developing breast cancer in her lifetime. In general, the older a woman is, the greater her risk of the disease.
- The best chance of surviving breast cancer comes from the early detection of cancerous tumors through regular clinical breast exams and mammograms. Reducing the risk of the disease's ever occurring, however, should be every woman's goal.

### Factors You Cannot Control

There are a number of factors beyond a woman's control that affect her risk of developing breast cancer. Understanding these may lead a woman to be more vigilant about those factors under her control and, if necessary, seek more frequent check ups or screening tests.

### AGE

Age is a well-established risk factor for breast cancer. In general, the older a woman is, the greater her risk of the disease. National data show that rates of breast cancer are low in women under forty, begin to increase after forty, and are highest in women over seventy (see Figure 5-4). Only after the age of about eighty does the risk stop increasing with age.

In a group of 100 women who are fifty years old, 9 will develop breast cancer before they reach the age of eighty. The 1 in 8 number that many women recognize is the lifetime risk of breast cancer. This means that for all adult women, 1 in 8 (or approximately 12 percent) is at risk of developing breast cancer in her lifetime. While a 12 percent lifetime risk is high for a serious disease like breast cancer, the lifetime risk of coronary heart disease is much higher (about 32 percent), and both coronary heart disease and lung cancer kill more women overall.

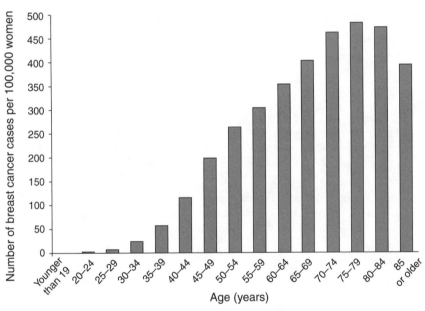

FIG. 5-4. Rates of breast cancer are low in women under forty, begin to increase after forty, and are highest in women over seventy. (Source: National Cancer Institute)

## FAMILY HISTORY AND GENETICS

It should come as no surprise that family history is linked to the risk of breast cancer. Most people realize that the risks of many diseases are associated with the experiences of their parents and siblings. In the Nurses' Health Study, we have found that having an immediate family member (mother or sister) who has been diagnosed with breast cancer approximately doubles the risk of the disease (see Figure 5-5). The age at which the mother was diagnosed, however, influenced the level of risk as well. The younger the mother was when she was diagnosed with the disease, the higher her daughter's risk of developing breast cancer. A woman whose mother was diagnosed before age forty has a large increase in risk, while a woman whose mother was diagnosed after age seventy has only a moderate increase in risk.

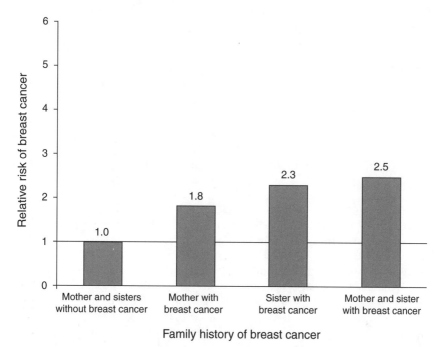

FIG. 5-5. The relative risk of breast cancer is higher in women whose mothers or sisters have been diagnosed with the disease. (Source: Nurses' Health Study)

The number of immediate family members with the disease also influences risk. When both a woman's mother *and* her sister had been diagnosed with breast cancer, we found that the risk of the disease increased to about 2.5 times that of a woman without a family history of the disease. Numerous other studies have also found a similarly strong relationship.

*Genetics.* Family members usually have very similar lifestyles and therefore may have similar "environmental" risk factors for breast cancer—such as weight, activity level, and alcohol intake. While this may account for the increased risk of breast cancer experienced by some families, in some cases genetics likely plays a large role.

Much has been written in scientific journals and reported in the media recently on inherited genetic mutations that greatly increase the risk of developing breast cancer. Two of the most well-known examples are BRCA 1 and

BRCA 2 (which stands for BReast CAncer gene 1 and 2). Studies have found that women who have the BRCA 1 mutation have approximately 15 times the risk of developing breast cancer compared to women without the BRCA 1 mutation. A BRCA 2 mutation appears to impart a slightly lower risk. Women found to have a breast cancer gene mutation, as well as other high risk women, have certain options that may help lower their risk of getting breast cancer or at least increase their chances of identifying the disease early when it is most treatable. (See Dr. Nancy Rigotti's advice for high risk women at the end of this chapter.)

Although genetic mutations like BRCA 1 are powerful predictors of who will get breast cancer, such mutations do not account for a large portion of

## Breast Cancer Gene Mutations—The Concept of Penetrance and the Option of Genetic Testing

The risk associated with gene mutations such as those in BRCA 1 or 2 is often expressed in terms of their penetrance. Penetrance describes the percentage of women with a mutation who actually go on to develop the disease over a certain period of time. A penetrance of 100 percent would mean that every single woman with the mutation would get breast cancer by age seventy. Studies have found that the overall penetrance of BRCA 1 is about 50 to 60 percent by the age of seventy. This means that 50 to 60 percent of the women with the BRCA 1 mutation are likely to develop breast cancer by the age of seventy.

Because of the very high risk associated with the BRCA 1 and 2 gene mutations, women with a strong family history of breast cancer (that is to say, multiple immediate family members with the disease) may want to consider genetic testing to determine whether or not they have the mutation. Many hospitals and medical centers now have genetic counselors on staff who can talk through the risks and benefits of being tested for the mutations.

Although there is an easily administered test for the BRCA mutations, it is important for women to weigh the risks and benefits before deciding to be tested. The primary benefits of testing center on a woman knowing for sure one way or the other about her genetic status. For women found to have a gene mutation, the guessing is finally over and they can now take concrete steps to protect themselves from the disease. For women without a mutation, they can rest easier that that specific risk factor is not hanging over their heads. Genetic testing, though, is not without its risks. In addition to the anxiety and worry a positive result can have on a woman (and her family), a major concern with testing is the confidentiality of the process. Though rare and against the law, a breech in this confidentiality can open a woman up to both insurance and employment discrimination, even based solely on the fact that she was tested for the mutation—regardless of the results.

breast cancer cases. It is estimated that only 5 to 10 percent percent of breast cancers can be attributed to inherited gene mutations, an approximation in line with our experience in the Nurses' Health Study.

## BENIGN BREAST DISEASE

The term *benign breast disease* is often used to describe a wide range of noncancerous conditions that can affect the breast. In the Nurses' Health Study, we have found that two specific types of benign breast disease—hyperplasia and radial scars—increase the risk of developing breast cancer. Other benign breast conditions, such as cysts and fibroadenomas, do not appear to influence risk.

*Hyperplasia.* Hyperplasia is a noncancerous condition where cells begin to multiply in the breast ducts or lobules. Supporting the results of smaller studies, we have found in the Nurses' Health Study that women with cases of hyperplasia confirmed by a biopsy have a moderate to large increase in the risk of developing breast cancer compared to women without hyperplasia. The greatest increase in risk is found in one specific type of hyperplasia, in which the multiplying cells look abnormal (atypical hyperplasia). Hyperplasia in which the multiplying cells still look normal (hyperplasia without atypia) results in a modest increase in risk.

*Radial Scars.* Like hyperplasia, histologic radial scars are a type of benign breast disease that is identified only on breast biopsy. They are usually microscopic in size and are not scars as most people think of them. The name refers to the type of tissue that makes up the condition and not to a scar that results from a healed cut or injury. Previous studies of radial scars have had varied findings, with some showing a link to an increased risk of breast cancer and some showing no link at all. When we examined the association of radial scars with breast cancer in the Nurses' Health Study, we found that women with radial scars had about twice the risk of developing breast cancer as women without. The size and number of radial scars also affected risk: the larger and more numerous the radial scars, the greater the risk of developing breast cancer.

## BREAST DENSITY

The density of a woman's breasts has been shown in many studies to be strongly related to the risk of breast cancer. Breast density is most often assessed by mammogram and depends on the proportion of fat and tissue that make up a woman's breasts. When the X-rays used in a mammogram take an image of the breast, fat appears dark and tissue appears light. Breasts with a high density have a relatively high proportion of tissue and low proportion of fat. Breasts with a low density have a relatively low proportion of tissue and high proportion of fat. We are currently assessing this issue in the Nurses' Health Study and hope to have results soon. Of note, one very large cohort study found that women with the most dense breasts had approximately 5 times the risk of breast cancer compared to women with the least dense breasts. And as breast density increased, so did the risk of the disease (see Figure 5-6).

Right now, breast density is not being regularly used to assess women's risk of breast cancer, but it may become standard practice in the future.

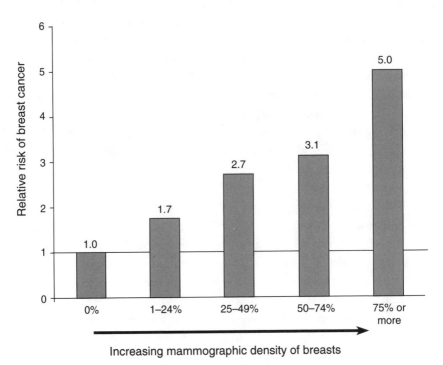

FIG. 5-6. The relative risk of breast cancer increases steadily as breast density as seen on a mammogram increases. (Source: Breast Cancer Detection Demonstration Project)

## RADIATION EXPOSURE IN CHILDHOOD OR ADOLESCENCE

Exposure to high doses of radiation to the chest in childhood or adolescence has been consistently linked to an increased risk of breast cancer in later adulthood. Although not specifically evaluated in the Nurses' Health Study, other studies have found that women who were exposed in their youth to atomic bomb blasts (in Hiroshima or Nagasaki, Japan) or radiation therapy for disorders like Hodgkin's disease or tuberculosis had 2 to 4 times the risk of breast cancer compared to women who were not exposed to such radiation. The greatest risk is generally in those women who were very young when exposed, and the risk decreases as the age at the exposure increases. Women over forty who have been exposed to high doses of radiation to the chest have only a small increase in risk.

That breast cancer risk is highest in those women who were exposed to radiation when very young illustrates the importance that early life may play in breast cancer risk. Breast tissue during this time may be more susceptible to elements that can cause cells to become cancerous later in life.

It is still unclear how exposure to low dose radiation, such as that received from an X-ray or mammogram, influences the risk of developing breast cancer. It is possible that there is some small risk associated with such procedures, but the health benefits they provide greatly outweigh any potential increase in breast cancer risk.

## PERSONAL HISTORY OF CANCER

Just as family history can affect the risk of breast cancer, so can a personal history of cancer. Women who have been previously diagnosed with cancer in one breast are at increased risk of developing cancer in the other breast. Studies other than the Nurses' Health Study that have assessed the issue have found the risk to be increased two- to fourfold for women previously diagnosed with breast cancer (including ductal carcinoma in situ) compared to those without a previous diagnosis.

Having a personal history of lobular carcinoma in situ—which is usually not treated after diagnosis, just closely followed—also increases the risk of cancer. Women with this condition are 7 to 10 times more likely to develop breast cancer than women without the condition.

A history of other cancers can also increase the risk of breast cancer. Studies have shown that women who have been diagnosed with colon or ovarian cancer have a slightly increased risk of developing breast cancer as well. The likely explanation for this is that the three cancers share some of the same genetic or lifestyle factors that are key to cancer development.

## ETHNICITY

Not all groups of women in the United States are equally impacted by breast cancer. Latina, Asian American, and American Indian women tend to have the lowest risk of breast cancer in the United States, and white women tend to have the highest risk—followed closely by Hawaiian American and African American women. For breast cancer occurring before midlife, however, African American women are at highest risk. This is likely due, at least in large part, to differences in the ages at which white women and African American women first give birth. While having children is protective against breast cancer overall, giving birth to the first child after thirty is actually linked to a modest increase in the risk of breast cancer in the short term. Since African American women tend to give birth for the first time earlier than white women, they may experience this increase in breast cancer risk earlier in life, pushing their rates of breast cancer before midlife past those of white women. Across the entire lifetime, though, these differences in reproductive behaviors seem to benefit African Americans, whose lifetime risk of breast cancer is lower than that of whites.

Unfortunately, as overall rates of breast cancer are leveling off or slightly decreasing in white women, they continue to increase in African American women.

Jewish women are another ethnic group at increased risk of breast cancer. Particularly affected are Ashkenazi Jewish women—Jews who immigrated from central or eastern Europe. One likely reason is that Ashkenazi Jews have an unusually high rate of BRCA 1 and 2 gene mutations compared to the national average.

## HEIGHT

There is a substantial amount of evidence that height is associated with the risk of breast cancer both pre- and postmenopause. In the Nurses' Health Study, we found that risk was slightly increased in all women who were 5 feet 3 inches or taller compared to those under 5 feet 3 inches. In another large cohort study, the risk of breast cancer in postmenopausal women was found to increase steadily with height (see Figure 5-7). The tallest women in the study had a little more than twice the risk of the disease compared to the shortest women.

Height is generally thought to reflect, at least in part, the quantity and quality of the diet in childhood. Well fed children generally have more rapid, bigger growth spurts than children fed poor diets. This may contribute to breast cancer risk because such rapid growth can increase the chance that the DNA in some breast cells will become permanently damaged, which can lead to cancer later in life. One other possibility is that levels of a hormone called insulin-like growth factor are higher in taller children than in shorter children. In some studies (including ours), high levels of insulin-like growth factor have been linked to an increased risk of breast cancer.

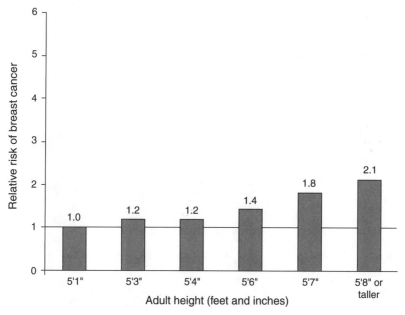

FIG. 5-7. The relative risk of breast cancer increases with height. (Source: Van den Brandt et al.)

## Factors You Can Control

It is important to know how all of the factors related to breast cancer make up a woman's risk. However, when given a choice, most women would prefer to focus on those things they have control over and can change for the better. These so-called modifiable factors are discussed in this section and range from alcohol intake to use of postmenopausal hormones.

Aside from a small number of factors related to diet, most of the modifiable factors are thought to affect the risk of breast cancer by influencing levels of female hormones (such as estrogen and progesterone) in the body. Estrogen is believed to be a key promoter of breast cancer development, and findings from the Nurses' Health Study have helped support this conclusion. We found that postmenopausal women with the highest blood levels of certain estrogens had almost double the risk of breast cancer compared to women with the lowest levels. Most strikingly, in a subset of women who had never used postmenopausal hormones (hence, their blood hormone levels could be better measured), those with the highest blood estrogen levels had almost four times the risk of developing breast cancer (see Figure 5-8). This increase in risk is similar in size to that between blood cholesterol levels and heart disease.

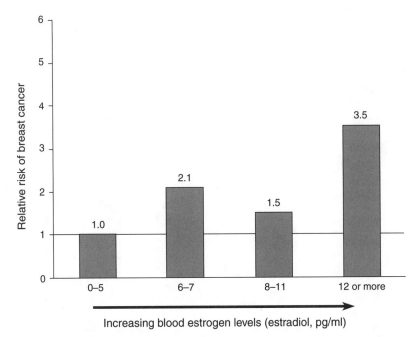

FIG. 5-8. The relative risk of breast cancer is increased in postmenopausal women with increased blood levels of estrogen. The risk is particularly apparent in those women who have never used postmenopausal hormones. Even though this figure shows that the relative risk in the third category (8–11 pg/mL) is lower than that in the second (6–7 pg/mL), the overall trend shows a substantial increase in breast cancer risk as blood estrogen levels increase. (Source: Nurses' Health Study)

## DIET

When asked if the food we eat plays an important role in breast cancer development, most people would respond with a definite yes. In reality, however, very few aspects of diet have been linked to breast cancer risk.

*Vitamin A, Carotenoids, and Fruits and Vegetables.* A number of studies have linked a low intake of vitamin A and carotenoids, such as beta-carotene, with an increased risk of breast cancer. Found in high amounts in green and yellow vegetables and certain fruits, vitamin A is important for cell growth, and carotenoids are powerful antioxidants that can help protect cells from the damaging effects of oxygen free radicals in the body. In the Nurses' Health Study, we found that premenopausal women who had a modest to high total intake of vitamin A from food had a 10 to 30 percent lower risk of the disease compared to women with the lowest intake. This reduction in risk was even more pronounced in premenopausal women with a family history of breast cancer: a 60 percent lower risk for those women with the highest intake of vitamin A compared to those with the lowest. This finding, though, was unexpected and needs to be explored further.

Similarly, when we assessed carotenoids, we found that, compared to premenopausal women with the lowest intake of certain carotenoids (beta-carotene, lutein, and zeaxanthin), those with greater intake had a slightly lower risk of breast cancer. No link was found between either carotenoids or vitamin A and breast cancer in postmenopausal women.

Because people eat foods and not specific nutrients, we have also assessed the link between fruits and vegetables and breast cancer risk. What we found was very similar to the relationship seen with vitamin A: premenopausal women who ate modest to high amounts of fruits and vegetables (over two servings per day) had a slightly lower risk of breast cancer than women who ate the least amount of fruits and vegetables (less than one serving). Again, no link was found in postmenopausal women.

When researchers combined our study results with those of seven other large studies, they found similar results: total intake of fruits and vegetables had very little effect on the risk of breast cancer. However, specific types of fruits and vegetables, such as those rich in carotenoids, do appear to reduce risk modestly, primarily in premenopausal women.

*Dietary Fat.* Eating high amounts of total fat in adulthood appears to have little, if any, effect on the risk of developing breast cancer. In the Nurses' Health Study, we found that, compared to women with a moderate fat intake, women with a high fat diet did not have a greater risk of developing breast cancer. Similarly, women who ate little fat (20 percent or less of total calories) did not have a lower risk of the disease compared to women who ate a moderate amount. These findings corroborate those of an analysis that pooled together the data from a number of large cohort studies (including the Nurses' Health Study). This analysis found that neither a high fat diet nor a low fat diet was related to the risk of breast cancer (see Figure 5-9).

Most Americans today get about 33 percent of their total calories from fat. In the Nurses' Health Study, the women in the cohort eat a diet ranging from approximately 20 percent of total calories from fat, to approximately 50 percent. Because very few of the women eat very low amounts of fat (10 to 15 percent of total calories), we cannot assess how this extremely low intake influences breast cancer risk. It seems, though, that even very low fat intake may not provide protection from the disease. A large case-control study performed in China found no link between fat intake and the risk of breast cancer, even though some women ate a diet containing less than 15 percent of total calories

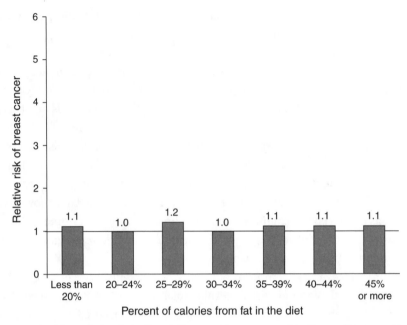

FIG. 5-9. Total fat intake has little, if any, influence on breast cancer risk. (Source: Hunter et al.)

from fat. The analysis that pooled data from a number of studies also found no protection from a very low fat diet (under 15 percent of total calories from fat). Upcoming results from the Women's Health Initiative will provide additional information on the relationship between breast cancer and a low fat diet in postmenopausal women.

Despite there being no apparent link between total fat intake and breast cancer, there may be a link between the type of fat women consume and their risk of the disease. High intake of monounsaturated fat (found in olive and canola oil) has been found in some studies to lower the risk of breast cancer. In the Nurses' Health Study, we have had mixed findings on this issue, with our most recent data showing no relationship between specific types of fat and the risk of breast cancer. One possible reason that our findings contradict those of some others may have to do with the source of the monounsaturated fat. Most of the studies that have shown monounsaturated fats to protect against breast cancer have been performed in Europe and specifically evaluated olive oil intake. In the Nurses' Health Study, animal products (such as red meat and cheese) have been the primary source of monounsaturated fats. That the fat comes from such different food sources could account for the difference in findings.

Although our data from the Nurses' Health Study provide information about how fat intake in midlife relates to breast cancer risk, we cannot address how fat intake in adolescence or early adulthood relates to the risk of the disease. Other studies are currently examining these issues, including our Nurses' Health Study II.

## FACTORS THAT AFFECT ESTROGEN LEVELS

Many modifiable factors can increase the level of estrogen in the body, and therefore increase the risk of breast cancer. Examples of such factors include gaining substantial weight as an adult; being overweight and physically inactive after menopause; drinking modest amounts of alcohol; or using postmenopausal hormones.

*Overweight and Weight Gain.* Studies that have assessed the effect of weight on the risk of developing breast cancer have found that it affects women differently at different ages.

PREMENOPAUSAL WOMEN. In the Nurses' Health Study, when we examined weight's association with breast cancer risk in premenopausal women, we found that as weight increased, the risk of breast cancer decreased. Even though being overweight premenopause lowers the risk of breast cancer, younger women should not take this as carte blanche to gain weight. First, being overweight does not provide premenopausal women with any substantial protection against dying from the disease. This may be due, in part, to the fact that overweight women are often diagnosed with the disease at a more advanced stage than leaner women, making treatment less effective. Second, almost 80 percent of breast cancer cases develop in postmenopausal women, and any weight gained in the premenopausal years will likely track into the postmenopausal years, where it can increase the risk of the disease.

POSTMENOPAUSAL WOMEN. When we assessed postmenopausal women, we found that results differed substantially from those of premenopausal women. For a subgroup of postmenopausal women—those who had never used postmenopausal hormones—obesity was linked to a moderate increase in breast cancer risk. For all other postmenopausal women, there was no link between weight and the risk of developing breast cancer.

Weight *gain,* however, was linked to an increase in risk for all postmenopausal women. Those women who had gained more than 45 pounds since age eighteen had a small increase in risk of developing breast cancer (see

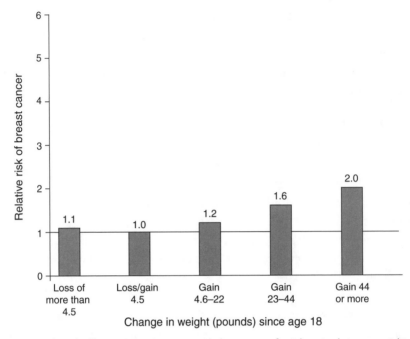

FIG. 5-10. The risk of breast cancer increases with the amount of weight gained since age eighteen. The increase in risk is even more apparent in women who have never used postmenopausal hormones. (Source: Nurses' Health Study)

Figure 5-10). For women who had gained more than 45 pounds but had never used postmenopausal hormones, breast cancer occurred twice as often as in those who experienced little weight gain as adults.

Being overweight is thought to increase the risk of breast cancer after menopause primarily by increasing levels of the hormone estrogen. Although a woman's ovaries stop producing estrogen after menopause, her fat tissue converts estrogen precursors to estrogen. The more weight put on after menopause, the more estrogen that is produced—a point the Nurses' Health Study helped confirm. This relation of weight to hormone levels explains why breast cancer risk in overweight postmenopausal women appears to be more pronounced in those who have never taken postmenopausal hormones. The amount of estrogen contained in postmenopausal hormones far outweighs that produced by the fat tissue in overweight and obese women. Therefore, the full effect of weight on breast cancer risk can become masked when a woman uses postmenopausal hormones. It is not that taking postmenopausal hormones eliminates the risk of breast cancer associated with being overweight; it is that using hormones likely hides the effect of weight on risk.

Other large cohort studies assessing the link between weight and breast cancer in pre- and postmenopausal women have had results similar to ours.

*Body Shape.* Body shape also seems to influence the risk of breast cancer in postmenopausal women. Women who are apple-shaped—those who tend to carry extra weight around the waist—seem to be at higher risk of breast cancer than women who are pear-shaped—those who tend to carry extra weight in their hips and thighs. Similar to the results of other studies, we found that postmenopausal women with the largest waist sizes have about a 35 percent greater risk of breast cancer compared to those with the smallest waist size. As with overall weight, the full effect of waist size on breast cancer risk may be obscured by the use of postmenopausal hormones. When we included only women who had never used postmenopausal hormones, the increase in risk was even greater: women with the largest waist sizes (36 to 55 inches) had about a 90 percent greater risk of breast cancer compared to those with the smallest waist size (15 to 28 inches).

*Physical Activity.* Numerous studies have examined the relationship between physical activity and breast cancer risk, but results to date have been somewhat inconsistent. This variability in findings likely relates to the different approaches researchers use to assess a woman's level of physical activity, which can be difficult to measure accurately.

In the Nurses' Health Study, we found that the effect of physical activity seems to depend on a woman's stage of life. Postmenopausal women who engaged in at least one hour of physical activity a day were 15 to 20 percent less likely to develop breast cancer than women who were sedentary. When we studied premenopausal women, we saw no clear association between amount of physical activity and risk of the disease. However, most other studies with premenopausal women have seen an association.

Physical activity may help lower the risk of breast cancer in postmenopausal women by helping curb weight gain, which in turn helps keep estrogen levels in check. In young girls, physical activity may have the added benefit of putting off the age at which a girl first has her period, therefore reducing lifetime exposure to estrogen.

*Alcohol.* Although news that moderate alcohol intake can lower the risk of coronary heart disease has been welcomed with enthusiasm by many, drinking alcohol does not come without accompanying risks as well—especially for women. The results of many studies have consistently shown that alcohol intake can increase the risk of breast cancer. An analysis evaluating data from five large cohort studies (including the Nurses' Health Study) showed that women who drank two or more drinks a day—whether beer, wine, or hard liquor—were 40 percent more likely to develop breast cancer than women who did not drink any alcohol. In our own analysis of the Nurses' Health Study data, we found that even fewer than 2 drinks per day could increase risk. Compared to women who did not drink, those who drank about half a drink to one drink a day had a small increase in the risk of breast cancer, and those who drank more than one drink a day had a moderate increase in risk (see Figure 5-11).

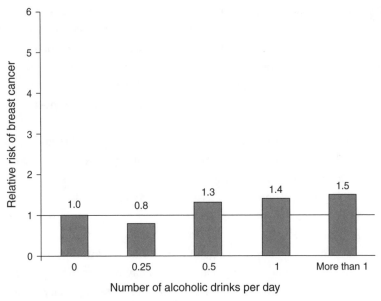

FIG. 5-11. The relative risk of breast cancer begins to increase with as little as half a drink per day. (Source: Nurses' Health Study)

There are a number of ways that alcohol may affect breast cancer risk. In addition to possibly lowering the level of vitamin A in the body, it has been demonstrated in some studies (including the Nurses' Health Study) that alcohol consumption may be linked to increased blood levels of estrogen. Alcohol may also hamper the body's ability to use folate, a vitamin that may help protect against tumor growth. Interestingly, we found in the Nurses' Health Study that the risk of breast cancer associated with one drink or more a day was lower in those women with a high intake of folate compared to those with a low intake. This finding, however, still needs to be confirmed.

For more information on the risks and benefits of alcohol, see Chapter 20.

*Postmenopausal Hormones.* A large number of U.S. women take postmenopausal hormone therapy to alleviate the short-term symptoms and longer-term health effects of menopause. While such hormone therapy appears to be beneficial in many ways—lowering the risk of osteoporosis and possibly coronary heart disease and colon cancer—it also increases the risk of breast cancer in certain users.

After menopause, when a woman's ovaries stop producing estrogen, postmenopausal hormone therapy is a key source of estrogen in those women choosing to use it. After examining many different aspects of the link between breast cancer risk and postmenopausal hormones, we have found in the Nurses' Health Study that risk is substantially increased only in those women who are currently using postmenopausal hormones *and* have been using them long term (over 5 years). Women who are long-term current users have an approximately 50 percent greater risk of developing breast cancer than women who did not use postmenopausal hormones (see Figure 5-12), and, in general, the longer women use hormones, the greater the risk.

Because postmenopausal hormones that contain only estrogen have been shown to increase the risk of cancer of the uterus, more and more women are

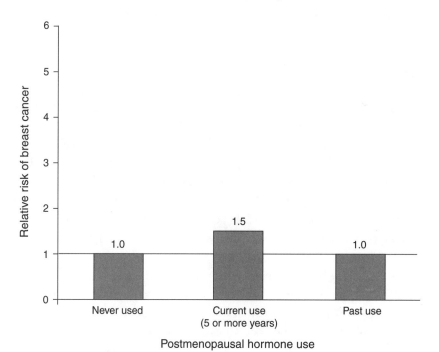

FIG. 5-12. The risk of breast cancer is increased in those women who currently use postmenopausal hormones *and* have been doing so for five or more years. Short-term use (under five years) of hormones does not seem to increase risk. And even for long-term users who stop, the risk drops to that of someone who never used hormones. (Sources: Nurses' Health Study)

choosing to take hormones that contain both estrogen and progestin. It was initially thought this combined therapy might reduce the excess risk of breast cancer linked to postmenopausal hormones. However, we in the Nurses' Health Study—along with others—have found that the risk of breast cancer was actually higher in those women using estrogen and progestin than in those using estrogen alone.

The findings from the Nurses' Health Study assessing postmenopausal hormones and breast cancer risk are very similar to those of numerous other reports, including a very large analysis based on over fifty international studies. Though the details are complicated, the bottom line message about post-menopausal hormone therapy and breast cancer is fairly simple.

- Women who use postmenopausal hormones for less than five years do not seem to be at significantly increased risk of breast cancer.
- Those who use hormones for more than five years are at an increased risk *while* they are on the hormones, and their risk increases the longer they use them. Once they stop, however, their risk returns to that of someone who has never used hormones. Formulations that contain estrogen and progestin increase risk more than formulations that contain estrogen alone.

Issues other than breast cancer, however, also need to be considered when deciding whether or not to use hormones after menopause. Several studies suggest that the risk of osteoporosis, coronary artery disease, and colon cancer can all be reduced with postmenopausal hormones. And some very preliminary data suggest that hormone therapy may possibly even lower the risk of Alzheimer's. Ultimately, a woman and her health care provider need to consider her risk of the various disorders before deciding what approach is best for her. Chapter 22 provides a detailed discussion of the potential risk and benefits of postmenopausal hormone use.

*Birth Control Pills.* The use of birth control pills moderately increases the risk of breast cancer in those women who are currently using them. In the Nurses' Health Study, we found that women who were currently taking the pill had a 50 percent increase in risk compared to women who had never used the pill. Women who had used the pill in the past (but were not doing so currently) did not show any increase in breast cancer risk. Moreover, how long a woman had been on the pill did not seem to change the results.

Although a number of other studies have found no association between use of the pill and an increased risk of breast cancer, a very large analysis that combined over 50 international studies corroborated our results, finding that current users of birth control pills had a small increase in breast cancer risk and that this excess risk slowly returned to zero ten years after stopping taking the pill (see Figure 5-13).

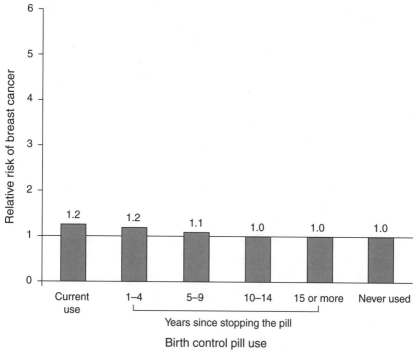

FIG. 5-13. Women have a slightly increased risk of breast cancer while they are taking birth control pills. Once they stop, however, their risk begins to decrease to that of women who have never used them. (Source: Collaborative Group on Hormonal Factors in Breast Cancer)

As with postmenopausal hormone therapy, there is a lot to consider when deciding whether or not to use the pill. Although the pill seems to slightly increase breast cancer risk in current users, it also has many benefits. In addition to preventing unwanted pregnancy, it lowers the risk of ovarian and endometrial cancers. Also, when women use the pill, it is during a time in life when their absolute risk of breast cancer is low, so even though a 50 percent increase in risk is substantial, it will actually result in only a few extra women developing breast cancer who otherwise would not have. Assessing such individual

## Women, Testosterone, and Breast Cancer

Many women in the United States are taking dietary supplements (for example, DHEA) that boost the level of the male hormone testosterone in the body, hoping to increase bone mass and sexual drive, especially after menopause. Some newer postmenopausal hormones even contain small amounts of testosterone. Unfortunately, there is now substantial evidence from a number of cohort studies that high blood levels of testosterone can significantly increase the risk of breast cancer. We found in the Nurses' Health Study that women with higher levels of testosterone had double the risk of the disease compared to women with lower levels. Therefore, it is prudent for all women—postmenopausal or not—to avoid such supplements and medicines, unless specifically prescribed by a health care provider.

risks and benefits and the impact they have on a woman's lifestyle is key to determining whether or not she uses birth control pills. Chapter 23 discusses these issues in greater detail.

### Reproductive Factors

Reproductive factors—such as age at first menstrual period (menarche), age at menopause, and age at first giving birth—have been linked to the risk of breast cancer in a wide range of studies. Much of the effect these factors have on breast cancer risk is thought to be related to their influence on levels of female hormones, such as estrogen, as well as on the maturation of the breast.

### AGE AT FIRST MENSTRUAL PERIOD (MENARCHE)

Girls in the United States are having their first menstrual periods (menarche) at an increasingly early age—with an accompanying elevation in breast cancer risk later in life. For many years, young age at menarche has been well established as a factor that increases the risk of breast cancer. In the Nurses' Health Study, we have found that women who were over thirteen when their periods began had a 35 percent lower chance of developing breast cancer than women whose periods started at age twelve or younger. A late age at menarche is thought to lower breast cancer risk by creating a shorter interval between the time a woman's period starts and the time she gives birth to her first child, reducing her exposure to the female hormones (such as estrogen and progestin) released during the menstrual cycle.

## AGE AT FIRST GIVING BIRTH AND NUMBER OF CHILDREN

For a number of reasons, more and more women are putting off starting a family. Unfortunately, beginning a family at a later age increases the risk of breast cancer. Numerous studies have found that the older women are when they give birth to their first child, the higher their risk of breast cancer. Our data from the Nurses' Health Study also show that women who have given birth have a lower risk overall than women who have not, and women who have more children have a lower risk than women who have fewer children. In addition, we have found that when women have more than one child, the spacing of births can influence risk. Women whose births were spaced closer in time have a slightly lower risk of breast cancer than women whose births were spaced further apart.

Our study and others have found that the risk of breast cancer associated with giving birth to a first child varies over a woman's life. Although the first birth lowers the risk of breast cancer in the long term, there is actually a short-term increase in risk for ten or more years immediately following the event. After this time, the risk begins to drop (see Figure 5-14).

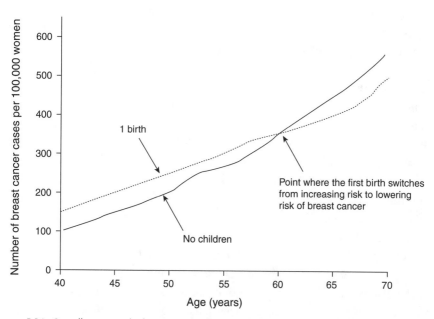

FIG. 5-14. Overall, women who have given birth one or more times have a lower risk of breast cancer than women who have never given birth. Initially, however, the first birth slightly increases risk of breast cancer. This excess risk disappears later in life, after which giving birth helps protect against breast cancer. (Source: Nurses' Health Study)

## The Role of Estrogen

- The female hormone estrogen is believed to be a key promoter of breast cancer development, so by controlling her estrogen levels, a woman may be able to influence her risk of breast cancer.
- Because being overweight increases estrogen levels in a woman's body, it can also increase the risk of breast cancer—but this result is age dependent; postmenopausal women who are overweight are at increased risk, while premenopausal women do not appear to be.
- The younger a woman is when she has her first menstrual period and the older she is at menopause, the longer her lifetime exposure to higher levels of estrogen and other female hormones that increase her risk of breast cancer.

In the short term, a first full-term pregnancy may increase the risk of breast cancer because of the high levels of hormones associated with fetal development that can promote a preexisting breast cancer. But pregnancy also confers long-term protection from the disease, possibly by causing changes to breast cells that make them less susceptible to becoming cancerous as well as by permanently lowering levels of estrogen in the body.

### BREAST-FEEDING

Breast-feeding has many benefits for mother and child, and it has been postulated for many years that it may reduce women's risk of breast cancer. Although there is still debate on the issue, a majority of studies have found that breast-feeding can lower women's risk of the disease, particularly for breast cancer that develops before menopause. In the Nurses' Health Study, we did not find a difference in breast cancer risk for premenopausal or postmenopausal women who had breast-fed. However, we were limited in our ability to assess the long-term effects of breast-feeding.

One possible reason that some studies show a benefit of breast-feeding and other do not may relate to the fact that women use breast-feeding in many different ways. Some use it as the only source of food for their infants, and some use it to supplement other modes of feeding. And over time, women may use a combination of these two approaches. The result is that two women who report that they have both breast-fed their child for six months may have, in fact, spent very different amounts of time actively breast-feeding. Better delineating the exact approaches women have used during their periods of breast-

## Prolactin and Insulin-like Growth Factors

Prolactin and insulin-like growth factor 1 are hormones that circulate naturally in the body. Prolactin plays an important role in breast development and lactation, while insulin-like growth factor 1 is a key hormone involved in human growth and development. Although these hormones are vital to maintain health, there is increasing evidence that women with higher levels may be at increased risk of breast cancer compared to those with lower levels. In the Nurses' Health Study, we found that women with higher prolactin levels had about twice the risk of breast cancer compared to those with lower levels. For insulin-like growth factor, we found that increased levels measured in premenopausal women were linked with a substantially increased risk of breast cancer, while higher levels of the hormone in postmenopausal women were not related to risk. This may suggest that insulin-like growth factor levels in adolescence or early adulthood are most important in determining the risk of breast cancer later in life. These findings need to be confirmed, however. Few studies other than the Nurses' Health Study have evaluated these relationships.

feeding—as we are currently doing in the Nurses' Health Study—may help clarify the relationship between breast-feeding and the risk of breast cancer. Aside from possibly protecting against breast cancer, breast-feeding also means fewer childhood infections, less work time lost to care for a sick child, and a quicker return to pre-pregnancy weight.

### AGE AT MENOPAUSE

Studies have long shown that women who go through early menopause, whether naturally or through surgical removal of the ovaries (oophorectomy), have a reduced risk of breast cancer. As with late age at menarche, early age at menopause is thought to decrease risk by shortening the lifelong exposure to the hormones released during the menstrual cycle. Our data from the Nurses' Health Study show that for every one-year increase in age at natural menopause, a woman's risk for breast cancer increases by 3 percent. This translates to an approximately 35 percent increase in risk for a woman going through menopause at age fifty-five or older compared to one going through it at forty-five.

### Unproven Factors and Factors Found to Have No Effect on Breast Cancer

Many factors discussed in the media and certain health circles are said to affect the risk of breast cancer but have not actually been proven to do so. Some of these may in the future be linked to breast cancer. Some, though, have been conclusively proven to have no influence on the risk of the disease. Here are some examples of these factors, many of which we have assessed in the Nurses' Health Study.

## ISOFLAVONOIDS AND SOY ESTROGEN

Isoflavonoids are specific types of estrogen that are found abundantly in soy products. In laboratory studies, isoflavonoids seem to protect breast cells from becoming cancerous by blocking the cancer initiating action of other estrogens. To date in the Nurses' Health Study, we have not studied this issue, primarily because exposure to isoflavonoids has historically been low in the United States. Since women have greatly increased their intake in recent years, we will be able to examine this thoroughly in the future. Results from the few studies that have looked at the issue have been mixed, with some showing a benefit and others showing no relationship. Before any conclusions can be drawn about the link (if any) between isoflavonoids, soy, and breast cancer, there must be more human studies on the topic.

## SELENIUM

Selenium is a substance found in food and nutrition supplements that has been shown in laboratory experiments to lower the risk of certain kinds of cancer in animals. When we assessed the link between selenium and breast cancer risk in the Nurses' Health Study, we found no association with the risk of disease in either premenopausal or postmenopausal women.

## ORGANOCHLORINE CHEMICALS

Organochlorine chemicals, found in certain pesticides and industrial chemicals, have often been discussed as potential risk factors for breast cancer because they have qualities similar to estrogen. Early studies suggested a link with breast cancer, but now it seems that organochlorines may have no effect on risk. When we examined a sub-sample of the Nurses' Health Study cohort, we found that blood levels of two specific organochlorine chemicals—DDE and PCBs—were not linked to breast cancer risk.

## HETEROCYCLIC AMINES

Heterocyclic amines are substances produced by cooking meat at high temperatures; they have been demonstrated to increase risk of cancer in laboratory experiments with animals. Heterocyclic amines appear in the greatest amount in meat that has been charred or flame-broiled. Though some studies have found a link between heterocyclic amines and breast cancer in humans—including the Iowa Women's Health Study—in an initial assessment in the Nurses' Health Study we found no link between the two.

## GINSENG

As with isoflavonoids, it is thought that the herb ginseng may help protect against breast cancer by blocking the cancer-initiating action of estrogen. Some laboratory studies have shown positive results, but few studies have been conducted in humans. We have yet to assess this issue in the Nurses' Health Study but hope to do so in the future.

## SMOKING

Because smoking lowers the age at which a woman enters menopause as well as affects the metabolism of estrogen, it has been thought that it may actually reduce the risk of breast cancer. However, we found in the Nurses' Health Study that smoking in adulthood had no influence on the risk of breast cancer. Smoking early in youth may modestly increase the risk of breast cancer, as some studies have suggested. However, we have not yet evaluated this in the Nurses' Health Study.

## HAIR DYES

Permanent hair dye contains substances called aromatic amines that have been shown in laboratory studies to increase the risk of breast cancer in some animals. In the Nurses' Health Study, we have repeatedly found no association between the use of permanent hair dyes and the risk of breast cancer.

## ABORTION

The association between abortion and breast cancer has been controversial in the past, but it now seems clear that abortion has no influence on the risk of the disease. As with other studies on the topic, our Nurses' Health Study II found no link between the two.

## OTHERS

Other factors that have not been proven to increase the risk of breast cancer include electromagnetic fields, antiperspirants/deodorants, and the use of bras. For each of these, there is no clear way biologically that they could increase the risk of the disease.

## Established and Probable Factors Associated with the Risk of Breast Cancer

| RISK FACTOR | APPROXIMATE RISK* |
|---|---|
| *Established* | |
| Lobular carcinoma in situ | ↑↑↑↑ |
| Family history of breast cancer | |
| Mother diagnosed before age 40 | ↑↑↑ |
| Mother diagnosed after age 70 | ↑↑ |
| Sister diagnosed with breast cancer | ↑↑↑ |
| Mother *and* sister diagnosed with breast cancer | ↑↑↑ |
| Confirmed BRCA 1 or 2 | ↑↑↑↑ |
| Previous breast cancer | ↑↑↑ |
| High blood levels of estrogen | ↑↑↑ |
| Repeated high dose radiation to chest in childhood | ↑↑↑ |
| (the lower the age at exposure, the higher the risk) | |
| Breast density (high density vs. low density) | ↑↑↑ |
| Benign breast disease | |
| Intraductal hyperplasia | ↑↑ |
| Atypical hyperplasia | ↑↑↑ |
| Radial scars | ↑↑ |
| Height (5'5" or taller vs. 5'1" or shorter) | ↑↑ |
| Weight | |
| Being overweight after menopause | ↑↑ |
| Gaining more than 15 to 20 pounds in adulthood | ↑↑ |
| Alcohol intake (2 or more drinks per day) | ↑↑ |
| Postmenopausal hormone use (current or recent use for 5+ years) | ↑↑ |
| Late age at menopause (age 55 vs. 45 or younger) | ↑↑ |
| Late age at giving first birth | ↑↑ |
| No children | ↑↑ |
| Birth control pills (current or recent use) | ↑ |
| Early age at first period (age 12 vs. 14) | ↑ |
| *Probable* | |
| High intake of vitamin A and carotenoids | ↓ |

| | |
|---|---|
| Breast-feeding | ↓ |
| Regular physical activity | ↓ |

| | |
|---|---|
| *↑ Small increase in risk | ↓ Small decrease in risk |
| ↑↑ Moderate increase in risk | ↓↓ Moderate decrease in risk |
| ↑↑↑ Large increase in risk | ↓↓↓ Large decrease in risk |
| ↑↑↑↑ Very large increase in risk | ↓↓↓↓ Very large decrease in risk |

## WHAT IT ALL MEANS

As is apparent from the lengthy list of factors discussed above, breast cancer is a very complex disease. But the messages are relatively simple when it comes to the steps a woman can take to try to reduce the risk of breast cancer, and the good news is that these same steps also help prevent coronary heart disease, diabetes, and other chronic disorders.

• **Maintain a healthy weight and avoid substantial weight gain (more than about fifteen to twenty pounds) during adulthood.** Maintaining a healthy weight at every age protects women against breast cancer, even if they are not physically active. A healthy weight in childhood increases the age at which the first menstrual period occurs and slightly decreases the age at which menopause occurs: together, these two factors lead to a lower lifetime exposure to estrogen. Maintaining a healthy weight also appears to have some protective effects over and above its effects on the age at menarche and menopause.

• **Lead a physically active lifestyle.** Physical activity at every age protects women against breast cancer. When young girls are physically active, the age at which they experience their first menstrual period is delayed. This lowers their lifetime exposure to estrogen, and this in turn lowers their risk of breast cancer. Being physically active throughout life may directly reduce the risk of breast cancer after menopause, even in women who are not overweight. When physical activity leads to weight loss or prevents weight gain, that also protects you.

• **Eat a diet rich in fruits and vegetables.** Fruits and vegetables contain a number of substances that may help the body fight cancer, including vitamin A and carotenoids.

• **Drink less than one alcoholic drink a day on average.** A drink a day or more has been linked to an increase in breast cancer risk. There may be no safe level of alcohol consumption in relation to breast cancer risk, but moderate alcohol intake has been linked to a decreased risk of coronary heart disease.

Avoiding long-term use of postmenopausal hormones can also lower the risk of breast cancer, but because hormone use carries both risks and benefits, it is important for women to discuss this issue individually with their health care providers.

# WHAT I TELL MY PATIENTS ABOUT LOWERING THEIR RISK OF BREAST CANCER

DR. NANCY RIGOTTI

Ask one of my patients which disease she fears most, and chances are that she will answer breast cancer. Most women do. Breast cancer cuts right to the heart of our identity as women, and the constant stream of stories, research findings, and advice about breast cancer keeps the disease at the forefront of women's concerns. It can, in fact, be difficult for women *not* to fear breast cancer.

There are two and possibly three ways in which you can help to protect yourself from breast cancer:

- Adopt a healthy lifestyle.
- Get breast cancer screening tests, when indicated.
- If you are at unusually high risk of getting breast cancer, consider whether to use certain preventive treatments (such as taking the drug tamoxifin).

## Adopt a Healthy Lifestyle

We know less about how to prevent breast cancer than we do about preventing some other diseases like heart disease, but fortunately we do have effective tests that can find the disease early, when treatment has the best chance of cure. And although breast cancer is influenced by many factors that you cannot control, it is also influenced by factors you can control. Diet and physical activity, the main components of a healthy lifestyle, may also lower the risk of getting breast cancer.

### START EXERCISING

Most of my patients know that regular physical activity is good for their heart and bones. But most of them don't know that it also reduces their risk of developing breast cancer after they reach menopause. It's yet another reason to get moving. The Surgeon General recommends thirty minutes of moderate physical activity on most days of the week. You don't have to go to a gym to become physically active! You can do things like take a brisk walk, garden, bicycle with your children, or swim with a friend. If you feel you don't have time to fit another thirty minutes into your hectic day, then aim for three ten-minute periods of activity a day.

## Keep Your Weight Under Control

Your weight affects your risk of developing breast cancer after you reach menopause. If you have gained more than forty-five pounds since you were eighteen, you are at increased risk of developing breast cancer. To reduce your risk, try not to gain more than fifteen to twenty pounds during adulthood. You can do this by eating a healthy diet and remaining physically active.

## Eat Plenty of Fruits and Vegetables

Although you may be worrying about whether pesticides on the food you eat can cause breast cancer, you should really be thinking about what you're *not* eating. Americans are notorious for not eating enough fruits and vegetables. That's a shame, because fruits and vegetables contain substances that prevent normal cells from turning cancerous. The American Cancer Society recommends a diet that includes five servings of fruits and vegetables a day. So eat as many fruits and vegetables as you can manage every day. Put fruit on your cereal in the morning and lettuce on your sandwiches. Pack carrots, an apple, or a banana for a snack. Substitute a glass of orange juice for a cup of coffee at work. Try to eat vegetables or a salad every night with dinner. These small steps add up.

## Cook with Monounsaturated Fats

For years people worried that a high fat diet might increase the risk of breast cancer. Further studies have failed to confirm this. In fact, there is growing evidence that cooking with oils that are high in monounsaturated fats (found in olive oil and canola oil) may actually lower the risk of breast cancer. These oils have many other health benefits as well.

## Have Less Than One Alcoholic Drink per Day

Who hasn't heard by now that there may be some health benefits from drinking alcohol? There are some benefits to moderate drinking, which has been linked to a reduced risk of coronary heart disease. The problem is that many of these studies have been done in men, who metabolize alcohol differently than women. So the best advice is that, if you want to drink alcohol, drink less than one drink per day (or less than seven drinks per week). Any more and you may increase your risk of breast cancer.

## THINK CAREFULLY ABOUT POSTMENOPAUSAL HORMONES

The decision about whether to take postmenopausal hormones when you reach menopause is a complicated one. But when it comes to the impact on breast cancer risk, the issue is not so much whether to take hormones, but if you do, how long to continue it. Women who take hormones for less than five years following menopause do not appear to increase their risk of breast cancer. But taking hormones longer than five years may increase your risk. The picture is complicated by other issues, such as your individual risk of breast cancer based on family history and other factors. This is definitely an issue you should discuss with your health care provider.

## Get Regular Breast Cancer Screening Tests

In addition to taking steps to try to prevent the disease, all women, once they reach a certain age, should be screened regularly for breast cancer. Although screening tests, like mammograms and clinical breast exams, cannot help *prevent* the disease from developing, they can identify it early when it is most treatable. The earlier a cancer is found, the more likely it is that a woman can be treated successfully.

### MAMMOGRAMS

Mammograms are special X-rays of the breast. Virtually everyone agrees that you should get a yearly mammogram once you turn fifty and continue until you turn sixty-nine. After that, you should get a mammogram every one to two years. This is hands-down the best way to catch breast cancer early.

Almost everyone also agrees that if you have an unusually high risk of breast cancer, such as from a strong history of breast cancer in your mother or sisters, regular mammograms are probably valuable starting at a younger age. If my patient's mother or sister has had breast cancer, I'll advise annual mammograms for her starting at age forty, or ten years before the age at which the close relative was diagnosed with breast cancer, whichever age comes first.

The evidence to support having regular mammograms before age fifty is not nearly as good as the evidence that mammograms starting at age fifty save lives. There are a couple of reason why this is so. First, the risk of breast cancer in this age group is much smaller, and second, the test appears to be less accurate because younger women tend to have denser breasts (more tissue and less fat) than older women. This makes reading mammograms and detecting abnormalities more difficult: a negative or normal result may be reported in a woman who actually has breast cancer. Both of these factors make it more difficult to prove a benefit to screening mammograms for women under age fifty. Furthermore, more mammograms in women aged forty to forty-nine lead to positive or abnormal results that result in a biopsy showing there was no cancer, after all. Having an abnormal mammogram result is scary for a woman and her family, even if the biopsy shows that no cancer was present. The wisest course of action is to discuss the decision about mammography with your health care provider, who can help you to factor in your individual risk and arrive at the best decision for you.

For women ages seventy and over, there is currently not enough evidence for me or most health care providers to make any concrete recommendation about mammograms. However, because breast density decreases with age,

## Breast Cancer Screening Recommendations from Three Different Health Organizations

|  | AMERICAN CANCER SOCIETY | NATIONAL CANCER INSTITUTE | U.S. PREVENTIVE SERVICES TASK FORCE |
|---|---|---|---|
| **Mammography** |  |  |  |
| Age 40–49 | Every year | Every 1–2 years | Only if at increased risk |
| Age 50–69 | Every year | Every 1–2 years | Every 1–2 years |
| Age 70 + | Every year | Every 1–2 years | Based on provider recommendation |
| **Clinical Breast Exam** | Every 1–3 years between ages 20 and 39<br><br>Every year beginning at age 40 | Every year beginning at age 30 | Only if at increased risk for ages 40–49<br><br>Every 1–2 years for ages 50-69<br><br>Based on provider recommendation for ages 70 and over |
| **Breast Self-Exam** | Every month beginning at age 20 | No guideline | No guideline |

there appears to be no reason that mammography should be less effective in women as they advance into this age group, and the risk of breast cancer continues to rise over age seventy. A woman aged seventy or older should discuss the decision about whether to get regular mammograms with her health care provider. I generally recommend it for my patients who are otherwise in good health and who could withstand breast cancer treatment if it were necessary.

## CLINICAL BREAST EXAMS

A clinical breast exam is a physical examination of the breasts by a health care provider (most often a physician, but a nurse practitioner or nurse may also perform it). Clinical breast exams are most effective in women aged fifty to sixty-nine, but I advise my patients to have them every year, as part of their regular physical. As with other kinds of screening tests, experts disagree on the age at which you should start, or the frequency with which the exam should be done.

## BREAST SELF-EXAM

You have probably seen laminated breast self-exam cards made to hang in the shower that outline how to properly do a breast self-exam. The main advantage of this technique is that it enables you to become more familiar with your breast tissue so that you may notice any changes or even detect a lump. Breast self-exam is vigorously promoted by many health organizations as an effective way for women to find breast cancers that develop during the period between regular mammograms and clinical breast exams. Unfortunately, very little data actually support this claim. Neither the U.S. Preventive Services Task Force nor the National Cancer Institute recommend that women of any age regularly perform breast self-exam. I do not discourage my patients from doing breast self-exam, but I stress that it should never take the place of getting regular mammograms and clinical breast exams.

## When My Patient Has a High Risk of Getting Breast Cancer

### ESTIMATING THE RISK

Fortunately, most women are at average or low risk for the disease and do not need to take extra precautions—aside from leading a healthy lifestyle and getting regular screening tests. However, some women are at high risk and do need to consider taking special steps to protect themselves. We now have pretty good information on factors that increase your risk of getting breast cancer, even though the details are still being worked out.

You are clearly at a higher risk of getting breast cancer if you have *any one* of the following risk factors:

- A mutation in the BRCA 1 or BRCA 2 genes
- A mother who developed breast cancer before she turned sixty, or a sister or daughter who developed breast cancer
- Breast abnormalities (such as atypical hyperplasia) in the past
- Repeated exposure as a child or adolescent to high dose radiation

You also are at a higher risk of getting breast cancer if you have *several* of the following risk factors:

- Your first menstrual period was at a relatively young age (twelve or younger).
- You reached menopause at a relatively late age (fifty-five or older).
- You first gave birth later in life (age thirty or older).
- You have high estrogen levels in your blood.

For patients of mine who are at a relatively higher risk of getting breast cancer, I generally recommend that they consider getting regular mammograms and clinical breast exams starting at age forty, even though the value of this has not yet been proven conclusively.

## Tools That Help You Estimate Your Risk of Breast Cancer

Though imperfect, some computer and web-based tools are available to help women estimate their risk of breast cancer. The most widely distributed is the National Cancer Institute's Breast Cancer Risk Assessment Tool (http://bcra.nci.nih.gov/brc/q1.htm). Another tool has been developed based primarily on data from the Nurses' Health Study, and it is available at the website (www.health.harvard.edu).

## TREATMENT OPTIONS FOR UNUSUALLY HIGH RISK WOMEN

Some of my patients are at unusually high risk of breast cancer. Those who I tend to put in this category have a very strong family history or have been diagnosed with lobular carcinoma in situ or ductal carcinoma in situ. If you are at unusually high risk of breast cancer, you basically have two options to try to lower your risk: chemoprevention or prophylactic mastectomy.

*Chemoprevention.* This is the use of drugs to prevent breast cancer, and it is a very active area of research. Tamoxifen and raloxifene are two of the most promising chemoprevention drugs that are in a class called selective estrogen receptor modulators (SERMs). SERMs act by blocking estrogen from attaching to breast cells.

In a National Cancer Institute–funded clinical trial of tamoxifen that included over 13,000 women at high risk of breast cancer, women who took tamoxifen over a five-year period had about half the risk of developing invasive cancer as women who did not take the drug. Though their risk of breast cancer was lower, the women on tamoxifen also experienced increased rates of some serious side effects, including endometrial cancer and blood clots in the lung (pulmonary embolism) and large veins of the legs (deep venous thrombosis). Raloxifene works in a similar fashion to tamoxifen, and early reports on its effectiveness show that it reduces the risk of breast cancer by more than half. It also seems to have an added benefit over tamoxifen in that women taking raloxifene seem to suffer fewer serious side effects.

High risk women should certainly talk with their health care providers about the risks and benefits associated with taking a chemoprevention drug. Drugs like tamoxifen and raloxifene seem to have a substantial benefit for some high risk women over a relatively short time period. However, the long-term benefits (and risks) related to these drugs have yet to be determined.

*Prophylactic mastectomy.* This is a drastic procedure that involves the surgical removal of both breasts in order to reduce the chances that breast cancer will develop. In my judgment, it is rarely indicated. The one exception may be for women who have the BRCA 1 or BRCA 2 genes that increase the risk of breast cancer (and ovarian cancer). Their risk is sufficiently high that—as radical as it seems—removing the breasts may be the right thing to do. One study has found that a thirty-five-year-old woman with BRCA 1 or BRCA 2 mutations can gain three to five years of life by having the procedure. Still, you never can know whether this radical approach was justified in the individual, because you will never know if she would have developed breast cancer or not.

And although the procedure does afford substantial protection, it does not guarantee complete protection. Breast cancer can still develop in the small amount of tissue that remains after surgery. Because it is such a disfiguring procedure, if you are at high risk I think you should consider prophylactic mastectomy only after a careful discussion with your health care provider about all of the associated risks and benefits.

Yes. The thought of breast cancer is frightening. But all women should feel they have the power to take action against the disease. The lifestyle factors I've outlined may help lower the risk of breast cancer and regular screening can find it when it's most curable. Perhaps most heartening is the great progress we've made over the past twenty-five years in our understanding of the disease, and as research continues to advance at an astounding pace, each new year will bring with it further understanding of the causes of breast cancer as well as the ways my patients and I together can combat it.

# Lowering the Risk
# of Lung Cancer

## BACKGROUND

Lung cancer is the leading cause of cancer-related death in the United States, claiming the lives of more than 67,000 women each year. To date, scientists have had little success with the early detection and treatment of this disease. Most people who develop lung cancer die within five years after diagnosis. Although they are more likely to survive if their cancer is detected early, there is not a good screening test available and so this rarely happens. Only about 15 percent of all lung cancers are detected in the earliest, most treatable stage, and even then, the odds of survival barely exceed 50 percent.

Fortunately, lung cancer is preventable. For more than thirty years, scientists—and most people in the general public—have known that lung cancer is caused by smoking. Although the disease does occur in people who do not

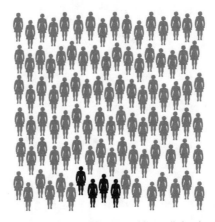

FIG. 6-1. In a group of 100 women who are fifty years old, 4 will develop lung cancer before they reach the age of eighty. (Source: National Cancer Institute)

smoke, more than 90 percent of cases are diagnosed in those who do. The best way to protect yourself from this disease is to never start smoking, and if you do, to quit for good as soon as possible.

## The Lungs and Lung Cancer

The lungs are part of an intricate network that delivers oxygen to the body and rids it of carbon dioxide (see Figure 6-2). Air is first inhaled through the nose or mouth and brought to the lungs through the trachea (or windpipe). The trachea divides into two tubes called bronchi and then into a branching system of ever-smaller tubes called bronchioles. The bronchioles eventually lead to a network of microscopic air sacs called alveoli, which are surrounded by millions of tiny blood vessels. Oxygen passes through the wall of the alveoli and enters the bloodstream. In exchange, carbon dioxide leaves the blood, enters the alveoli, and is exhaled through the lungs. The oxygen-rich blood then travels to the heart for distribution throughout the body.

Because the air we breathe is not pure, the lungs have an elaborate system for filtering out impurities before they reach the alveoli and damage them. For

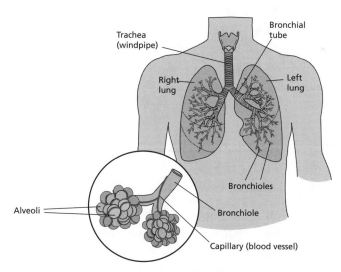

FIG. 6-2. Your lungs. Air is inhaled through the nose or mouth and moves through the trachea, through small bronchial tubes and even smaller bronchioles into millions of tiny air sacs (alveoli). Next to the alveoli are capillaries (blood vessels). The close proximity of the alveoli and capillaries allows carbon dioxide from the blood to be exchanged for oxygen in the lungs. Oxygen enters the lungs and then the blood, and carbon dioxide is released by the blood and exhaled through the lungs.

example, the lining of the bronchial tree produces a thick mucus that traps particles. In addition, the tubes of the bronchial tree are lined with tiny hairs called cilia that beat upward toward the trachea. These tubes carry mucus (and any particles that have been caught) up to the upper airways to be coughed or sneezed out. The last line of defense for the lungs is the white blood cells of the immune system. These are stationed in the lining of the bronchial tree and alveoli, where they can engulf particles and kill germs.

Despite the presence of this elaborate defense system, the lungs do not cope well with tobacco smoke and other dangerous pollutants. In smokers, the bronchi make too much mucus, which clogs the airways and makes it difficult to breathe. In addition, these pollutants can infiltrate the defense system of the lungs and lead to the development of lung cancer.

Most lung cancers start in the lining of the bronchi and are thought to develop over a period of many years. Although there are many different types of lung cancer, they are usually divided into two basic categories, based on the size of the cancer cells. About 20 percent of all lung cancers are small cell lung cancers. Although the cells of these tumors are small, they multiply rapidly to form large tumors and almost always spread to other parts of the body. The remaining 80 percent of lung cancers are non–small cell and include squamous cell cancer, adenocarcinoma, and large cell cancer.

The most common sign of lung cancer is a prolonged cough, sometimes with blood-tinged phlegm or shortness of breath. Other symptoms include chest pain, a raspy voice, loss of appetite, and repeated bouts of pneumonia. In more advanced disease, where the cancer has already spread to other parts of the body, the symptoms may include pain in the bones or neurological disturbances.

## LESSONS FROM THE NURSES' HEALTH STUDY AND OTHER STUDIES

### Factors You Cannot Control

Although smoking, the most important risk factor for lung cancer, is within your control, a number of other factors, like your family history, are not. The reason that you should know about these factors is simple: if you have them, and they put you at higher risk, you need to talk to your health care provider about them. You may want to be more vigilant about things you can control, like not smoking and limiting your exposure to passive smoke.

## AGE

In general, the older a woman is, the more likely she is to develop lung cancer. National data show that rates of lung cancer are low in women under age forty, begin to increase after forty, and are highest in women over age sixty-five (see Figure 6-3). Only after age seventy-five does the risk stop increasing with age.

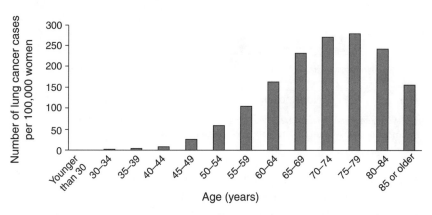

FIG. 6-3. The risk of lung cancer increases with age until age seventy-five. This is probably due to the accumulated effects of tobacco smoke and other pollutants. (Source: National Cancer Institute)

## FAMILY HISTORY

Although most people with lung cancer are smokers, the large majority of smokers never develop the disease. This suggests that some people might be more genetically susceptible to lung cancer than others. Several studies have supported this idea, showing that lung cancer does run in families. Having a family history of lung cancer appears to double—possibly even quadruple—a woman's risk of the disease. This excess risk is of particular concern for women who smoke, since they already have a very high risk of lung cancer (see Figure 6-4).

## EXPOSURE TO CHEMICALS IN THE WORKPLACE

Being exposed to certain chemicals in the workplace can greatly increase the risk of lung cancer. This is because some chemicals can damage the genetic structure of the lung cells, causing them to become cancerous. Workplace chemicals that have been linked to lung cancer include asbestos, arsenic, beryllium, chloromethyl ether, cadmium, chromium, mustard gas, radon, and nickel.

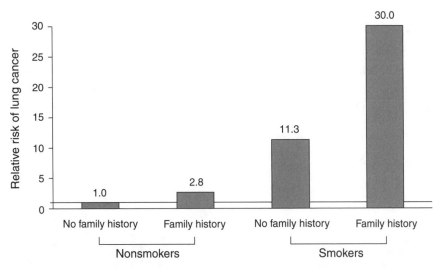

FIG. 6-4. Women with a family history of lung cancer have an increased risk of the disease. Those who smoke *and* have a family history are at very high risk. (Source: Horwitz et al.)

In addition, there are certain chemical processes that are linked to lung cancer. These include aluminum production, coal gasification, coke production, hematite mining, iron and steel founding, and painting.

## Exposure to Urban Air Pollution

Women who live in urban areas for at least ten years may have a slightly increased risk of lung cancer. This is probably due to particles and gases in the air resulting from car and truck exhausts and emissions from factories and power-producing facilities.

### Factors You Can Control

Although other factors are related to your risk of lung cancer, the one that has the most impact is one you can control: smoking.

## Smoking

For over thirty years, research has shown that cigarette smoking dramatically increases the risk of lung cancer. Although other factors have been linked to this disease, smoking is by far the most important, accounting for almost 90 percent of all lung cancers. Not surprisingly, when we looked at this issue in the Nurses' Health Study, we found a very strong relationship: the more cigarettes women smoked per day, the more likely they were to develop lung cancer

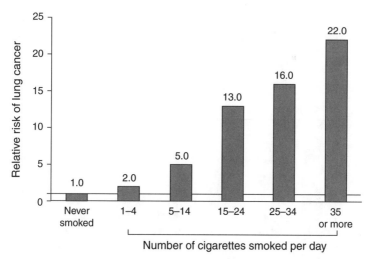

FIG. 6-5. The relative risk of lung cancer increases with the number of cigarettes smoked per day and is remarkably high for women who smoke two or more packs a day. (Source: Nurses' Health Study)

(see Figure 6-5). The risk was 22 times higher among women who smoked two packs a day compared to women who had never smoked.

Although some studies have suggested that "lite" cigarettes might not be as detrimental to women's health as regular cigarettes, we did not find this to be true in the Nurses' Health Study. On first glance, women who smoked low tar cigarettes did appear to have a lower risk of lung cancer than those who smoked regular cigarettes. However, women smoking lite cigarettes often attempt to compensate by smoking more cigarettes or inhaling more deeply. When we took into account the number of cigarettes that women smoked per day, we found that low tar cigarettes raised the risk of lung cancer just as much as regular cigarettes did.

Fortunately, the effect that smoking has on the lungs appears to be at least partially reversible. We found that within two years after a woman stops smoking, her risk of lung cancer begins to drop. After fifteen years of not smoking, her risk is almost equal to that of a woman who has never smoked (see Figure 6-6). This means that for virtually all women who smoke, it is never too late to benefit from quitting.

## EXPOSURE TO PASSIVE SMOKE

Women who do not smoke have an increased risk of lung cancer if they are repeatedly exposed to passive smoke (smoke from another person's cigarette). More than thirty studies, including the Nurses' Health Study, have shown a 25

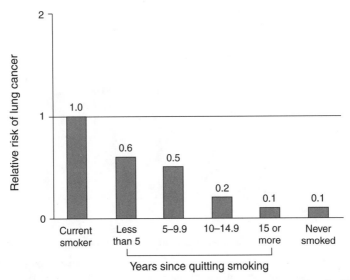

FIG. 6-6. After a woman quits smoking, her risk of lung cancer drops steadily. After fifteen years, it nearly equals the risk of a woman who has never smoked. (Source: Nurses' Health Study)

to 50 percent increase in the risk of lung cancer among nonsmoking women whose husbands smoke. The longer and more intense the exposure to passive smoke, the greater the risk. In a large analysis, researchers found that a non-smoker's risk of lung cancer was small if the spouse smoked less than ten cigarettes a day, but grew to be large if the spouse smoked more than a pack a day.

## EXPOSURE TO RADON IN THE HOME

Radon is an invisible, odorless gas that often leaks from the soil into the foundations of older buildings. The U.S. Environmental Protection Agency estimates that as many as 10 percent of all homes may have elevated levels of this gas. Although excessive exposure to radon (such as that incurred by uranium

## Cigars and the Risk of Lung Cancer

Cigars are often perceived as safer than cigarettes because the smoke is not inhaled as deeply into the lungs. However, there is solid evidence that cigars still increase the risk of lung cancer. In a large study conducted by the American Cancer Society, researchers found a fivefold increase in the risk of fatal lung cancer among men who smoked cigars. The effects of cigars have not been well studied in women, but there is no reason to think that they would be less harmful in women than they are in men.

miners) is known to be a major cause of lung cancer, it is not yet clear whether there is also an increased risk among people who live in buildings with high radon levels. In one of the largest studies to address this issue, researchers found a 50 percent increase in the risk of lung cancer among women who lived in a home with elevated radon levels for at least fifteen years. The higher the levels, the more likely women were to develop the disease.

## CAROTENOIDS

Found naturally in fruits and vegetables, carotenoids are a diverse group of substances that act as antioxidants; that is, they help prevent damage to the cells. Some of these substances can also be converted into vitamin A, which is essential for cell growth. Because of their antioxidant properties and vitamin A activity, carotenoids have long been thought to be linked to a lower risk of lung cancer. However, the details of this relationship are still being studied.

The carotenoid that has received the most study to date is beta-carotene. In the past decade, at least three randomized controlled trials have been conducted to test the effectiveness of beta-carotene in preventing lung cancer. In all of these trials, researchers assigned a daily supplement of beta-carotene to one group of participants and a daily placebo to the other group. They then followed the participants over time to see which group had lower rates of lung cancer: those on the supplements or those on the placebo. What they found was that the beta-carotene supplements offered no protection against lung cancer. This may be because beta-carotene alone is not as important as the combination of carotenoids that is found naturally in fruits and vegetables.

Studies now suggest that a wide range of carotenoids other than beta-carotene may offer protection against lung cancer. In the Nurses' Health Study, women who consumed the most carotenoids were 30 percent less likely to develop the disease than those who consumed the least. Alpha-carotene, lutein, lycopene, and beta-cryptoxanthin all appeared to be beneficial. These carotenoids can be found in most fruits and vegetables, with tomatoes being the best source of lycopene and carrots the best source of alpha-carotene.

## FRUITS AND VEGETABLES

Eating fruits and vegetables may modestly lower the risk of lung cancer among smokers and nonsmokers alike. This has been shown in several large cohort studies, including the Nurses' Health Study and the Iowa Women's Health Study. In our study, women who ate at least four servings of fruits and vegetables a day had a 20 percent reduction in their risk of lung cancer.

## Selenium

Selenium is a mineral found abundantly in seafood, meat, chicken, grains, and some vegetables. Because it is a key part of an important antioxidant enzyme and has been shown to inhibit cell growth, selenium has been studied extensively with respect to lung cancer. However, results to date have been inconsistent, and very few studies have included women.

Some studies on this topic have shown a higher risk of lung cancer among individuals with low levels of selenium in their bodies. However, smoking lowers the level of selenium in the body and also dramatically raises the risk of lung cancer. Thus, it is not yet clear whether individuals are at higher risk because of their low selenium levels or because of their cigarette use.

## WHAT IT ALL MEANS

Smoking is the most powerful cause of lung cancer. It is best to never start smoking, but if you do, quit for good as soon as possible. Within ten years, your risk of lung cancer will drop by half, and after another five years, it will be about the same as a woman your age who never smoked. Clearly, quitting smoking (or even better, not starting) remains the best way for you to prevent lung cancer. Eating a diet rich in fruits and vegetables may also offer modest protection, but it will not be enough to counterbalance the adverse effects of smoking.

## WHAT I TELL MY PATIENTS ABOUT LOWERING THEIR RISK OF LUNG CANCER

DR. CELESTE ROBB-NICHOLSON

When it comes to telling patients how to avoid lung cancer, the advice I offer is simple: if you smoke, quit. Smoking accounts for nine out of ten cases of lung cancer.

Following this advice is not so simple. Many patients have tried to quit before and failed many times. They're discouraged or depressed. They are often worried about gaining weight. Or they try to counteract the risks associated with smoking by living otherwise healthy lives: exercising regularly and eating a diet full of fruits and vegetables. But it doesn't matter. Smoking is far and away the most significant risk factor for lung cancer.

So if you smoke, quit. If you can't quit the first time, keep trying. Consider every possible quit-smoking technique, and force yourself to talk to your doctor about it. Don't brush it under the table and hope you will stop smoking by the time of your next office visit. See Dr. Rigotti's advice in Chapter 17 for strategies that may help you to quit, even if you've tried before.

If you don't smoke but your husband or partner does, you may also be at greater risk of lung cancer. So try to persuade your loved one to quit. If he or she is not able to, then at least limit the amount of passive smoke you and your children are exposed to in the house. Ask that your partner smoke outside, or in a designated room with a door that can be closed. Ask that he or she not smoke in the car if it is one that you share.

If you have lived in a city for more than ten years or if you work in an occupation that exposes you to carcinogens like asbestos, your risk of lung cancer is also increased. But these factors do not override smoking. Both increase your risk of lung cancer, and exposure to tobacco smoke will only increase it more.

## Established, Probable, and Possible Factors Associated with the Risk of Lung Cancer

| RISK FACTOR | APPROXIMATE RISK* |
|---|---|
| *Established* | |
| Smoking (5 or more cigarettes a day vs. none) | ↑↑↑↑ |
| Age (greater than 60 vs. less than 50) | ↑↑↑ |
| Parent or sibling diagnosed with lung cancer | ↑↑↑ |
| Exposure to chemicals in the workplace | ↑↑↑ |
| Exposure to radon in the home | ↑↑ |
| Exposure to passive smoke (living with a smoker vs. not living with a smoker) | ↑ |
| Exposure to urban air pollution | ↑ |
| *Probable* | |
| Carotenoids (high intake vs. low intake) | ↓↓ |
| *Possible* | |
| Low intake of selenium | ↑ |
| High intake of fruits and vegetables | ↓ |

*↑ Small increase in risk    ↓ Small decrease in risk
↑↑ Moderate increase in risk    ↓↓ Moderate decrease in risk
↑↑↑ Large increase in risk    ↓↓↓ Large decrease in risk
↑↑↑↑ Very large increase in risk    ↓↓↓↓ Very large decrease in risk

# CHAPTER SEVEN

# Lowering the Risk of Stroke

## BACKGROUND

Stroke is a feared disease, not only because it claims the lives of nearly 100,000 women each year but also because it is the leading cause of long-term disability in the United States. Say the word *stroke* and you are likely to picture people who need help completing life's daily tasks—eating, dressing, walking, and grocery shopping. And, unfortunately, this is not far from the truth. Of those who survive a first stroke—fully 30 percent of stroke victims die within one year after the event—nearly a third lose much of their personal independence, and over two-thirds experience problems on the job over the long-term. Possibly most disturbing—for family and friends as well—is stroke's effect on mental ability. Up to 25 percent of stroke survivors develop dementia following a stroke.

A stroke—also referred to as a cerebrovascular accident—occurs when the blood flow to the brain is disrupted because a vessel supplying it has either ruptured or become blocked. While men are slightly more likely to have a stroke

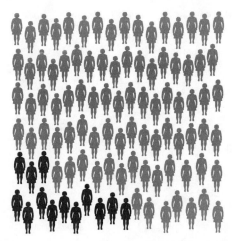

FIG. 7-1. In a group of 100 women who are fifty years old, 13 will develop a stroke before they reach the age of eighty. (Source: Grady et al.)

than women, women are much more likely to die from the event, possibly because they tend to develop the disease at an older age when the body is less able to handle the trauma. African Americans are also more likely than most other racial and ethnic groups to develop as well as to die from the disease.

The good news, though, is that a lot can be done to lower the risk of stroke. In the United States, the rate of death from the disease has dropped significantly since the 1960s, largely due to improvements in health care and decreasing rates or improved treatment of important stroke risk factors—such as high blood pressure (also known as hypertension), smoking, and poor diet.

## Different Kinds of Stroke: Ischemic and Hemorrhagic

Stroke is a form of cardiovascular disease, a group of disorders that also includes coronary heart disease and peripheral vascular disease. There are two main types of stroke: ischemic and hemorrhagic (see Figure 7-2). Ischemic strokes are by far the most common in the United States—accounting for 70 to 80 percent of all strokes—and occur when there is an interruption in the flow of blood to the brain, almost always due to a clot blocking a blood vessel. The remaining 20 to 30 percent are hemorrhagic strokes, which occur when a blood vessel in the brain ruptures and bleeds.

### ISCHEMIC STROKE

Ischemic stroke occurs when there is a blockage in one of the arteries that supplies blood to the brain. If the blockage lasts longer than about two hours, the part of the brain nourished by the artery dies. The exact effects of a stroke depend on the part of the brain that is affected and how long the blood vessel is blocked.

There are two main types of ischemic strokes: thrombotic and embolic. Like a heart attack, thrombotic stroke most often occurs when a buildup of fat and cholesterol (plaque) in a brain artery ruptures and a blood clot (thrombus) forms that blocks the blood supply to brain tissue.

Embolic stroke is the result of a blockage in an artery by a clot or fragment of plaque that is formed elsewhere in the body, often in the heart, and travels with the blood until it lodges in a small blood vessel in the brain. Clots and other debris that travel through the blood are called emboli. Embolic strokes are often linked to atrial fibrillation, a condition in which one of the chambers of the heart beats rapidly and irregularly. The fluttering motion allows blood to pool in the heart and form clots that can travel to the brain. Other heart diseases also greatly increase the risk of emboli, including coronary heart disease, valve disease, and congestive heart failure.

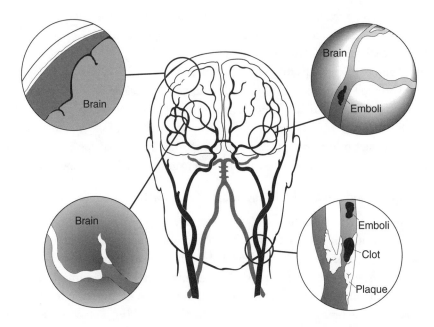

FIG. 7-2. Hemorrhagic strokes are caused by a rupture of a blood vessel in the brain. The subsequent accumulation of blood in or around the brain compresses both the brain tissue and other blood vessels that nourish brain tissue. When bleeding takes place inside the brain tissue, the stroke is called an intracerebral hemorrhage (*bottom left*). When a vessel on the surface of the brain bursts it is called a subarachnoid hemorrhage (*top left*). Ischemic strokes, such as an embolic stroke (*top right*) or a thrombotic stroke (*bottom right*), are caused by an interruption in blood flow to the brain. In an embolic stroke, a clot forms elsewhere in the body and travels through the circulatory system to the brain. It lodges in a small vessel and cuts off the supply of blood. In a thrombotic stroke, a vessel in the brain is progressively narrowed by a buildup of plaque. A clot eventually forms at the site of the narrowing, cutting off the blood supply.

*Transient Ischemic Attacks.* Strokes are often preceded, from days to months, by events called transient ischemic attacks (TIAs). Often referred to as ministrokes or precursors to stroke, TIAs result from a temporary interruption in blood flow to the brain. TIAs can occur when small pieces of debris—such as blood clots, cholesterol deposits, or other foreign matter—travel through the blood and lodge in the small blood vessels in the brain but dissolve before any permanent damage occurs. When the debris interrupts the flow of blood to brain tissue, the tissue temporarily stops functioning until the debris dissolves, which can cause sudden onset of many of the same symptoms of a full-blown stroke. Because TIAs are temporary events, symptoms typically last only a few hours and go away in less than twenty-four hours.

TIAs serve as a warning that a person could have a stroke in the future. Al-

# Don't Hesitate! Recognize the Symptoms of a Stroke and Get Care Immediately

It is exceptionally important for anyone having a stroke to receive medical care as quickly as possible. Similar to a heart attack, getting quick care for a stroke (which is sometimes referred to as a "brain attack") can minimize injury to the brain and even mean the difference between life and death. Anyone experiencing any of the symptoms below should seek care immediately.

## ISCHEMIC STROKE

The symptoms develop suddenly and can vary, depending on the size of the blockage, the region of the brain affected, and how quickly the blockage of the artery developed. Possible symptoms of ischemic stroke include:

- Sudden weakness on one side of the body in an arm, hand, or leg
- Sudden numbness on one side of the face or body
- Sudden dimness or loss of vision, particularly in only one eye
- Sudden difficulty speaking or sudden inability to understand what someone is saying
- Sudden dizziness or loss of balance
- Sudden headache

## HEMORRHAGIC STROKE

As with ischemic stroke, the symptoms of hemorrhagic stroke tend to develop suddenly and vary depending on where in the brain the stroke occurs. Possible symptoms of hemorrhagic stroke include:

- Sudden, excruciating headache
- Seizures
- Nausea and vomiting
- Sudden weakness on one side of the body in an arm, hand, or leg
- Sudden numbness on one side of the face or body
- Sudden dimness or loss of vision, particularly in only one eye
- Sudden difficulty speaking or sudden inability to understand what someone is saying
- Sudden dizziness or loss of balance
- Sudden loss of mental ability
- Loss of consciousness

most half of all people who have had an ischemic stroke have had at least one TIA some weeks or months before the event. Not all people who have TIAs, though, will have a stroke.

## HEMORRHAGIC STROKE

A hemorrhagic stroke, also called a brain hemorrhage or cerebral hemorrhage, occurs when a blood vessel in the brain ruptures, causing bleeding (hemorrhaging) into or around the brain. Brain damage can result from a hemorrhagic stroke because of lack of blood and oxygen to the tissues, as well as a buildup of pressure from the bleeding.

Although every stroke is serious, brain hemorrhages are often devastating because they are more likely to cause death. There are essentially two types of hemorrhagic stroke: intracerebral hemorrhage and subarachnoid hemorrhage. Where the bleeding occurs determines the type of stroke.

When bleeding takes place inside the brain tissue, the stroke is called an intracerebral hemorrhage. When a vessel on the surface of the brain bursts, it is called a subarachnoid hemorrhage—the only type of stroke more common in women than in men. While intracerebral hemorrhages usually occur in normal blood vessels that may have been weakened by a factor such as hypertension, subarachnoid hemorrhages tend to occur in abnormally shaped, weak-walled arteries in the brain. Subarachnoid hemorrhages also tend to be more serious than intracerebral hemorrhages. Because a subarachnoid hemorrhage causes bleeding into the area between the brain and the skull (called the subarachnoid space), pressure can build up and press upon a large area of the brain that controls vital functions.

## LESSONS FROM THE NURSES' HEALTH STUDY AND OTHER STUDIES

A great deal of research over the years has identified a number of factors that influence the risk of stroke. Although much of this research either has been done solely on men or has not separated out the results for women, there is an increasing amount of information about the causes of stroke specific to women. Studies like our Nurses' Health Study are helping to determine not only how female-specific factors—such as using birth control pills or postmenopausal hormones—affect the risk of stroke but also how factors common to both genders may affect the risk in women differently from that in men.

Because both stroke and coronary heart disease are cardiovascular diseases, they share many similar risk factors—hypertension, diabetes, and obe-

## Stroke: The Larger Picture

- A stroke occurs when the blood flow to the brain is disrupted because a vessel supplying it has either ruptured or is blocked.
- Approximately 30 percent of stroke victims die within one year after the event.
- Strokes are often preceded, from days to months, by events called transient ischemic attacks (TIAs), often referred to as ministrokes.
- Having an immediate family member (a parent or sibling) who has had a stroke or experienced TIAs greatly increases the risk of stroke.
- The single most important modifiable risk factor for stroke is hypertension. Women with hypertension have a large risk of stroke compared to women with normal blood pressure.

sity, for example. But it is not a perfect one-to-one relationship. Some factors that have a large influence on the risk of coronary heart disease, such as fat in the diet and blood cholesterol, either have no effect on stroke risk or affect it to a lesser degree than with coronary heart disease.

### Factors You Cannot Control

Age, family history, and race/ethnicity have an important influence on the risk of stroke. Even though you can't control these factors, it is still important to know how they might affect your risk of the disease so that you can be even more careful about those factors you can control.

### Age

The risk of stroke goes up dramatically as a person ages, with men having slightly higher rates than women for all ages. Rates are very low in those under age forty-five but steadily increase with age. After age forty-five, the risk of stroke essentially doubles with each successive decade. Approximately 72 percent of all stroke victims are aged sixty-five years or older.

### Family History

Having an immediate family member (a parent or sibling) who has had a stroke or experienced transient ischemic attacks approximately doubles the risk of stroke. A large study of middle-aged women in Finland found that the risk of stroke was 80 percent greater in women who had a parent who had a stroke than in women whose parents had not. Whether the increase in risk seen with family history is due to a genetic predisposition passed from generation to generation or is due to behaviors that are similar among family members—such as diet and smoking—is still not completely clear.

## RACE AND ETHNICITY

The risk of stroke varies by race and ethnicity (see Figure 7-3). African Americans tend to fare the worst of all minorities in the United States. Not only are African American women about twice as likely to have a stroke as white women, they also tend to have more severe strokes and to have them at younger ages. It is not clear whether this increase in risk is due to genetic predisposition or to lifestyle factors. African American women are more likely than white women to possess important risk factors for stroke—such as hypertension, obesity, and diabetes.

In contrast, Latina, American Indian, and Asian American women tend to have a slightly lower risk of stroke than white women. It should be noted, though, that Asian Americans and Asians living in Asia generally have very different risks for the disease, most likely due to differences in lifestyle between the two

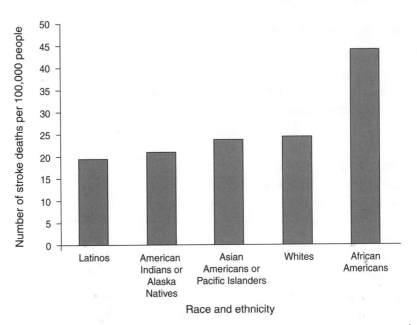

FIG. 7-3. The rate of death from stroke varies with race and ethnicity. Mexican Americans tend to have the lowest rates, followed by American Indians, Asian Americans, and whites. African Americans have the highest rates overall. (Source: National Center for Health Statistics)

countries. While Asian Americans have a relatively low risk of stroke, Asians who live in Asia—where stroke is a leading killer—tend to have a high risk.

### Factors You Can Control

You can control most of the known risk factors for stroke, providing an excellent opportunity to lower your risk of the disease. These modifiable factors range from behaviors you can adopt to medical conditions you can have treated and controlled. The single most important modifiable risk factor for stroke is hypertension.

### BLOOD PRESSURE

Hypertension is a major risk factor for stroke (see Chapter 4 for more information on hypertension). The increased blood pressure that defines the condition can raise the risk of stroke by injuring and weakening artery walls. An injury to an artery wall can start the process of atherosclerosis, and a weakened artery wall is more likely to burst and bleed, especially when blood pressure is very high.

## Systolic and Diastolic Blood Pressure

Blood pressure is reported as two numbers—systolic blood pressure and diastolic blood pressure. Systolic blood pressure—the higher of the two numbers—measures the force of the blood (in millimeters of mercury [mm Hg]) as your heart is contracting and pumping blood. Diastolic blood pressure—the lower of the two numbers—measures the force of the blood as your heart rests in between beats. Although blood pressure varies with age, for most people the optimal blood pressure is a systolic blood pressure of 120 mm Hg or lower and a diastolic blood pressure of 80 mm Hg or lower. Hypertension is a systolic blood pressure of 140 mm Hg or greater or a diastolic of 90 mm Hg or greater.

When we assessed blood pressure in the Nurses' Health Study, we found that women with hypertension have a large risk of stroke, nearly three times that of women with normal blood pressure. Other studies have had results similar to ours and have also been able to show that the risk of stroke steadily increases as blood pressure increases. For every 9-point increase in systolic blood pressure or every 5-point increase in diastolic blood pressure, the risk of stroke increases by about a third.

One specific type of hypertension—isolated systolic hypertension—is very common in women, especially as they age. In the condition, only systolic blood pressure is elevated, while diastolic remains normal. A number of studies, including the Framingham Heart Study, have found that isolated systolic hypertension approximately triples the risk of stroke.

With treatment, however, the increases in risk linked to hypertension can be almost totally reversed. Studies of drug treatment have shown that lowering isolated systolic hypertension—for example, from 165/90 to 149/90—can reduce the risk of stroke by over 35 percent and that a 6 mm Hg drop in diastolic blood pressure—for example, from 130/100 to 130/94—can lower risk by up to 45 percent.

But medication is not always necessary to treat hypertension. Lifestyle changes—such as eating a healthier diet, getting more physical activity, and losing weight (if necessary)—are often the first approach used to bring blood pressure under control. Such changes also have a beneficial effect on the risk of coronary heart disease and several types of cancer.

## SMOKING

Smoking raises the risk of many serious disorders, and numerous studies show that its adverse effect on stroke is no different. In the Nurses' Health Study, we found that, compared to women who have never smoked, those who currently smoke are almost three times more likely to experience a stroke of any type. And the more cigarettes the women smoked per day, the higher their risk. When we assessed the different kinds of stroke, we found that smoking had a particularly large influence on the risk of subarachnoid hemorrhage, with the risk nearly fivefold higher in current smokers compared to those who had never smoked.

Smoking can raise the risk of stroke in many ways. It promotes atherosclerosis, increases short-term blood pressure, and makes it more likely that blood will clot.

The good news: the increased risk linked to smoking appears reversible. For all types of stroke, we found that the risk of the disease dropped by 25 percent only one to two years after a woman had stopped smoking. Five or more years after quitting, the risk of a former smoker nearly equaled that of someone who had never smoked.

## HEART DISEASES AND TIAs

Mentioned earlier, transient ischemic attacks and certain heart diseases can greatly increase the risk of stroke. While having such disorders is not directly under a person's control, getting treatment for the conditions and making healthy lifestyle changes is.

*Transient Ischemic Attacks (TIAs).* TIAs are a very important warning sign for stroke. The small clots that cause TIAs are often precursors to a larger clot that may cut off a large amount of blood flow and cause severe permanent brain damage. Overall, the risk of stroke is about 5 times greater in someone who has had a TIA compared to someone who has not, and the risk is greater closer to the time of the TIA. The first year following a TIA, a woman's risk of stroke is exceptionally high.

Under the care of a physician, anyone who has experienced TIAs can take steps to lower the risk of a stroke. Drugs to prevent blood clots, such as aspirin and warfarin (Coumadin), are almost always recommended. In some instances, surgery may be an option to remove the severe buildup of atherosclerosis in the large arteries of the neck—the carotid arteries—from which blood clots could break lose. Called carotid endarterectomy, this surgery can significantly lower the risk of death from stroke.

*Atrial Fibrillation.* Atrial fibrillation greatly increases the risk of stroke—approximately 6 times in those with the condition compared to those without. The irregular beating of the atria—the upper chambers of the heart—that defines the condition can cause blood to pool, promoting the formation of clots, which can then travel to the brain and get lodged in an artery, cutting off the blood supply. Approximately 15 percent of all strokes are directly linked to atrial fibrillation, and the risk is greatest in women who have other risk factors for stroke, such as age over seventy, coronary heart disease, and hypertension. A woman who experiences atrial fibrillation but is otherwise healthy generally has only a small increase in her risk of stroke. Nevertheless, most women with atrial fibrillation should take some form of drug that hampers the formation of blood clots. Physicians usually recommend that women at higher risk of stroke take the prescription drug warfarin (Coumadin), which can lower the risk of stroke due to atrial fibrillation by up to 70 percent. Women at lower risk may be advised to take aspirin.

*Heart Attack.* A heart attack can increase the risk of stroke by weakening the pumping action of the heart or causing an irregular heartbeat, both of which can cause blood clots to form; these clots can then travel to the brain. The risk of a stroke is highest in the first month following a heart attack, but remains elevated for years afterward. A heart attack can also be a sign that a person is prone to atherosclerosis, which increases the likelihood that they will also develop plaque in the large arteries of the neck—called carotid artery stenosis. Plaque in the carotid arteries can cause clots to form, break off, and travel to the brain. Following a heart attack, the regular use of aspirin is often recommended—from a fourth of a tablet to one full one (325 milligrams) a day—to help lower the risk of a stroke as well as of another heart attack.

*Other Heart Conditions.* A number of other heart conditions, such as valve disease and congestive heart failure, can also increase the risk of stroke, usually by increasing the likelihood that clots will form and travel through the bloodstream to the brain.

## DIABETES

There are two main types of diabetes, and both significantly increase the risk of stroke. The most common type of diabetes by far is adult-onset diabetes, also referred to as type 2 or non-insulin-dependent diabetes mellitus. Adult-onset diabetes develops most often in adults and especially in people who are overweight. A woman with adult-onset diabetes can often control her blood sugar with lifestyle changes and/or oral medicine. The other type of diabetes is juvenile-onset diabetes, also referred to as type 1 or insulin-dependent diabetes mellitus, which most often develops before the age of thirty. A woman with juvenile-onset diabetes requires insulin injections to control her blood sugar.

In the Nurses' Health Study, we found that women with adult-onset diabetes had 2.5 to 3 times the risk of stroke compared to women without diabetes. One of our most striking findings was the extent to which diabetes magnified the risk of stroke when a woman also had other risk factors for stroke. We found that women who had diabetes and also smoked or also had hypertension or were also obese had approximately 12 times the risk of stroke compared to women without these risk factors.

How does diabetes increase the risk of stroke? The high level of sugar in the blood that characterizes the condition can not only increase the tendency of blood to clot but also injure the walls of arteries in the neck and brain, which can lead to the buildup of atherosclerosis. In addition, diabetes is associated with hypertension, obesity, and poor cholesterol levels, which can increase the risk of stroke as well.

The best way for people with diabetes to lower their risk of stroke is by taking steps to manage the risk factors that interact with diabetes to greatly magnify risk. These include avoiding smoking, controlling blood pressure and blood cholesterol, and maintaining a healthy weight. In addition to lifestyle changes, certain medications may also be helpful, such as aspirin, cholesterol-lowering drugs, and angiotension-converting enzyme (ACE) inhibitors.

## Weight

Outside of the Nurses' Health Study, only one other cohort study—the Framingham Heart Study—has found that being overweight increases the risk of ischemic stroke in women. What we specifically found in the Nurses' Health Study is that overweight women have a moderate increase in risk compared to lean women, while those who are obese have a large increase in risk (see Figure 7-4). How much a woman currently weighs, though, is not the only aspect of weight that increases the risk of stroke. Gaining weight also raises risk. We found that women who put on twenty-two to forty-four pounds as adults had a 70 percent increase in their risk of ischemic stroke compared to women with a stable adult weight. For those who gained more than forty-four pounds, the risk was even greater. Weight gain, however, did not seem to increase the risk of hemorrhagic stroke.

Although we have not yet studied the issue, some studies have found a link between body shape and stroke. A large Swedish study found that women who carried the most weight around their middles had a greater risk of stroke than women who carried the most weight in their hips and thighs.

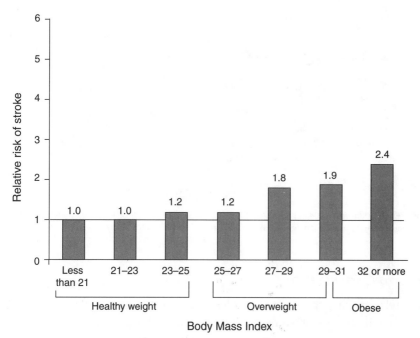

FIG. 7-4. The risk of stroke increases as weight increases. See Appendix C for information on calculating body mass index. (Source: Nurses' Health Study)

Obesity, weight gain, and being apple-shaped may promote stroke in many ways, including raising the risk of many important stroke risk factors, such as diabetes, hypertension, high blood cholesterol, and coronary heart disease.

## PHYSICAL ACTIVITY

The few studies that have examined the relationship between physical activity and stroke have consistently shown that even moderate amounts of activity can protect against the disease. In the Nurses' Health Study, we found that women who walked for at least one hour a week at a brisk pace were 30 percent less likely to have a stroke than sedentary women (see Figure 7-5). The quicker a woman's walking pace, the lower her risk. Physical activity likely reduces the risk of stroke by its wide-ranging effect on many stroke risk factors. Regular physical activity can aid weight loss; lower the risk of diabetes, hypertension, and high blood cholesterol; and inhibit the formation of blood clots.

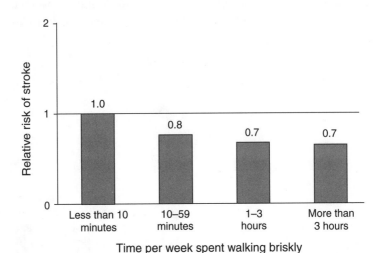

FIG. 7-5. Women who walk at a brisk pace (more than 3 miles per hour) for at least one hour a week receive moderate protection against stroke. (Source: Nurses' Health Study)

## BLOOD CHOLESTEROL

The relationship between blood cholesterol level and the risk of stroke is complex and, in the case of women, a little unclear. To date, only a few studies have assessed the issue in women, and those that have, have had mixed results. What the studies in men have suggested, though, is that the relationship between the risk of stroke and blood cholesterol depends on the type of stroke being stud-ied: high levels of blood cholesterol approximately double the risk of ischemic stroke, while low levels approximately triple the risk of hemorrhagic stroke.

It is not exactly clear why the effect on risk varies depending on the type of stroke. For ischemic stroke, it is likely that high levels of blood cholesterol pro-mote atherosclerosis in the larger arteries of the neck and brain as well as in the coronary arteries. How low blood cholesterol might increase the risk of hemorrhagic stroke is less well understood. Some scientists speculate that since cholesterol is necessary for the normal lining of arteries, low levels may make them more fragile and likely to burst.

While hemorrhagic stroke is a serious and often fatal event, it is much less common in the United States than ischemic stroke. For this reason, it seems prudent for all women to take steps to keep their blood cholesterol levels under control. The potential increase in the risk of hemorrhagic stroke linked to low-normal blood cholesterol levels is outweighed by the drop in the risk of is-chemic stroke—not to mention coronary heart disease. This is especially so in the United States, where very low blood cholesterol levels (those under 160 mg/dL) are relatively rare.

In fact, studies have shown that using drugs to lower blood cholesterol—even in women with average levels—can lower the overall risk of stroke. Stud-ies of drugs called statins (such as lovastatin and pravastatin) that lower LDL cholesterol—the "bad" cholesterol—found that when blood cholesterol levels dropped, so did the risk of stroke. One study of women who had previously had a heart attack found that pravastatin lowered the risk of stroke by more than 30 percent compared to women taking a placebo. And while an increase in the risk of hemorrhagic stroke might be expected because of the drop in cholesterol level due to the statin drugs, many of the recent studies have found the risk of hem-orrhagic stroke actually stays the same or even drops slightly with statin use.

## Alcohol

Alcohol is an important risk factor for stroke, although, as in the case of blood cholesterol, it can affect the risk of hemorrhagic and ischemic stroke differ-ently. For high levels of intake (more than two drinks a day), the message is clear: alcohol greatly increases the risk of both types of stroke. However, at moderate (one-half to two drinks a day) or low levels (less than a half a drink a day) of alcohol intake, the relationship becomes more complex. As with heart disease, a moderate amount of alcohol seems to significantly lower the risk of ischemic stroke, possibly by improving blood cholesterol levels or decreasing the risk of blood clots. In contrast, there does not appear to be any safe amount of alcohol intake when it comes to hemorrhagic stroke. Moderate and even low intake can increase the risk of the disease, and the more a woman drinks, the higher her risk. In addition to inhibiting clotting, alcohol also increases blood pressure, blood flow to the brain, and the chance of having irregular heartbeats, all factors that make it more likely that a blood vessel in the brain will burst and bleed.

In the Nurses' Health Study, we found that, compared to women who did not drink, those who drank approximately one drink a day had a 40 percent lower risk of stroke overall (see Figure 7-6) and a 50 percent lower risk of ischemic stroke. Because the women in our study generally reported that they drank very little, we do not have information on the effect of high alcohol intake on stroke risk. Other cohort studies, however, have shown that, compared to nondrinking women, heavy drinkers approximately double their risk of ischemic stroke.

In contrast, when we assessed hemorrhagic stroke, we found that women had to drink only one to nine drinks per week to more than double their risk of the disease. Such a finding helps illustrate the complexity of the alcohol-health relationship. Although there are clear benefits to moderate drinking, there are also some serious risks. For a detailed discussion of alcohol consumption, see Chapter 20.

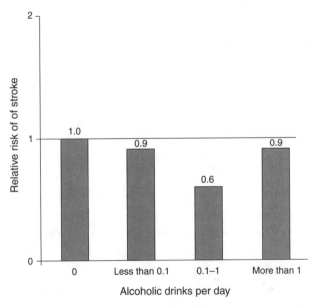

FIG. 7-6. The risk of total stroke (both ischemic and hemorrhagic combined) goes down with moderate alcohol consumption. (Source: Nurses' Health Study)

## DIET

Although many different types of food have been proposed as risk factors for stroke, only two are currently supported by the science: fruits and vegetables, and whole grains.

*Fruits and Vegetables.* Just about any publication discussing food and health suggests that we should all eat at least five servings of fruits and vegetables every day to improve our health. In addition to lowering the risk of disorders ranging from hypertension to certain cancers, eating a diet rich in fruits and vegetables also seems to lower the risk of stroke. In the Nurses' Health Study— one of the first large, detailed studies to assess this issue in women—we found that eating five or more servings of fruits and vegetables a day could lower the risk of ischemic stroke by as much as 30 percent (see Figure 7-7). Citrus fruits (such as oranges and lemons), cruciferous vegetables (such as broccoli and cauliflower), and green leafy vegetables (spinach and kale) seemed particularly beneficial.

How do fruits and vegetable protect against stroke? Although it is not completely clear, fruits and vegetables contain a number of nutrients that may help lower the risk of the disease: potassium, which can help lower blood pressure; folate, which can help lower levels of the atherosclerosis-promoting pro-

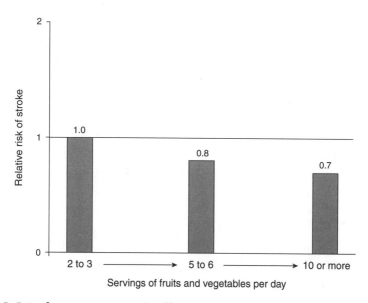

FIG. 7-7. Eating five or more servings a day of fruits and vegetables lowers the risk of ischemic stroke. (Source: Nurses' Health Study)

tein homocysteine; antioxidants, which can help prevent the oxidation of LDL cholesterol; and fiber, which can lower the risk of diabetes, high blood cholesterol, and the formation of blood clots. Although not all studies are completely consistent on the issue, the potential to lower the risk of stroke provides one more reason to eat a diet rich in fruits and vegetables.

*Whole Grains.* A diet rich in whole grain foods—such as dark bread, whole grain breakfast cereal, cooked oatmeal, wheat germ, brown rice, and bran—may lower the risk of ischemic stroke. Compared to refined grains like white flour, whole grains tend to be richer in nutrients (such as fiber, folate, and vitamin E) that may help protect against stroke. In the Nurses' Health Study, we found a 30 to 40 percent reduction in the risk of ischemic stroke among women who ate at least one serving of grains a day. (A serving of grains is equivalent to a slice of wheat bread or a cup of brown rice.) We also found that refined grain foods (like white bread and muffins) offered little to no benefit. Simply substituting whole grain cereal for refined cereal at breakfast may help women lower their risk of ischemic stroke.

## ANTIOXIDANT VITAMINS—A, C, AND E

Although the evidence is not yet conclusive, certain vitamins—the antioxidants A, C, and E—may help lower the risk of stroke. Antioxidants help protect cells and tissue from damage by oxygen free radicals. These free radicals can oxidize LDL cholesterol, a chemical change that makes the cholesterol more likely to injure artery walls and promote atherosclerosis. Antioxidant vitamins may help prevent the oxidation of LDL, avoiding atherosclerosis and lowering the risk of ischemic stroke.

Studies of this issue have had mixed results to date, and it is not yet clear whether women should—in addition to eating a balanced and varied diet—take vitamin supplements to lower their risk of stroke. Results from two large randomized controlled trials of women, due out in one to two years, should help clarify the exact relationship between antioxidant vitamins and the risk of stroke.

## HOMOCYSTEINE

A number of studies have linked high blood levels of the protein homocysteine with an increased risk of stroke. High levels of this protein may promote blood clots and injure artery walls, which can start the process of atherosclerosis that eventually leads to a stroke. One large study based on a sample of the U.S. population found that individuals with the highest levels of homocysteine in their

## Stroke: Weighing the Risks

- Compared to women who have never smoked, those who currently smoke have a large risk of stroke. Fortunately, five or more years after quitting smoking, the risk of a former smoker nearly equals that of someone who has never smoked.

- Women who have diabetes in combination with other risk factors for stroke, such as smoking, hypertension, and obesity, have an exceptionally high risk of stroke compared to women without these risk factors.

- Women who put on twenty to forty-five pounds as adults have a moderate increase in their risk of ischemic stroke compared to women with a stable adult weight.

- Women who walk at a brisk pace for at least two and a half hours a week have a moderately lower risk of stroke than sedentary women.

- Compared to women who do not drink, those who drink approximately one drink per day have a moderate drop in the risk of stroke overall and a large drop in the risk of ischemic stroke.

- Women who eat five or more servings of fruits and vegetables a day have a moderately lower risk of ischemic stroke compared to women eating three servings a day.

- Among men and women with a history of stroke or TIAs, those who regularly take aspirin have a slightly lower risk of stroke compared to those not taking aspirin.

- Women taking birth control pills—particularly the older, higher dose pills—have an increased risk of stroke; however, after a woman stops taking the pill, her risk of stroke drops to equal that of a woman who has never used it.

- Compared to women with the lowest intake of calcium, those getting at least a modest amount of calcium have a moderately lower risk of ischemic stroke.

blood had more than double the risk of stroke of those with the lowest levels of homocysteine, and the risk increased with increasing homocysteine level.

While a number of factors can influence homocysteine level, diet seems to be an important way to maintain low blood levels of the protein. Getting enough vitamin $B_6$, vitamin $B_{12}$, and folate—from food or vitamin supplements—can keep homocysteine levels low. Not getting enough of these vitamins can make it rise.

### ASPIRIN

For its ability to lower the risk of death from cardiovascular disease—especially in those who have already had a heart attack or stroke—aspirin is increasingly being viewed as a low cost wonder drug. By hampering the ability of blood to clot, aspirin reduces the chances that clots will develop or get lodged in an artery in the brain, causing an ischemic stroke.

One large study of aspirin and cardiovascular disease that combined the results of over 170 trials found that among men and women with a history of stroke or TIAs, those who regularly took aspirin had an approximately 25 percent lower risk of stroke compared to those not taking aspirin. One-fourth to one full aspirin (325 milligrams) taken once a day seemed to provide the most benefit.

But what about women wanting to prevent a first stroke? Unfortunately, it is still unclear whether aspirin use can lower the risk of stroke in women who have not had TIAs or a previous stroke. In the Nurses' Health Study, we found that it could, but many other studies on this topic have found no link between regular aspirin use and a lower risk of a first stroke. When we assessed the issue, we found that women who took one to six aspirins a week had a small reduction—approximately 15 percent—in the risk of a first stroke compared to women who took no aspirin at all.

Despite its many benefits, aspirin use is not without side effects, some of which can be very serious. One such serious side effect is an increased risk of hemorrhagic stroke. While hampering clotting is beneficial for ischemic stroke, it has the opposite effect on hemorrhagic stroke because it increases the likelihood of bleeding. In our study, we found that women who took fifteen or more aspirins a week had double the risk of hemorrhagic stroke compared to women who did not take any aspirin. It is important, though, to keep this risk in perspective. A doubling of risk may seem large, but when compared to the possible benefits of aspirin in lowering the chances of heart attack and ischemic stroke, the risk of hemorrhagic stroke linked to aspirin use is relatively small. A large study that combined the results of sixteen randomized trials on aspirin and cardiovascular disease—largely containing high risk men—found that while aspirin use was linked to 137 fewer cases of heart attack for every 10,000 people, it was linked to only 12 extra cases of hemorrhagic stroke. Unfortunately, the study did not present separate findings for the women included in the trials.

## BIRTH CONTROL PILLS

The use of older, high dose birth control pills (see Chapter 23)—used most often by women in the United States from the early 1960s through the mid-1970s—has been shown in many studies to increase the risk of stroke, especially among smokers and those over age thirty-five. The high doses of hormones contained in the older pills were thought to promote the formation of blood clots. Even with these high dose formulations, though, the risk of stroke was elevated only in women currently using the pill. We found in the Nurses' Health Study that after women stopped taking the pill, the risk of stroke slowly dropped to equal that of women who had never used birth control pills.

Because most of the women in our study who used birth control pills likely took the older, higher dose formulations, we do not have any information on the risk of stroke linked to the newer, lower dose pills. This issue is currently being studied by other researchers, but the available evidence suggests that there is only a small to moderate increase in risk while women are on the pill. As with the high dose pill, any risk linked to the low dose pill would likely disappear after a woman stops using it. Regardless, the risk of stroke is already very low among women of childbearing age—those who would be taking birth control pills. Therefore, any increase in risk linked to the pill would still result in only a small number of extra cases of stroke.

## POSTMENOPAUSAL HORMONES

A large number of U.S. women take postmenopausal hormones to alleviate the short-term symptoms and longer-term health effects of menopause. In addition to its many benefits—such as lowering the risk of osteoporosis and possibly coronary heart disease—postmenopausal hormone use also has some risks, such as an elevated risk of breast cancer and possibly stroke.

The evidence of its effect on stroke, however, is far from conclusive, with some studies showing that it can increase risk and others showing that it can decrease risk. When we assessed the issue in the Nurses' Health Study, we found only a weak relationship between postmenopausal hormone use and the risk of stroke. Compared to women who never used hormones, women taking the highest doses had a slightly elevated risk. With women today tending to take lower dose formulations, it is not totally clear what their risk may be. Preliminary results from the Women's Health Initiative show that women on these lower dose formulations have a higher risk of stroke (and other cardiovascular events) during the first two years of use compared to women taking a placebo. However, as the study progresses, it seems that the rate of stroke and other cardiovascular events is equaling out between the women on hormones and the women on placebos. Conclusive evidence from this trial will be available in 2005.

## OTHER RISK FACTORS

Though not as well established, a number of other factors may increase the risk of developing stroke. However, more evidence is needed before it is known if, and precisely how, these factors influence stroke risk.

*Dietary Fat.* Even though it has such an important influence on the risk of coronary heart disease, fat in the diet does not appear to have a strong link to stroke. Because certain types of fat increase the risk of developing atherosclerosis, it seems logical that these same fats would increase the risk of stroke. However, the studies have not shown this. Many have found no link between dietary fat and stroke, and others have suggested that high amounts of fat may lower the risk of dying from a stroke. These counterintuitive results are likely due to dietary fat having a different effect on the risk of hemorrhagic stroke than on the risk of ischemic stroke. Among other influences, a high fat intake can increase blood cholesterol levels, which can lower the risk of hemorrhagic stroke while at the same time increase the risk of ischemic stroke. Future studies that specifically address the different types of stroke as well as the different types of fat should help clarify this issue.

*Calcium and Potassium.* Because a number of studies have shown that a high intake of calcium and potassium may lower the risk of hypertension, there is speculation that it may also lower the risk of stroke. To date, though, there have been a relatively small number of studies on the subject. Even rarer is information on women. When we assessed this issue in the Nurses' Health Study, we found that a low intake of calcium and possibly potassium could increase the risk of ischemic stroke. Compared to women with the lowest intake of calcium (less than half of the recommended dietary allowance for a fifty-year-old woman), those getting at least a modest amount of calcium had a 20 to 30 percent lower risk of ischemic stroke (see Figure 7-8). Though the evidence was less solid, potassium seemed to have a similar relationship to the risk of stroke: only women with the lowest intake seemed to be at increased risk. More research needs to be done before any definite recommendation can be made about calcium and potassium intake in relation to the risk of stroke.

*Other Factors.* A number of other potential risk factors are also being studied, but as with dietary fat, calcium, and potassium, more information is needed before it is known exactly how they influence the risk of stroke. Some of these potential risk factors include:

- Emotional stress, anger, and aggression
- Infection and inflammation
- Excess protein in the urine (proteinuria)
- Height

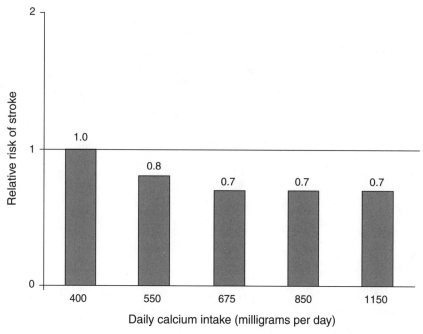

FIG. 7-8. Low calcium intake may increase the risk of ischemic stroke. (Source: Nurses' Health Study)

## WHAT IT ALL MEANS

Although stroke is a very serious and potentially disabling disorder, you can do a lot to try to lower your risk. The most important action you can take is to keep your blood pressure under control. If it is high, see a health care provider regularly and take steps to bring it down to normal. If it *is* normal, take steps to keep it there. If you have TIAs, heart disease, diabetes, or high blood cholesterol, you should try to control and be treated for these conditions. Lifestyle factors are equally important. As with coronary heart disease, simple changes in your life can significantly lower your risk of stroke: avoid smoking, be physically active, and eat a healthy diet. Beyond lowering the risk of stroke, these key lifestyle changes can lower the risk of heart disease, diabetes, and certain cancers, as well as improve quality of life.

## Established, Probable, and Possible Factors Associated with the Risk of Total Stroke (Ischemic and Hemorrhagic Stroke Combined)

| RISK FACTOR | APPROXIMATE RISK* |
|---|---|
| *Established* | |
| Heart conditions and transient ischemic attacks | ↑↑↑↑ |
| Age (greater than 65 vs. under 45) | ↑↑↑ |
| Ethnicity (African American vs. white) | ↑↑↑ |
| High blood pressure | ↑↑↑ |
| Smoking (current vs. never) | ↑↑↑ |
| Diabetes | ↑↑↑ |
| Weight | |
| Being overweight | ↑↑↑ |
| Gaining more than 22 pounds in adulthood | ↑↑ |
| Having a large waist (35 inches or larger) | ↑↑ |
| Family history of stroke (parent or sibling with a stroke vs. no family history) | ↑↑ |
| Poor blood cholesterol levels | ↑ |
| Regular physical activity (3 hours per week vs. none) | ↓↓ |
| Low dose aspirin—for lowering the risk of stroke in women with a history of ischemic stroke (however aspirin use can increase the risk of hemorrhagic stroke significantly) | ↓↓ |
| Alcohol intake (1 or fewer drinks per day vs. none) (even a low intake of alcohol, though, can increase the risk of hemorrhagic stroke significantly) | ↓ |
| *Probable* | |
| Homocysteine (high blood levels vs. low blood levels) | ↑↑↑ |
| Birth control pills—older, high-dose formulations (current or recent use vs. never used) | ↑ |
| Fruits and vegetables (high intake vs. low intake) | ↓↓ |
| Whole grain foods (high intake vs. low intake) | ↓ |
| *Possible* | |
| Birth control pills—newer, low dose formulations (current or recent use) | ↑ |

| | |
|---|---|
| Postmenopausal hormones (current use vs. never used) | ↑ |
| Low dose aspirin—for lowering the risk of a first stroke | ↓ |
|    (however, aspirin use can increase the risk of hemorrhagic stroke significantly) | |
| High intake of vitamins A, C, and E | ↓ |
| High calcium and potassium intake | ↓ |

| | |
|---|---|
| *↑ Small increase in risk | ↓ Small decrease in risk |
| ↑↑ Moderate increase in risk | ↓↓ Moderate decrease in risk |
| ↑↑↑ Large increase in risk | ↓↓↓ Large decrease in risk |
| ↑↑↑↑ Very large increase in risk | ↓↓↓↓ Very large decrease in risk |

# WHAT I TELL MY PATIENTS ABOUT LOWERING THEIR RISK OF STROKE

DR. CAROL BATES

Strokes often come on suddenly and without warning. Once a stroke has started, you cannot prevent it. However, by getting immediate medical attention, you can get treatments that may limit the damage that it does. Some people do have transient warning symptoms (TIAs) that precede strokes. Treatment of these TIAs can prevent strokes. Knowing the symptoms of stroke and TIAs and immediately seeking treatment in response to those symptoms is imperative. The most common symptoms are listed on page 123.

Although strokes come on out of the blue, the abnormalities that lead to them have been building up over many months and years. During those years, you can take action to protect yourself. Here's what you can do:

1. **If you have hypertension, take steps to reduce it.** This is the *single most important thing* you can do to reduce your risk of having a stroke. Hypertension is common; the older women get, the more likely they are to have hypertension.

   So for starters, have your blood pressure checked regularly. You can have this done most accurately at your annual physical exam. And if your health care provider finds your blood pressure is high, discuss strategies to reduce it. These include improving your diet and increasing your physical activity, and then taking blood pressure medication if these initial strategies don't work.

2. **Stop smoking.** Smoking increases your risk of stroke, as well as your risk of heart disease, lung cancer, and many other serious disorders. For strategies on how to stop smoking, see Chapter 17.

3. **If you have experienced TIAs or have an irregular heart rhythm called atrial fibrillation, talk with your health care provider about whether you should take blood thinners.** Transient ischemic attacks, or TIAs, are often referred to as ministrokes. Fortunately, you recover fully from TIAs, but they are a warning sign: the chance you will have a full stroke in the future is much higher if you have had a TIA in the past.

   The irregular heart rhythm called atrial fibrillation also greatly increases your risk of having a stroke. Blood clots tend to form in the chambers of the heart called the atria. These clots can pass out into the bloodstream and lodge in an artery that feeds your brain.

   If you have had a TIA, or suffer from atrial fibrillation, talk with your health care provider about whether you should take aspirin or drugs like warfarin (Coumadin). These blood-thinning medicines can greatly reduce your risk of having a stroke.

4. **Try to avoid developing diabetes, or manage your disease carefully if you have it.** Diabetes increases your risk of stroke. The most important thing you can do to prevent adult-onset diabetes is to maintain a healthy weight. Have your blood sugar levels checked periodically, particularly if you have risk factors for diabetes.

5. **Eat better and exercise more.** We all tend to gain weight as we grow older, but if you have gained a significant amount—twenty-two pounds or more since you were eighteen—then you face an increased risk of stroke. The more weight you gain, the more the risk increases. To lose weight, increase your level of physical activity and eat a diet lower in fat and higher in fruits, vegetables, and fiber. Even taking a brisk half-hour walk five days a week will reduce your risk of a stroke. And the more you increase your level of physical activity, the more you will reduce your risk of stroke.

6. **Drink alcohol in moderation, or don't drink at all.** The benefits and risks of alcohol are quite complex and are still being investigated. Having a drink a day will likely reduce your risk of coronary heart disease and ischemic stroke, the most common type of stroke. At the same time, having a drink a day will increase your risk of hemorrhagic stroke. This type of stroke is, fortunately, much less common

than an ischemic stroke, but it tends to strike earlier in life and be more deadly. Moderate consumption of alcohol may also increase your risk of breast cancer. Because excess alcohol consumption can cause numerous health problems, I generally don't advise non-drinkers to start drinking alcohol as a preventive measure. If you do drink alcohol, do so in moderation—no more than a drink a day.

7. **Keep your blood cholesterol levels healthy.** Many of the studies looking at the link between blood cholesterol levels and stroke have been done in men, leaving some uncertainty about the link in women. But other studies have reported that the medications used to lower blood cholesterol in women will also reduce their risk of stroke. Since keeping your blood cholesterol levels under control will reduce your risk of other diseases, particularly coronary heart disease, it makes sense to have your cholesterol levels checked regularly (every five years beginning at age twenty, more often if your levels are high). If your cholesterol levels are high, then changes in your diet and level of physical activity should help reduce them. If not, ask your health care provider about medication.

8. **Eat plenty of fruits and vegetables.** Eating five or more servings of fruits and vegetables a day decreases your risk of stroke as well as hypertension and certain cancers. Many people find this amount overwhelming, but you can usually work five servings a day into your diet by planning ahead and making substitutions.

9. **Make sure you are getting enough vitamins in your diet, especially vitamin $B_6$, $B_{12}$, and folic acid.** Although the jury is still out on whether you should take a daily vitamin supplement to reduce your risk of stroke, we do know that vitamins $B_6$ and $B_{12}$, as well as folic acid, will reduce your blood levels of homocysteine. This protein seems to increase the risk of stroke.

10. **Talk with your health care provider before you take birth control pills or postmenopausal hormones, but both should be safe.** Older forms of birth control pills, which contained much higher levels of hormones, increased women's risk of stroke. But the types of birth control pills used since the mid-1970s have a lower dose. Although studies of what effect these pills will have on your risk of stroke are still under way, any risk they pose appears to be slight. The same is true of postmenopausal hormones. But to be on the safe side, talk through all the risks with your health care provider.

# CHAPTER EIGHT

# Lowering the Risk of Diabetes

## BACKGROUND

Diabetes mellitus is a huge health problem in the United States. Approximately 16 million people have the condition, only half of whom know it and are able to take active steps to control it. Characterized by a high level of sugar in the blood, diabetes can have many serious consequences—from heart disease and stroke to blindness and amputation—especially if left untreated. Women are especially impacted by the disease. Not only are women more likely to develop diabetes than men are, they are also more likely to suffer certain complications from the disease, such as coronary heart disease. Many ethnic groups are also more likely to be affected by diabetes. African Americans, Latinos, American Indians, and Asian Americans all have higher rates than whites (see Figure 8-2). As with many serious disorders discussed in this book, though, there are many things you can do to lower your risk of developing diabetes in adulthood.

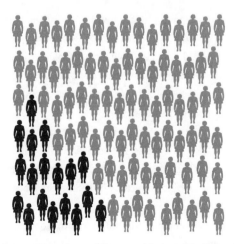

FIG. 8-1. In a group of 100 women who are fifty years old, about 18 will develop diabetes before age eighty. Rates are higher in African Americans and Hispanics. (Source: NIDDK)

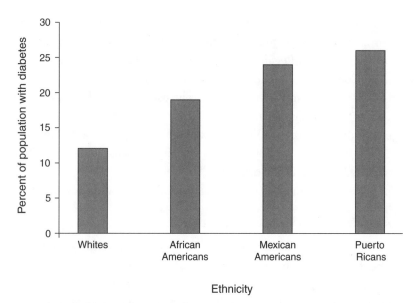

FIG. 8-2. The rate of diabetes varies with ethnicity. Whites have the lowest rate, with most other ethnic groups having higher rates. (Source: NIDDK)

## Blood Glucose and Diabetes

Glucose, a simple form of sugar, is very important to the body. It is the preferred energy source for most tissues, and maintaining normal levels of glucose in the blood is key to the body functioning optimally.

The body's primary source of glucose is food that contains carbohydrates—starches and sugars. After a meal, the body converts starches and sugars to glucose, which then enters the bloodstream and raises blood glucose levels. In response to this increase in glucose levels, an organ in the abdomen called the pancreas releases the hormone insulin. Insulin allows the glucose in the blood to enter the body's cells, where it is either used immediately for energy or stored for use at a later time. As the glucose is taken up by the tissues, its level in the blood drops. When the blood glucose level drops back down to normal, insulin is released at a much lower rate.

Diabetes develops when there is a buildup of glucose in the blood because the body cannot transfer the glucose to its tissues. This can occur for a couple of reasons—either the body can't make enough (or any) insulin or the tissues become resistant to the insulin (insulin resistance), meaning they stop responding as they should to the insulin that the body produces. Sometimes both problems exist at once. Regardless, the end result is the same: the level of glucose in the blood rises to higher than normal levels.

Problems maintaining normal blood glucose levels tend to develop over time. Rather than having normal blood glucose levels one day and diabetes the next, blood glucose levels will slowly rise over months or years. Slightly elevated levels indicate a condition called impaired glucose tolerance. Significantly elevated levels indicate diabetes.

There are two main types of diabetes, juvenile-onset and adult-onset.

## JUVENILE-ONSET (TYPE 1) DIABETES

Juvenile-onset diabetes, also referred to as type 1 or insulin-dependent diabetes, most often develops before the age of thirty and is the less common of the two, accounting for only 5 to 7 percent of diabetes cases. A person with juvenile-onset diabetes produces little or no insulin due to a defect that develops in the pancreas, which can cause blood glucose levels to rise to very high levels if the diabetes is uncontrolled.

The excess glucose passes through the kidneys and is excreted in the urine—usually in very high amounts. Not only will someone with uncontrolled juvenile-onset diabetes have to urinate frequently, he or she will also feel constantly thirsty because of the need to replace the fluids lost through urination. This high output of sugar-rich urine goes to the root of the term *diabetes mellitus*. Diabetes means "running through," and mellitus means "sweet."

In uncontrolled juvenile-onset diabetes, the cells of the body recognize that they are not getting enough glucose (because there is no insulin to help glucose enter the cells). In an attempt to compensate, the body makes glucose (in a form the cells can use) in the liver as well as from fat stores throughout the body. However, this comes with a price. Acids called ketones, which are byproducts of the conversion of fat to glucose, get released into the blood and can accumulate to dangerous levels.

The combination of high glucose-rich urine output, dehydration, and the buildup of acids in the blood can result in a serious condition called diabetic ketoacidosis, which can cause nausea, vomiting, mental confusion, and, in serious cases, coma and even death. It occurs most often in younger diabetics and is frequently a first sign that a child has developed juvenile-onset diabetes.

Despite their inability to make their own insulin, people with juvenile-onset diabetes can control their blood sugar levels with insulin injections. Not only is the vigilant control of blood sugar levels essential to avoid the immediate effects of very high blood glucose—such as ketoacidosis—but it may also lower the risk of developing the long-term problems associated with the disease. One large study found that people with juvenile-onset diabetes who tightly controlled their blood sugar levels could significantly lower their risk of both kidney and eye disorders over a ten-year period.

## ADULT-ONSET (TYPE 2) DIABETES

Adult-onset diabetes, also referred to as type 2 diabetes or non-insulin-dependent diabetes, is by far the most common type of diabetes, accounting for about 90 to 95 percent of cases. It develops most often in adults, especially in people who are overweight. Although children and adolescents develop the disease more rarely than adults, it is becoming increasingly common in these age groups in the United States, most likely due to rising rates of obesity and sedentary lifestyles in the young.

In general, adult-onset diabetes does not affect blood sugar levels to the same extent as juvenile-onset diabetes. For people with adult-onset diabetes, the primary problem is that the tissues resist the effect of insulin, and thus the glucose does not move into the cells as it normally would. To compensate for this inefficient transfer of glucose into cells, the pancreas makes more insulin. While this works in the short term, insulin resistance usually worsens over time, forcing the pancreas to produce increasing amounts of insulin to try to bring blood sugar levels down to a normal level. Eventually, the pancreas becomes exhausted from producing such large amounts of insulin, and the cells that make the insulin fail, after which they make only small amounts of the

## Many Different Names, but Just Two Main Types of Diabetes

The two main types of diabetes go by a variety of names. Juvenile-onset diabetes, which most often develops before the age of thirty, also goes by the names *type 1 diabetes* and *insulin-dependent diabetes*. Adult-onset diabetes, which usually develops in adults but is becoming an increasing problem in youth, also goes by *type 2 diabetes* and *non-insulin-dependent diabetes*.

## Diabetes: The Larger Picture

- Diabetes is the fourth leading cause of death in the United States, accounting for approximately 180,000 deaths each year.
- Diabetes develops when there is a buildup of glucose in the blood because the body cannot transfer the glucose to its tissues. The two main types of diabetes are juvenile-onset (type 1) diabetes and adult-onset (type 2) diabetes.
- Adult-onset diabetes is by far the most common type, accounting for about 90 to 95 percent of cases.
- Women are especially affected by diabetes. They are both more likely to develop the disease than men and more likely to suffer from certain complications, including coronary heart disease.
- Lifestyle changes, such as being physically active, maintaining a healthy weight, and eating the type of diet that does not drastically increase blood sugar levels, are the first line of defense in fighting adult-onset diabetes.
- Coronary heart disease, kidney failure, blindness, foot ulcers, and nerve disease are some of the more serious complications of diabetes.

hormone. Because insulin levels are no longer high enough to compensate for the resistance of the tissues, blood sugar levels rise and diabetes results.

While adult-onset diabetes has many serious, long-term effects on the body, only rarely does a person with adult-onset diabetes develop diabetic ketoacidosis. There is usually enough natural insulin in the system to keep blood sugar to a level that avoids the ketone buildup that leads to acidosis.

As with juvenile-onset diabetes, controlling blood sugar levels is also essential for those with adult-onset diabetes. Certain drugs can help bring blood sugar under control (for example, oral medication or insulin), but the first line of defense in fighting adult-onset diabetes is often through changes in lifestyle—being physically active, maintaining a healthy weight, and eating the type of diet that does not drastically increase blood sugar levels and that may improve the body's sensitivity to insulin. These lifestyle changes will also lower the risk of other diseases, including coronary heart disease and certain cancers.

### COMPLICATIONS OF DIABETES

Like high blood pressure (also called hypertension) and obesity, diabetes is a far-reaching condition that causes problems throughout the body. In addition to increasing the risk of diseases that affect the large blood vessels (such as coronary heart disease and stroke), diabetes also affects the small blood vessels,

## Recognizing the Symptoms of Diabetes

As with heart disease and stroke, identifying and treating diabetes is very important. However, many people are not aware of the symptoms of diabetes and may therefore not seek out the medical care they need. Women experiencing any of the symptoms listed below should contact a health care provider.

### JUVENILE-ONSET (TYPE 1) DIABETES

Symptoms of juvenile-onset diabetes tend to develop fairly rapidly and can include:

- Increased thirst and urination
- Constant hunger
- Unexpected weight loss
- Blurred vision
- Coma (in instances where the diabetes goes undiagnosed and untreated)

### ADULT-ONSET (TYPE 2) DIABETES

Symptoms of adult-onset diabetes tend to develop more slowly than those of juvenile-onset diabetes and can include:

- Feeling tired or ill
- Frequent urination (especially at night)
- Unusual thirst
- Unexpected weight loss
- Blurred vision
- Frequent infections
- Slow healing of sores

resulting in an increased risk of microvascular complications, including kidney failure, blindness, foot ulcers and nerve disease. Infections are more common in people with diabetes as well. Most of these conditions result from the extra strain placed on organs and blood vessels by high levels of blood glucose and insulin (in those with adult-onset diabetes).

All told, diabetes has a staggering impact on health. It is the fourth leading cause of death in the United States, accounting for approximately 180,000 deaths each year. A person with diabetes is about twice as likely to die prematurely than someone without the disease, and studies estimate that a middle-aged person with diabetes dies five to ten years earlier than a person of the

## Cardiovascular Disease and Diabetes

Diabetes is a very powerful risk factor for cardiovascular disease, especially in women. Women with diabetes have 2.5 to 3 times the risk of stroke and 3 to 7 times the risk of coronary heart disease as women without the disorder. Following a heart-healthy lifestyle can reduce the risk of heart disease and stroke in diabetics and is very similar to the lifestyle that lowers the risk of diabetes. Especially important is controlling the main cardiovascular disease risk factors—blood cholesterol, blood pressure, weight, and smoking; all of these interact with diabetes to greatly magnify the risk of both heart disease and stroke. In addition to lifestyle changes, though, medications that lower blood pressure, such as angiotension-converting enzyme (ACE) inhibitors, and blood cholesterol, such as the statins, are often necessary to lower risk. Regular aspirin use also benefits some patients.

same age without diabetes. Although the exact numbers are not clear, women are thought to lose more years of life due to diabetes than men. Diagnosing diabetes early and vigilantly controlling blood sugar levels reduce the risk of developing many of these complications. But, obviously, the best approach is to avoid diabetes altogether.

## LESSONS FROM THE NURSES' HEALTH STUDY AND OTHER STUDIES

Diabetes is clearly a disorder with serious consequences, especially if it goes uncontrolled. The good news about diabetes, though, is that most cases could be avoided. Studies show that adult-onset diabetes—by far the most common type—is largely related to lifestyle factors, such as obesity, lack of physical activity, and poor diet. As important as lifestyle is, however, it is not the sole contributor to the risk of the disease. Other factors are also important, including some you have no control over, such as age, family history, and ethnicity.

Unlike adult-onset diabetes, there is currently no known way to lower the risk of juvenile-onset diabetes, which seems to be caused by an as yet unknown combination of genetic and environmental factors. However, the prevention of juvenile-onset diabetes remains an active area of research, and several medications are currently being tested that may help lower the risk of the disease.

## Factors You Cannot Control

### AGE

As with many other disorders, the risk of diabetes goes up with age. Generally very low in those under age thirty, the risk of diabetes increases very quickly as people advance to middle and old age (see Figure 8-3). Currently, in the United States, approximately 6 percent of women age forty-five to sixty-four and 10 percent of women age sixty-five and over have been diagnosed with diabetes. At most ages, women tend to have a slightly higher rate of the disease than men.

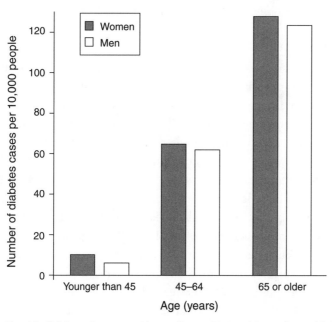

FIG. 8-3. The risk of diabetes increases with age. (Source: National Center for Health Statistics)

### ETHNICITY

The rate of diabetes in the United States varies greatly depending on ethnic group. Compared to whites, most other ethnic groups are at an increased risk of the disease. African Americans and Latinos tend to have about twice the risk of diabetes as whites. At even greater risk are American Indians, of which some populations have more than 10 times the risk of whites. The Pima Indians of Arizona are particularly affected by the disorder. A full 50 percent of adult Pima Indians suffer from adult-onset diabetes.

Although there is not a great deal of information on the rates of diabetes in Asian American populations, certain groups appear to be at increased risk of the disease. Studies done in the 1970s and '80s found that Japanese Americans living in Hawaii and on the West Coast of the United States had rates of diabetes higher than the national average for whites.

Lifestyle factors—such as obesity and poor diet—common to members of a particular ethnic group are thought to account for part of the differences seen in the risk of diabetes. But even when we and other researchers have taken these factors into account, differences between ethnic groups persist, pointing to a possible interplay between genetics and other risk factors (both known and unknown) as a reason for the variations in risk.

## FAMILY HISTORY

Family history is an important predictor of the risk of diabetes. Individuals with at least one immediate family member (brother, sister, parent) with diabetes have a large increase in their risk of the disease compared to someone with no affected family members. Similar to ethnicity, family history likely affects risk by a combination of lifestyle and genetics. Family members often have similar behaviors—such as how much they exercise and what kind of food they eat—that can cause them to have similar risks of diabetes. Yet studies that have taken lifestyle factors into account still find that family history has a large impact on the risk of diabetes, probably through genetic factors that get passed on from generation to generation. In the Pima Indians, a group that appears to be genetically susceptible to diabetes, one study found that individuals with two diabetic parents had 4 times the risk of diabetes as those with no family history, even after lifestyle factors were taken into account.

This does not mean, though, that someone with a family history will inevitably get diabetes. Genetics and lifestyle together make up a person's risk of the disease. And overall, factors such as obesity and physical activity seem to contribute more to the risk of diabetes than family history alone.

### Factors You Can Control

Lifestyle factors play a large role in diabetes, and much of the work we have done in the Nurses' Health Study has focused on identifying such factors in hopes of providing women the means to lower their risk of the disease. While each of these lowers the risk of diabetes by themselves, three—healthy weight, healthy diet, physical activity—are particularly important because they interplay with each other. Healthy diet and physical activity alone can lower risk, but

## Diabetes: Weighing the Risks

- Women over sixty-five and women with a family history of diabetes have a large risk of diabetes compared to women under forty-five and women without a family history.

- Women who are overweight, even just slightly, are at increased risk of diabetes. The heavier a women is, the greater her risk. Obese women have a very high risk compared to lean women.

- Women who gain substantial weight in adulthood, even if they stay in the healthy weight range, are also at increased risk of diabetes. The more weight gained, the higher the risk. Women who have put on forty-five pounds since age eighteen have an exceptionally high risk of diabetes compared to women with a stable weight.

- Women who smoke have a moderately greater risk of diabetes than those who have never smoked.

- Women eating a diet filled with high glycemic index foods (foods that convert quickly to glucose when digested) have a large risk of diabetes compared to those eating a diet that limits high glycemic index foods (see Appendix C).

they can also help with maintaining a healthy weight, the most important predictor of diabetes risk.

### WEIGHT, WEIGHT GAIN, AND BODY SHAPE

Approximately 80 percent of those diagnosed with adult-onset diabetes in the United States are obese—for example, 173 pounds or more for a woman who is 5 feet 4 inches or 197 pounds or more for a women who is 5 feet 8 inches. Yet it is not only the very heavy who are at increased risk. Simply being overweight or at the upper end of the healthy range as defined by federal guidelines also increases risk. In the Nurses' Health Study, we found that the risk of diabetes rose steadily with weight (see Figure 8-4). Obese women had the highest risk, nearly 16 times that of lean women, but even women in the upper part of the healthy range had a large increase in risk, about 3 times that of lean women.

How much a person weighs, however, is only one aspect of weight that affects the risk of diabetes. Body shape and weight gain are also important. Women who carry their weight around their waists (often called apple-shaped) tend to have a greater risk of diabetes compared to women who carry their weight in their hips and thighs (often called pear-shaped). We found that risk steadily increased as women's waist size increased (see Figure 8-5). Those

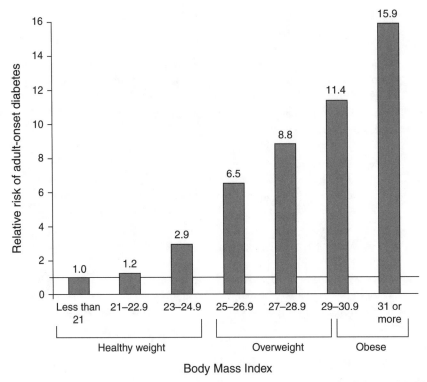

FIG. 8-4. As weight increases, so does the risk of developing adult-onset (type 2) diabetes. The risk is large even for women in the upper part of the healthy range and is exceptionally high in overweight and obese women. (Source: Nurses' Health Study)

women with waist sizes of thirty-five inches or more had a very large risk of the disease, 5 to 6 times that of women with small waists.

We also found that gaining weight or losing weight as an adult can have a major influence on the risk of diabetes. Women who put on twelve or more pounds from the time they were eighteen were twice as likely to develop diabetes as women whose weight remained steady. And the more weight gained, the higher a woman's risk. Women who gained more than forty-five pounds during adulthood were over 12 times as likely to develop the disease. The good news: weight loss had the opposite effect. Women who took off twelve to eighteen pounds had an almost 50 percent drop in their risk of diabetes compared to women whose weight remained steady. Women who lost more than eighteen pounds benefited even more.

An important finding from our study is that a woman's current weight seems to have a much greater influence on her risk of diabetes than what she weighed in the past, suggesting that both weight loss and weight gain have a

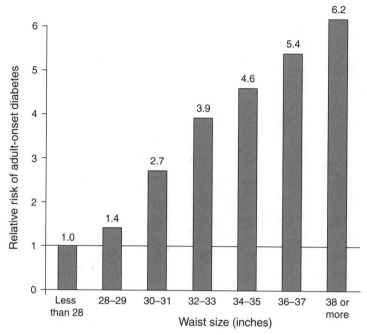

FIG. 8-5. As waist size increases, so does the risk of developing adult-onset (type 2) diabetes. The risk is very large for women with waists 35 inches or larger. (Source: Nurses' Health Study)

---

### In the Nurses' Own Words . . .

I have always tried to get the answer forms back to you as soon as possible, realizing that my answers will serve to advance health care in other women. When filling in the answers, many times I realized that I needed to incorporate into my life some of the things that I was being asked to answer. I have tried to eat better and keep a watch on weight gain. . . . Because of some of the results of this study, I have been able to make easier decisions concerning health matters with my doctor. I look forward to continuing in this study.

—From GS

---

fairly immediate influence on the risk of diabetes. This means that a woman who loses weight and keeps it off will lower her risk of the disease relatively quickly.

## PHYSICAL ACTIVITY

Physical activity not only lowers the risk of diabetes but also helps control blood sugar levels in those who already have the disease. It does this in two ways.

First, activity helps people achieve and maintain a healthy weight. Second, it increases the ability of tissues to take up glucose from the blood.

In the Nurses' Health Study, we have confirmed what many other studies have previously suggested—that physical activity provides moderate protection against diabetes, and that the more active women are, the lower their risk of the disease (see Figure 8-6). We also found, though, that it is not necessary to run marathons to get benefit from physical activity. A modest increase in activity level with something as simple as walking can lower the risk of the disease, even if a woman has been sedentary her whole life. In addition, walking can be just as protective against diabetes as such vigorous activities as running or aerobics. Women in our study who walked briskly (approximately three miles per hour) for three hours a week or exercised vigorously for one and a half hours per week each had a 40 percent lower risk of diabetes. The more time women spent walking, and the faster they walked, the lower their risk.

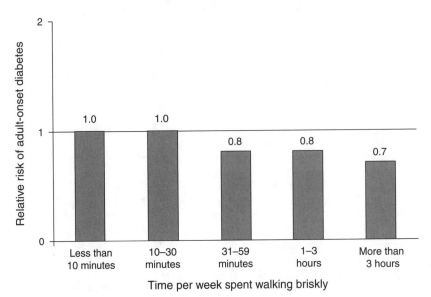

FIG. 8-6. Women who walk at a brisk pace (more than 3 miles per hour) for at least 3 hours a week receive moderate protection against diabetes. (Source: Nurses' Health Study)

## DIET

From the early 1900s, scientists have linked diet to diabetes. Despite such a long history, researchers are still trying to uncover exactly what aspects of the food we eat increase the risk of diabetes. Currently, there is solid evidence for eating too many calories, eating too many foods with a high glycemic index (foods that are quickly converted to glucose), and getting too little fiber, magnesium, potassium, and calcium.

*Total Number of Calories.* Given that obesity is such a strong risk factor for diabetes, it seems obvious that how much food a person eats—the total number of calories he or she eats in a day—would relate to diabetes. Ultimately, it is an imbalance in the number of calories a person eats and the calories he or she burns that leads to weight gain. With a large number of people in the United States consistently eating more calories than they burn, obesity is an increasingly large problem. From 1991 to 1998, a span of just nine years, the percentage of obese women in the United States rose from 12 to 18 percent.

Translated, this means that nearly one out of every five women in the United States is obese. If the trend continues and obesity becomes even more common, diabetes will as well.

Although there appears to be an obvious link between calories and diabetes, only a few studies have actually been able to demonstrate the relationship. The interplay of many different factors can make it difficult to tease out the exact relationship between the two. An imbalance of calories leads to obesity, but a high calorie intake does not necessarily mean that someone eats too much. Often, a high calorie intake means someone is physically active, which promotes a healthy weight and lowers the risk of diabetes. Getting enough information to accurately take all these factors into account can be difficult and may be the reason only a few studies have found a link between calories and diabetes. In the Nurses' Health Study, we found a weak relationship between total calories and the risk of diabetes in obese women. Those women who ate the most calories had a 35 percent higher risk of the disease compared to those who ate the least.

*Glycemic Index.* Not all foods affect blood glucose levels in the same way. Some foods have what is called a high glycemic index and are converted much more quickly than others into glucose, which can quickly raise blood glucose levels. Eating a lot of high glycemic index foods (such as white rice and white bread) increases the need for insulin, which the body produces in large amounts to try to clear the high levels of glucose in the blood. Over time, this increase in insulin production can increase the risk of diabetes. In the Nurses' Health Study, we found that those women who ate the most foods with a high glycemic index had a 50 percent greater risk of diabetes compared to those women who ate the least (see Appendix C for the glycemic index of selected foods).

*Fiber.* A number of studies have shown that fiber can help lower the demand for insulin in patients who already have diabetes and may also lower the risk of initially developing the disease. A high intake of fiber may help avoid spikes in blood glucose levels by slowing down the conversion of certain foods into glucose during digestion. Fiber can essentially make a high glycemic index food act more like a medium or low glycemic index food. This reduces the demand for insulin, which lowers the risk of diabetes.

In the Nurses' Health Study, we found that, compared to women eating the least amount of fiber, those eating the most had a 20 percent lower risk of developing adult-onset diabetes. Most of this benefit, though, seemed to be from one particular type of fiber: cereal fiber, the kind found in whole grain foods. Compared to women eating the least amount of cereal fiber, those eating the most were nearly 30 percent less likely to develop diabetes (see Figure 8-7).

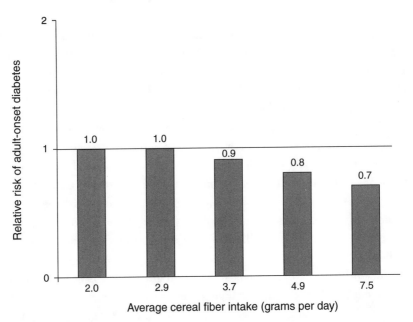

FIG. 8-7. As intake of cereal fiber increases, the risk of adult-onset diabetes decreases. (Source: Nurses' Health Study)

*Minerals (Magnesium, Potassium, and Calcium).* These minerals have been shown in certain studies to have a beneficial effect on insulin production and blood sugar levels, which may help lower the risk of developing diabetes. When we assessed these minerals in the Nurses' Health Study, we found that women getting the greatest amounts of each had a 30 to 40 percent lower risk of diabetes than women getting the least. Eating a healthy diet is the best approach to increasing intake of these minerals. Although supplements are an easy way

| Foods rich in magnesium, potassium, and calcium | | |
| --- | --- | --- |
| MAGNESIUM | POTASSIUM | CALCIUM |
| Whole grains | Whole grains | Milk |
| Nuts | Nuts | Yogurt |
| Legumes | Meats | Cheese |
| Bitter chocolate (cocoa) | Fruit (especially bananas, | Nuts |
| Leafy plants (such as spinach) | oranges, and avocados) | Whole grains |

to boost intake, there is no evidence that they do a better job at lowering the risk of diabetes than a nutrient-rich diet.

It is important to remember that eating a healthy diet—rich in fiber, nutrients, and low glycemic index foods—also means not getting more calories than needed. Maintaining a healthy weight is key to lowering the risk of diabetes as well as many other conditions.

## SMOKING

In addition to smoking being a cause of lung cancer, asthma, emphysema, chronic bronchitis, and cardiovascular disease, there is evidence that it may also increase the risk of diabetes. Most large cohort studies done to date have found a link between the two. In the Nurses' Health Study, we found that women who smoked twenty-five or more cigarettes a day had a risk of the diabetes that was 50 percent greater than that of those who had never smoked. Smoking may raise the risk of the disease in a number of ways. It has been shown to lower insulin levels and increase blood glucose levels. Smoking also increases the chances of developing an apple-shaped body type, which is linked to a higher risk of diabetes.

Smoking also magnifies the risk of cardiovascular disease in women who already have diabetes. We found that smokers with diabetes had about 3 times the risk of coronary heart disease and stroke compared to nonsmokers with diabetes. This increase is quite significant, given that diabetes alone tends to impart a threefold risk of cardiovascular disease. Add the combined risk of smoking and diabetes, and the increase in risk becomes very high, further highlighting the importance of stopping smoking and bringing diabetes under control.

## The Good News

- Losing weight (if necessary) is the single best way to lower the risk of diabetes. Even a small amount of weight loss has benefit, and the more weight lost, the bigger the drop in risk.
- Simply walking can lower the risk of diabetes. Women who walk briskly for three hours a week have a moderately lower risk of diabetes compared to sedentary women.
- A high fiber diet can lower the risk of diabetes. Fiber can essentially make a high glycemic index food act more like a medium or low glycemic index food. Women with a high intake of cereal fiber (found in whole grains) have a moderately lower risk of diabetes compared to women with a low intake.
- Some minerals may help lower risk. Women getting the greatest amounts of magnesium, potassium, and calcium have a moderately lower risk of diabetes than women getting the least.

### GESTATIONAL DIABETES

About 3 to 5 percent of women are diagnosed with diabetes during pregnancy—known as gestational diabetes. Although not an extremely serious condition (especially when it is controlled), it can result in certain problems for both mother and child. One of the most common results of gestational diabetes is larger babies. The extra glucose in the diabetic mother's blood freely passes to the baby, whose tissues take it up and store it mainly as fat. Large babies can complicate birth, slowing the process and making it more likely that women will have cesarean sections. And some studies suggest that babies born to women with gestational diabetes may also have problems with blood sugar control and may later in life be more likely to experience obesity and adult-onset diabetes.

Gestational diabetes and adult-onset diabetes are closely linked diseases, and one of the most important implications for a woman with gestational diabetes is that she is at increased risk of developing adult-onset diabetes. Studies have shown that up to 40 percent of women with gestational diabetes will develop adult-onset diabetes within twenty years of their pregnancy. In the Nurses' Health Study, when we assessed the contributors to gestational diabetes, we found that many of the major risk factors for adult-onset diabetes were also risk factors for gestational diabetes. These included:

- Increasing age
- Family history
- Nonwhite ethnicity
- Obesity and pre-pregnancy weight gain
- Smoking

Following the same steps to lower the risk of adult-onset diabetes—such as maintaining a healthy weight, being physically active, and eating a healthy diet—should also lower the risk of gestational diabetes. Women diagnosed with gestational diabetes should view it as an opportunity to make healthy lifestyle changes that lower their risk of developing adult-onset diabetes in the future.

## POLYCYSTIC OVARY SYNDROME

Polycystic ovary syndrome is a condition that affects about 5 percent of women in their childbearing years. It is characterized by highly irregular menstrual cycles associated with higher than normal levels of male hormones, called androgens. Polycystic ovary syndrome may increase the risk of heart disease and endometrial cancer as well as diabetes. It is associated with increased insulin resistance, the first step toward developing adult-onset diabetes. Compared to a woman without polycystic ovary syndrome, a woman with the condition has about 2.5 times the risk of diabetes.

## OTHER RISK FACTORS

It is still unclear how certain factors—such as postmenopausal hormones, birth control pills, and fat in the diet—influence the risk of diabetes. To date, there is not enough information to say with confidence that such factors either are or are not linked to the disease. Time and further study, however, should help clarify each factor's relationship to the risk of developing diabetes.

*Postmenopausal Hormones.* Small, short-term studies have suggested that using postmenopausal hormones may adversely affect insulin and blood glucose levels. It is unclear, though, whether the effect these hormones have in the short term actually translates to an increased risk of diabetes. Only a small number of cohort studies have assessed this issue, most of which—including the Nurses' Health Study—have found no increase in risk among women who use hormones.

*Birth Control Pills.* As with postmenopausal hormones, studies have shown that using birth control pills can adversely impact insulin and blood glucose levels. However, studies that have explored whether birth control pills actually increase the risk of diabetes have had varied results. In the Nurses' Health Study, we found that women who had used older, high dose birth control pills had a very slight—only 10 percent—increase in the risk of the disease compared to women who had not used the pill. In the younger group of women participating in the Nurses' Health Study II, however, we found no link between the pill and diabetes, possibly because the younger women in the study use newer, lower dose versions of the pill.

*Having Children.* Because insulin resistance can develop during the course of pregnancy, some have wondered if having children increases the risk of developing diabetes in the long term. While some studies have found a link and others have not, many of these studies were small and did not follow women over time. When we assessed the issue in the Nurses' Health Study, we found that there was no overall link between number of births and the risk of diabetes.

For a small subgroup of women, though—those who have experienced gestational diabetes—pregnancy may increase risk. There is evidence that women who have had gestational diabetes and then have another pregnancy afterward increase their risk of adult-onset diabetes approximately 2.5 to 3 times that of women who did not have another pregnancy. Women who develop gestational diabetes may have problems with insulin production that get magnified with each pregnancy, increasing their risk of adult-onset diabetes.

*Fat in the Diet.* The total amount of fat in the diet does not seem to be linked to the risk of diabetes. While many international and small studies have found a link between high fat intake and diabetes, most large cohort studies—including the Nurses' Health Study—have not. Some different types of fat, however, may be linked to risk. We found that a high intake of trans unsaturated fat—found in high amounts in stick margarine and many snack foods—increased the risk of adult-onset diabetes. In contrast, we also found that a high intake of vegetable fat could lower the risk of diabetes by as much as 40 percent, comparing women with the highest intake to those with the lowest. And there is some evidence that monounsaturated fat—found largely in olive and canola oil—may help improve the sensitivity of tissues to insulin.

## WHAT IT ALL MEANS

You have control over many of the factors that can significantly lower your risk of adult-onset diabetes, all of which are also an important part of a generally healthy lifestyle. Topping the list are maintaining a health weight, being physically active, and eating a healthy diet. If you are forty-five or over, it is also important that you see a health care professional to have your blood glucose level checked every three years. You may need to be tested at a younger age if you have one or more of these risk factors for diabetes:

- Family history of diabetes—mother, father, brother, or sister with the condition.
- Overweight
- High blood pressure
- Poor cholesterol levels or high triglyceride level
- Nonwhite ethnicity
- Given birth to a baby over nine pounds

For those people at high risk of diabetes, a study is currently under way to measure the relative benefits of diet and exercise or medication in preventing the disease.

## WHAT I TELL MY PATIENTS ABOUT LOWERING THEIR RISK OF ADULT-ONSET DIABETES

DR. NANCY RIGOTTI

In my experience, not many patients worry about their risk of developing diabetes. Yet many of them should. People with diabetes have a dramatically increased risk of heart disease and other disabling conditions like blindness and kidney failure. The most common type of diabetes, adult-onset diabetes, is becoming more common, and women are more likely to develop it than men.

Fortunately, there are ways to reduce your risk of developing diabetes. And much of what you do to reduce your risk will also protect you against coronary heart disease and some types of cancer.

### Maintain a Healthy Weight

Four out of five women who are diagnosed with adult-onset diabetes are obese. As discussed earlier in this chapter, every aspect of weight—how much

## Established, Probable, and Possible Factors Associated with the Risk of Diabetes

| RISK FACTOR | APPROXIMATE RISK* |
|---|---|
| *Established* | |
| Weight | |
|     Being overweight | ↑↑↑↑ |
|     Gaining 12 to 18 pounds in adulthood | ↑↑ |
|     Gaining 22 pounds or more in adulthood | ↑↑↑↑ |
|     Having a large waist (35 inches or larger) | ↑↑↑↑ |
| Age (greater than 65 vs. under 45) | ↑↑↑ |
| Family history of diabetes (parent or sibling with diabetes vs. no family history) | ↑↑↑ |
| Ethnicity (African American, Latino vs. white) | ↑↑↑ |
| Total calories (too many for energy needs) | ↑↑ |
| Regular physical activity | ↓↓ |
| *Probable* | |
| High glycemic index foods (high intake vs. low intake) | ↑↑↑ |
| Smoking | ↑↑ |
| Fiber intake (high intake vs. low intake) | ↓↓ |
| *Possible* | |
| Polycystic ovary syndrome | ↑↑↑ |
| High trans fat intake | ↑↑ |
| High calcium, magnesium, and potassium intake | ↓↓ |
| Birth control pills use—older, high dose formulations | ↑ |

| | |
|---|---|
| *↑ Small increase in risk | ↓ Small decrease in risk |
| ↑↑ Moderate increase in risk | ↓↓ Moderate decrease in risk |
| ↑↑↑ Large increase in risk | ↓↓↓ Large decrease in risk |
| ↑↑↑↑ Very large increase in risk | ↓↓↓↓ Very large decrease in risk |

you weigh, how many pounds you've gained since you were eighteen, and even if you store your weight around your middle as opposed to in your hips and thighs—will all influence your risk of developing diabetes.

So the best step you can take to reduce your risk is to maintain a healthy

| IF YOUR BMI IS | YOUR WEIGHT IS | TRY TO |
|---|---|---|
| 18.5–24.9 | Healthy | Maintain it |
| 25–29.9 | Overweight | Lose weight |
| 30 or over | Obese | Lose weight |

weight throughout your life. To determine whether your weight is considered healthy or not, do the following three things:

1. Calculate your body mass index (BMI), using the steps outlined in the BMI chart in Appendix C.
2. Figure out how much weight you've gained since you were eighteen. If you have gained even twelve pounds, you are twice as likely to develop diabetes as someone who has not gained weight, so you should lose weight or at least try not to gain anymore. If you have gained more than forty-four pounds, you have 12 times the risk of someone who has maintained a steady weight, and you should definitely try to reduce your weight.
3. Determine your body shape by looking in a mirror or measuring your waist. If you are apple-shaped or have a waist size of 35 inches or larger, then you are at increased risk for diabetes.

The best way to maintain a healthy weight is to eat less and become more physically active.

## Become More Physically Active

In addition to helping you lose weight, regular exercise also helps you to metabolize blood sugar more readily. You don't have to join a gym to become more physically active. In fact, the best way to increase your activity level is to follow these three guidelines:

1. Integrate more activity into your daily life.
2. Do something you enjoy (walk, bike, swim—or whatever you prefer)
3. Start slowly and build gradually.

### Eat a Healthy Diet

Eat lots of fruits, vegetables, fiber, and whole grains, and reduce your consumption of high-calorie and high-fat foods. Because diabetes develops when glucose levels in the blood rise too high, eat fewer foods that are converted more quickly into glucose than others. The substitution chart below may help you:

| INSTEAD OF THIS (RELATIVELY HIGH GLYCEMIC INDEX) | TRY THIS (RELATIVELY LOW GLYCEMIC INDEX) |
| --- | --- |
| White bread for sandwiches (69) | 100% stoneground wheat bread (53) |
| White rice (72) | Brown rice (66) |
| Raisins (65) | Pear (41) or apple (39) or cherries (22) |
| Low fat ice cream (50) | Yogurt (33) |
| Cornflakes (80) | Bran cereal (51) |

### If You Smoke, Quit

Smoking not only increases your chances of developing diabetes, it also raises your risk of lung cancer, coronary heart disease, and a number of other serious illnesses. See Chapter 17 for tips on how to quit smoking.

### Have Your Blood Glucose Levels Checked

If you are at average risk of diabetes, consider having your blood glucose level checked at age fifty and every few years after that. You can have this done during your annual physical.

If you are overweight, if any of your parents or siblings have diabetes, if you have given birth to a baby that weighed more than nine pounds, or if you have other risk factors for diabetes, consider having your glucose levels checked at a younger age. Talk with your health care provider.

# CHAPTER NINE

# Lowering the Risk
# of Colon Cancer

## BACKGROUND

Despite being one of the most common cancers diagnosed in American women, colon cancer remains largely unheard of. Although it is often called a silent killer because it progresses with few symptoms, it has also earned this title for another reason: fear and embarrassment have traditionally kept women (and their health care providers) from talking about colon cancer, and this silence has contributed to thousands of deaths. Only now are women beginning to take advantage of and share the vast amount of information available about protecting themselves from this disease.

Colon cancer is currently the third leading cause of cancer death in American women, claiming nearly 25,000 lives each year. However, it need not occupy such a high rank among the leading causes of death and illness in the

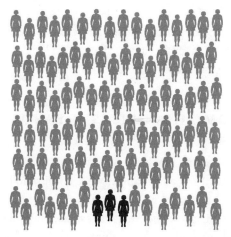

FIG. 9-1. In a group of 100 women who are fifty years old, 3 will develop colon cancer before they reach the age of eighty. (Source: National Cancer Institute)

United States. It is preventable through the same healthy lifestyle that also prevents heart disease, stroke, and a variety of other cancers. This lifestyle involves regular checkups, a healthy diet that includes multivitamins, daily doses of physical activity, and no smoking. With so many potential ways to lower their risk, why shouldn't women be talking about colon cancer?

## The Colon and Colon Cancer

The colon is a part of the digestive system and, together with the rectum, makes up the large intestine (or large bowel). It is about six feet long and has a muscular wall with an inner lining of gland-like cells. Its primary function is to absorb the liquid from the waste that has passed from the small intestine and then store the waste in solid form until it is released from the body.

In a process that is relatively well understood, cancer tends to develop slowly in the colon (see Figure 9-2). It starts when a single cell on the inner lining of the colon wall becomes abnormal and then reproduces to develop a small clump of similar cells. These cells can grow into a small visible lump, called a polyp, that is often shaped like a grape or mushroom. Although many different types of polyps can grow in the colon, only one type—called an adenomatous polyp—has the potential to become cancerous. It does so by invading the mucous lining of the colon wall. The cancerous cells then destroy what is left of the polyp and extend into the muscular wall of the colon. Fortunately, this transformation from polyp to cancer is relatively rare, given how common adenomatous polyps are.

About a quarter of all women have adenomatous polyps by age fifty, and half have them by age sixty-five. Fortunately, less than 5 percent of all adenomatous polyps will become cancerous and those that do usually take five years and sometimes much longer. Because they take so long to transform, polyps can usually be caught and removed before they ever have the opportunity to become malignant.

## LESSONS FROM THE NURSES' HEALTH STUDY AND OTHER STUDIES

Aside from lung cancer and smoking, we know more about preventing colon cancer than we do about any other cancer. We know how to find the polyps that can turn into colon cancer, and we understand many of the factors that influence whether polyps will grow and turn into cancer. Though some of these factors are beyond your control (such as your age and family history), most are

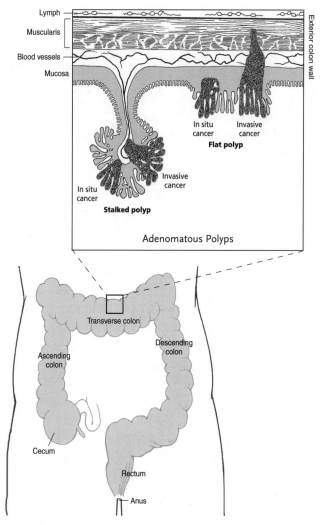

Lymph
Muscularis
Blood vessels
Mucosa
Exterior colon wall

In situ cancer
Invasive cancer
**Flat polyp**

Invasive cancer
In situ cancer
**Stalked polyp**

Adenomatous Polyps

Transverse colon
Descending colon
Ascending colon
Cecum
Rectum
Anus

FIG. 9-2. Colon cancer almost always develops from a small growth (polyp) on the inner lining of the colon. Polyps are very common and usually do not grow or become cancerous. However, one particular type of polyp (adenomatous polyp) has the potential to become cancerous by invading the mucous lining (mucosa) of the colon wall. The cancer cells then destroy what is left of the polyp and extend into the muscular wall (muscularis) of the colon.

related to behaviors you can change (such as physical activity and diet). By knowing how each of these factors affects your risk, you can take appropriate steps to protect yourself from colon cancer. Ultimately, this is a disease that most women can prevent.

## Colon Cancer: The Larger Picture

- Contrary to popular belief, colon cancer is just as common in women as it is in men.
- It is one of the most preventable forms of cancer and, when detected early, is almost always treatable.
- Almost all colon cancers arise from small noncancerous growths called adenomatous polyps.
- These polyps can be detected and removed before they have the chance to become cancerous.

### Factors You Cannot Control

Some factors that influence your risk of colon cancer—like your family history—simply cannot be changed. But this does not mean that you don't have control over your risk of this disease. There is still a lot you can do to protect yourself, and talking to your health care provider about screening should be at the top of your list. Women with particular medical and family histories usually need to be tested for colon cancer at a younger age and more frequently than most women.

### AGE

Although colon cancer does occur in younger women, more than 90 percent of cases are diagnosed in those over age fifty. After that age, the rate of colon cancer doubles—and sometimes even triples—with each additional decade of life (see Figure 9-3). For example, in a group of 100,000 women ages fifty to fifty-five, about 27 women will be diagnosed with colon cancer. In a similarly sized group of women ten years older (ages sixty to sixty-five), about 80 will be diagnosed.

### FAMILY HISTORY

Several studies, including the Nurses' Health Study, have shown conclusively that colon cancer runs in families. Whether this is due to shared genetic traits among family members or a similarity in lifestyles is not yet clear. Most likely, it is a combination of the two.

Having a family member with either colon cancer or rectal cancer doubles a woman's risk of colon cancer. Although it does not seem to matter which specific relative had the disease (mother, father, or sibling), it does matter how

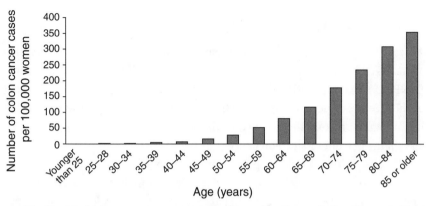

FIG. 9-3. The risk of colon cancer increases steadily after age fifty. (Source: National Cancer Institute)

many relatives were diagnosed and how old they were at the time of diagnosis. Having two relatives with colon cancer quadruples a woman's risk of the disease (see Figure 9-4). In addition, women whose relatives were diagnosed before age forty-five have a higher risk of colon cancer—and are more likely to develop the disease at an early age themselves—than women whose relatives were diagnosed after age forty-five.

Having a family history of adenomatous polyps may also increase a woman's risk of colon cancer. In one study, researchers found a moderate increase in risk among women whose parents or siblings had adenomatous polyps. Risk was particularly high if the family members were diagnosed with polyps before age fifty.

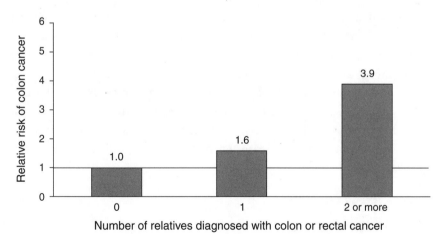

FIG. 9-4. The risk of colon cancer is increased in women with a family history of colon or rectal cancer and is particularly high in those with two or more affected relatives. (Source: Nurses' Health Study)

## SPECIFIC GENETIC SYNDROMES

At least two genetic syndromes predispose women to colon cancer: familial adenomatous polyposis (FAP) and hereditary nonpolyposis colorectal cancer (HNPCC). FAP and HNPCC affect approximately 0.02 percent and 5 percent of the American population, respectively. Although both of these syndromes impart a great risk on those who are affected by them, overall they account for less than 5 percent of all colon cancers.

Women with FAP develop adenomatous polyps when they are in their teens and have hundreds to thousands of polyps by their twenties and thirties. They have an almost 100 percent chance of developing colon cancer by age fifty. Women with HNPCC don't have an unusually large number of polyps, but they too tend to develop colon cancer at a relatively young age. Though this condition can be detected by genetic screening, it is often identified by the following family history: (1) Three or more relatives, one of whom is a parent, sibling, or child of the other two, have been diagnosed with colon or rectal cancer. (2) Colon or rectal cancer has affected family members from at least two different generations. (3) At least one relative was diagnosed with colon or rectal cancer before age fifty. Women with these genetic syndromes should be followed by a specialist and may require special screening and treatment.

## INFLAMMATORY BOWEL DISEASE

Inflammatory bowel disease is characterized by inflammation of the intestines. It includes both ulcerative colitis, in which the inner lining of the colon is inflamed, and Crohn's disease, in which the deeper layers of the colon wall or other portions of the intestinal tract are inflamed. The longer a woman suffers from an inflammatory bowel disease, the more likely she is to develop colon cancer. Although bowel disease does impart a substantial risk on those who are affected by it, overall it accounts for less than 1 percent of all colon cancers. Notably, the more common irritable bowel syndrome (a disorder characterized by crampy pain, gassiness, bloating, and a change in bowel habits) is not an inflammatory bowel disease and is not associated with an increased risk of colon cancer.

### Factors You Can Control

The majority of colon cancers (about 75 percent) occur in women who do not have a family history of the disease, a genetic syndrome, or a personal history of inflammatory bowel disease. This suggests that most colon cancers are within a woman's control and can be prevented through lifestyle changes. Some of these changes—like taking a daily multivitamin—are most effective if you adopt them early in life and maintain them for a long period of time, while others—like getting screened and being active—probably have a more immediate impact.

Regardless of your age, there are always steps you can take to lower your risk of colon cancer.

## SCREENING TESTS

Of all the behaviors that can potentially reduce the risk of colon cancer, getting screened is the single most important one for women over age fifty. Screening tests for colon cancer offer twice the benefits of screening tests for other diseases. First, just as mammograms can detect early stages of breast cancer, tests for colon cancer can detect the disease in its earliest, most treatable stages. When colon cancer is found before it has spread to other parts of the body, it is more than 90 percent curable. When it is not found, however, chances of long-term survival drop dramatically—to about 9 percent.

The added benefit of colon cancer screening is that it can actually prevent cancer from developing. When a woman is screened for colon cancer, her health care provider is really looking for both colon cancer *and* adenomatous polyps. If these polyps are found, they can be removed immediately—before they even have the opportunity to become cancerous. In this way, screening tests for colon cancer lower not only a woman's risk of dying from the disease but also her risk of developing it.

There is substantial evidence to support the benefits of colon cancer screening among women over age fifty. Getting screened regularly can cut women's risk of fatal colon cancer by at least 33 percent. This is about the same level of protection that mammography offers against breast cancer. Yet very few women actually get screened for colon cancer, especially compared to the number who get screened for breast cancer. Research indicates that if as many American women were screened for colon cancer as are screened for breast cancer, the rate of colon cancer would be half what it is today.

## PHYSICAL ACTIVITY

Physical activity has been more consistently linked to a lower risk of colon cancer than any other behavior. There are at least two possible reasons for this. First, when a woman is physically active, waste moves through her colon more quickly, and this may reduce the exposure of the colon wall to any carcinogens

# Screening Tests for Colon Cancer

Although there is usually only one screening test available for any one disease (like mammography for breast cancer or Pap smears for cervical cancer), there are four to choose from for colon cancer: fecal occult blood tests, flexible sigmoidoscopy, barium enema, and colonoscopy. Each of these tests has been shown to be effective in detecting adenomatous polyps and early stage cancers in women over the age of fifty. However, there is still debate about which one is most effective.

## FECAL OCCULT BLOOD TESTS EVERY YEAR

Some polyps and cancers in the colon bleed, but in such small amounts that the blood cannot be seen by the naked eye. Fecal occult blood testing involves checking a sample of your stool for the presence of hidden (or occult) blood. If blood is found, you will need to have your colon examined directly via colonoscopy (see below). This will help confirm the source of the bleeding.

While it can be unpleasant to take a sample of your stool, doing this test every year is worth the effort: it can cut your risk of fatal colon cancer by 33 percent. It is the least invasive test for colon cancer screening and the only one you can do in the privacy of your home.

## FLEXIBLE SIGMOIDOSCOPY EVERY FIVE YEARS

The term *sigmoidoscopy* refers to a visual examination of the sigmoid colon (the lower third of the colon). Prior to the test, you will need to clear out your colon. There are various ways to do this, but most involve drinking only clear liquids and using a laxative or enema before the test.

For the test, you will need to go to a medical office or hospital. A long, thin, flexible tube will be inserted into your rectum and advanced into your colon. This tube has a tiny video camera and a light on the end that allows your health care provider to look for polyps and cancerous growths in your colon. If you have a polyp or a growth that looks cancerous, your health care provider might take a small tissue sample (biopsy) during the test or recommend that you have a more thorough exam, called a colonoscopy (see below).

Despite being invasive and possibly uncomfortable, flexible sigmoidoscopy is relatively painless and it can save your life: having this test once every five years cuts your risk of fatal colon cancer by 33 percent.

## BARIUM ENEMA EVERY TEN YEARS

This test involves having a series of X-rays to see if there are any abnormal growths in your colon. About twenty-four hours before the test, you will need to clear out your colon. Again, there are various ways to do this, but most involve drinking only clear liquids and using a laxative or enema before the test. When it's time for the test, you'll need to go to a hospital or medical office. A fluid called barium will be passed into your colon through a small tube in your rectum. X-rays are then taken, with the barium highlighting any growths in your colon. If a polyp or growth is seen on the X-rays, you will need to have your entire colon examined with a colonoscopy (see below).

Overall, this test can be uncomfortable and embarrassing, but it can save your life: having a barium enema cuts your risk of fatal colon cancer by 50 percent.

## COLONOSCOPY EVERY TEN YEARS

Having a colonoscopy is like having a flexible sigmoidoscopy, with some very important exceptions. First, the tube used in a colonoscopy is longer than in a sigmoidoscopy, which means that the health care provider can search the entire colon for polyps and cancers, not just the lower third. As a result, this test is probably more effective. Second, if any growths are found during colonoscopy, they can be removed on the spot (which is why this test often serves as a follow-up to other tests). Finally, you will be sedated during the colonoscopy, since it is more invasive than flexible sigmoidoscopy.

## SUMMARY OF SCREENING

By choosing any *one* of the four screening options discussed above, you can substantially reduce your risk of dying from—or possibly even developing—colon cancer. The variety of options gives you the opportunity to choose, along with your health care provider, which test is most appropriate for you. If you have a family history of colon or rectal cancer, a genetic syndrome, or a personal history of inflammatory bowel disease, talk to your health care provider about how often you need to have these tests.

in the waste. Second, being active may lower a woman's level of blood insulin, which in high amounts may stimulate abnormal cell growth in the colon.

In the Nurses' Health Study, we found that physical activity cut women's risk of colon cancer and adenomatous polyps in half. We also found that walking can be as effective in preventing colon cancer as vigorous activity. Walking at a normal to brisk pace (about three miles an hour) for one hour a day provides the same amount of protection against colon cancer as doing more strenuous activity, like jogging, cycling, or swimming, for half an hour a day (see Figure 9-5). If all women added half an hour of walking to their daily routine, more than 15 percent of all colon cancers could be prevented.

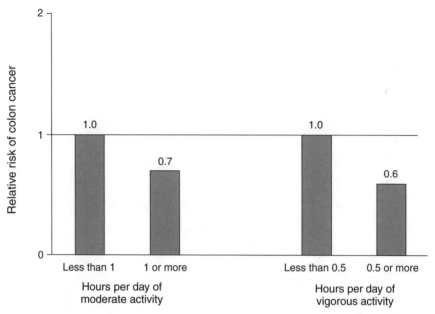

FIG. 9-5. Moderate physical activity for an hour a day provides approximately the same protection against colon cancer as vigorous activity for half an hour a day. (Source: Nurses' Health Study)

## RED MEAT

Most studies that have examined the link between red meat (including beef, pork, and lamb) and colon cancer have seen a strong relationship: eating red meat frequently can double the risk of colon cancer. However, each study has its own definition of "frequently," which can make it difficult to tell how much meat is too much. What we have found in the Nurses' Health Study is that women who eat red meat once a week are at slightly increased risk, while those who eat it once a day are at much greater risk (see Figure 9-6).

Researchers are not yet sure how red meat increases the risk of colon cancer. Some think it is because of the saturated fat found abundantly in red meat, but there is little evidence to confirm this. Researchers are now focusing on the possibility that red meat might generate cancer-causing chemicals (or carcinogens) when it is cooked at high temperatures. These carcinogens would come into direct contact with the colon wall when the meat is digested.

## MULTIVITAMINS CONTAINING FOLIC ACID

Many women have heard of folic acid because of the protection it offers against birth defects. In fact, all women of childbearing age are advised to take vitamins that contain at least 400 micrograms of folic acid. Now, data from two

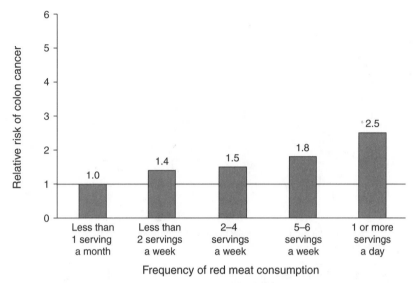

FIG. 9-6. The more meat women eat, the higher their risk of colon cancer. (Source: Nurses' Health Study)

studies suggest that vitamins with folic acid might also reduce the risk of colon cancer.

Folic acid is the synthetic form of the vitamin folate, which is found naturally in a variety of fruits and vegetables. Many studies have suggested that eating folate-rich vegetables might also reduce the risk of colon cancer. However, recent evidence suggests that women can lower their risk of colon cancer more by taking a daily multivitamin with folic acid than by eating a diet rich in folate. In one study, women who used daily multivitamins were 50 percent less likely to develop colon cancer than women who never used multivitamins. In the Nurses' Health Study, we found an even larger protective effect for long-term multivitamin use. Women who used multivitamins for at least fifteen years were 75 percent less likely to develop colon cancer than women who never took multivitamins (see Figure 9-7). Those whose diets were high in folate but who never took multivitamins did not have a substantial reduction in colon cancer risk.

Why would the folic acid in vitamins offer better protection against colon cancer than the folate found naturally in food? Folic acid in food is absorbed in the gut more readily than folate is, since folate has to be broken down before it can be absorbed. As a result, a woman would have to eat about 800 micrograms of natural folate to obtain the amount of folic acid (400 micrograms) found in a multivitamin. That translates into roughly eight servings of fruit or four to six cups of cooked vegetables a day. Few women consume that much

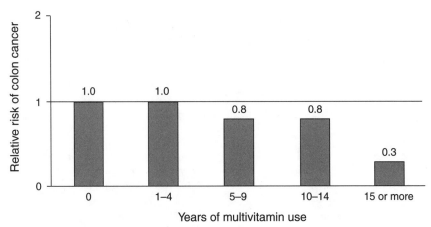

FIG. 9-7. The risk of colon cancer is greatly reduced among women who have taken multivitamins for fifteen or more years. (Source: Nurses' Health Study)

natural folate through their diet alone. Thus, while it is wise to continue eating foods that are naturally high in folate since they contain many other health-promoting nutrients, doing so is probably less effective than using multivitamins when it comes to reducing the risk of colon cancer.

## WEIGHT

Being overweight or obese has been linked consistently to an increased risk of colon cancer in women. In the Nurses' Health Study, we found that obese women were about 50 percent more likely to develop colon cancer than lean women (see Figure 9-8). Similar results were reported in the Iowa Women's Health Study, where researchers found an increased risk even among women who were only moderately overweight.

Obesity may also affect women's risk of adenomatous polyps. We observed a 50 percent increase in the risk of polyps among obese women and women whose waists measured at least 35 inches. The reason for this relationship is not yet clear, but it may have to do with the effect of weight on insulin. Obesity can lead to higher levels of insulin in the blood, which might in turn promote abnormal cell growth in the colon.

## SMOKING

Colon cancer can be added to the already long list of diseases related to smoking. Although not all studies are consistent, a growing body of evidence suggests that smoking can increase the risk of colon cancer, particularly if a woman starts smoking early in life and continues for more than twenty years.

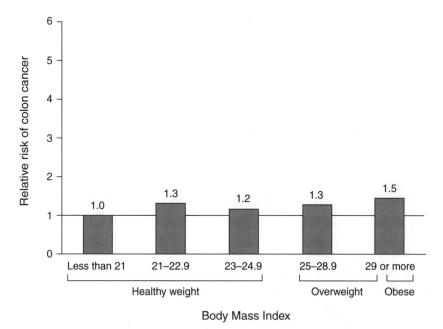

FIG. 9-8. Obesity increases the risk of colon cancer. See Appendix C for information on calculating body mass index. (Source: Nurses' Health Study)

In the Nurses' Health Study, we found that the risk of colon cancer did not increase until thirty-five years after a woman had started to smoke more than ten cigarettes a day. At that point, whether she had quit or not, she was twice as likely to develop the disease as a woman who had never smoked. We also found that smoking increased the risk of adenomatous polyps much faster than it did the risk of colon cancer. Within twenty years after a woman started smoking, her risk of polyps went up. The more cigarettes she smoked per day and the longer she smoked, the higher her risk.

These results suggest that tobacco actually initiates the development of colon cancer. It may cause cells to grow abnormally, which may then lead to small adenomatous polyps. These polyps may progress to larger polyps, and finally, after a period of several decades, to cancer. Thus, a substantial period of time may pass between the time a woman takes up smoking and the time that she develops the disease.

Unlike the relationship of smoking with other cancers, smoking's effects on the colon appear irreversible: women who quit smoking still have an increased risk of colon cancer decades later. Women who smoked early in life should thus take special effort to engage in behaviors known to reduce the risk of colon cancer, such as routine screening, physical activity, and multivitamin use. It is also important to prevent adolescents from starting to smoke.

## ALCOHOL USE

Only a handful of long-term studies have examined the relationship between moderate alcohol consumption and the risk of colon cancer. To date, results have been inconsistent. Several studies have shown that alcohol does not alter colon cancer risk, while others have demonstrated a modest increase in risk. Overall, the epidemiologic evidence suggests that alcohol probably does increase the risk of colon cancer. This may be because alcohol has an effect on folate levels, which in turn may influence the risk of colon cancer.

## ASPIRIN

An increasing amount of evidence suggests that aspirin may lower the risk of colon cancer. Although the reason for this is not yet known, it may be that aspirin blocks the production of certain chemicals that then indirectly inhibit the growth of tumors.

Early studies on aspirin and colon cancer generally found no relationship, probably because they assessed only short-term aspirin use (five years or less). More recent studies suggest that it may take at least ten years of regular aspirin use before women receive any protection against colon cancer. In one study, researchers found a very large reduction in risk among people who took aspirin regularly for at least ten years, but no benefit among those who took it for less time. In the Nurses' Health Study, we found that the longer women took aspirin, the less likely they were to develop colon cancer. Women who took at least two adult tablets (325 milligrams) a week for twenty years received the greatest protection.

Although aspirin may reduce the risk of colon cancer, it does have other effects on women's health that need to be considered (see Chapter 24). For example, it may protect against heart disease but increase the risk of hemorrhagic stroke and intestinal bleeding. These competing risk and benefits make it necessary for women to consult with their health care providers before beginning a program of long-term aspirin use.

## POSTMENOPAUSAL HORMONES

During menopause, there is a drastic drop in the amount of estrogen being produced by the ovaries. This decline in estrogen production can cause a variety of menopausal symptoms, including hot flashes, vaginal dryness, and insomnia. To alleviate these symptoms and to lower the risk of osteoporosis, many women supplement their natural supply of estrogen by taking post-menopausal hormones (see Chapter 22). There is now evidence that this practice may also lower the risk of colon cancer. Although the reason for this is not yet clear, it has been suggested that exogenous estrogens (such as those from postmenopausal estrogen pills) can slow the production of bile acids and lower the level of the growth hormone IGF-I. Both IGF-I and bile acids are known to stimulate cancerous growth in the colon.

We examined the relationship between postmenopausal hormones and colon cancer by combining the results of eighteen epidemiologic studies on the topic. We found that while women are on postmenopausal hormones, they are about 35 percent less likely to develop colon cancer than women who have never taken postmenopausal hormones. However, once women stop taking the therapy, the protection they received diminishes and eventually disappears altogether.

Of course, there is more to consider than colon cancer risk when deciding whether or not to use postmenopausal hormones. In addition to offering short-term protection against colon cancer, postmenopausal hormones reduce the risk of osteoporosis. However, they may also raise the risk of breast cancer. Ultimately, a woman and her health care provider must assess her risk of these various diseases before deciding what approach is best for her.

## Birth Control Pills

Many studies have shown that birth control pills reduce the risk of colon cancer, but the results have typically not been strong enough to suggest a definitive relationship. This may be because most studies evaluated the effects of short-term pill use. As with aspirin and multivitamins, the pill may need to be used for an extended period of time before its use affects a woman's risk of colon cancer. In the Nurses' Health Study, we found that women had to take the pill for at least eight years before receiving any substantial protection against colon cancer.

As with postmenopausal hormones, birth control pills can have a variety of effects on a woman's health. For example, taking the pill reduces the risk of endometrial and ovarian cancer, in addition to protecting against unwanted pregnancies. However, it may also increase the risk of breast cancer and deep vein clots in the legs. These competing risks and benefits make it necessary for women to consult with their health care providers before going on the pill.

## Vegetables and Fiber

Although smaller studies have long suggested that eating vegetables and fiber might lower the risk of colon cancer, larger studies have not confirmed this. In fact, they are suggesting there is probably no link at all. In two randomized controlled trials, researchers found that the risk of polyps (precursors to colon cancer) was the same among those who ate a fiber-rich diet and those who did not. A number of large cohort studies, including the Nurses' Health Study, have shown similar results.

Although a vegetable- and fiber-rich diet does not appear to protect women against colon cancer, it is still recommended for its many other benefits, including protection against coronary heart disease.

## CALCIUM

Although results have not been entirely consistent, several studies have shown that calcium might offer protection against colon cancer. In the Iowa Women's Health Study, researchers found a direct relationship between calcium and the risk of colon cancer: the more calcium women consumed per day, the less likely they were to develop the disease. Notably, this was true only for women who did not have a family history of colon cancer.

This relationship has also been studied in at least one randomized controlled trial. In that trial, all of the participants already had an adenomatous polyp, and researchers were studying which group would be less likely to develop a second polyp: those on a daily dose of calcium or those on a placebo. They found that the group on calcium was 25 percent less likely to develop a polyp than the group on placebo.

## VITAMIN D

Although results to date are mixed on the topic, there is some evidence that a high intake of vitamin D can lower the risk of colon cancer. In the Nurses' Health Study, we found that women who had the highest intake of vitamin D (over 550 IU) from food and supplements had a 60 percent lower risk of the disease compared to women with the lowest intake. It is not exactly clear how vitamin D might lower the risk of colon cancer, but some studies show that it can inhibit the rapid growth of cells in the colon.

## WHAT IT ALL MEANS

Colon cancer is a common, fatal disease that can be detected early and even prevented by routine screening. In addition, scientists have identified a large number of behaviors that are related to the risk of colon cancer and are easily modifiable (see the table below). The most important ones that you can adopt to lower your risk of colon cancer, without raising your risk of other complica-

## Colon Cancer: Weighing the Risks

You can substantially lower your risk of colon cancer by:

- Getting regular screening tests after the age of fifty (or earlier if you have a family history or personal history related to the disease)
- Walking for one hour a day
- Taking a daily multivitamin
- Maintaining a healthy weight
- Eating a diet that is low in red meat
- Not smoking
- Limiting alcohol intake

Your risk of colon cancer may also be increased by factors beyond your control, including:

- A family history of colorectal cancer or adenomatous polyps
- A personal history of inflammatory bowel disease
- A genetic syndrome

tions or diseases, include getting screened regularly, engaging in regular physical activity, taking a daily multivitamin, and maintaining a healthy weight.

## WHAT I TELL MY PATIENTS ABOUT LOWERING THEIR RISK OF COLON CANCER

DR. CAROL BATES

When it comes to preventing colon cancer, there is a lot of good news to share with my patients. This is a type of cancer that usually develops slowly, which means that there is time to take steps to prevent it or at least to catch it before it becomes serious. We also know more about how to prevent colon cancer than we do about preventing many other types of cancer. And some of the factors that cause colon cancer are things that we can control—physical activity, diet, and vitamins.

The bad news is that few of my patients want to talk about colon cancer. Women seem less aware of its risks than the risks of breast, ovarian, and cervical cancer. There seems to be some squeamishness about the disease or the methods used to detect it. That is a shame, because colon cancer is the third

## Established, Probable, and Possible Factors Associated with the Risk of Colon Cancer

| RISK FACTOR | APPROXIMATE RISK* |
|---|---|
| *Established* | |
| Age (greater than 60 vs. less than 50) | ↑↑↑↑ |
| Genetic syndrome (FAP or HNPCC) | ↑↑↑↑ |
| Parent or sibling diagnosed with colon cancer or rectal cancer | ↑↑↑ |
| Parent or sibling diagnosed with adenomatous polyps | ↑↑↑ |
| Personal history of inflammatory bowel disease | ↑↑↑ |
| Red meat (1 serving a week vs. none) | ↑↑ |
| Colon cancer screening | ↓↓ |
| Physical activity (1 hour of walking a day vs. none) | ↓↓ |
| *Probable* | |
| Greater weight (obese vs. lean) | ↑↑ |
| Alcohol intake (4 drinks a week vs. none) | ↑↑ |
| Multivitamins use (15 years of use vs. none) | ↓↓↓ |
| Aspirin (20 years of use vs. never used) | ↓↓ |
| Postmenopausal hormones (current use vs. never used) | ↓↓ |
| Birth control pills (more than 8 years of use vs. never used) | ↓↓ |
| *Possible* | |
| High vegetable intake | ↓↓ |
| High calcium intake | ↓↓ |
| High vitamin D intake | ↓↓ |

| | |
|---|---|
| *↑ Small increase in risk | ↓ Small decrease in risk |
| ↑↑ Moderate increase in risk | ↓↓ Moderate decrease in risk |
| ↑↑↑ Large increase in risk | ↓↓↓ Large decrease in risk |
| ↑↑↑↑ Very large increase in risk | ↓↓↓↓ Very large decrease in risk |

leading cause of cancer death among women in the United States. It doesn't have to be that way. Here are some ways to reduce your risk of colon cancer.

## Undergo Regular Screenings

If you are over fifty, this is the single most important step you can take to reduce your chances of developing colon cancer. Regular screening for women over fifty reduces the risk of colon cancer by 33 percent. Not only does screening detect colon cancer in its earliest stages, when it is most readily treated, it can also actually prevent the disease by removing abnormal growths, known as polyps, before they have a chance to develop into cancer.

If you feel embarrassed at the thought of undergoing these tests, you are not alone. Many women are. One way to get over that is to think about the benefits of screening. Another is to recognize that your physician and the other health care providers are experienced at these procedures and perform them frequently.

Some of these tests are uncomfortable. Many of my patients dislike the preparation for the examinations, which require dietary restrictions and the use of laxatives or enemas to empty the colon. Preparation is important so that any abnormalities can be seen more clearly. It is hard to prepare for these tests, but it is worth it.

As has been discussed on page 176, there are four different screening methods available. Some should be used every year, others only periodically. For patients of average risk, I recommend flexible sigmoidoscopy every five years plus fecal occult blood tests every year. For patients with a family history of colon cancer or adenomatous polyps, I recommend colonoscopy before age fifty. For those reluctant to undergo any procedure, I recommend fecal occult blood testing and continue to discuss the other options annually.

## Increase Your Physical Activity

If you are like most of my patients, you find it hard to become more physically active. You may be busy with work and family, have a sedentary job, or live in an area where you have to drive to most of your destinations. Even so, there are ways to build physical activity into your daily life. And if you do so, you may reduce your risk of developing colon cancer by as much as 50 percent. Even moderate physical activity, such as taking a brisk one-hour-long walk, can be as protective as more strenuous activity. So what can you do? Here are a few tips that have worked for my patients:

- Find an activity that you enjoy. It is much easier to continue a pattern of exercise if you enjoy what you are doing.
- Take a walk at lunch time with a friend. Walk as fast as you can while continuing normal conversation.
- Exercise with your children. Bicycling, soccer, and skating are only some of the options. You will also help your children develop healthy habits; after all, you are an important role model.

- Take a class in tai chi, yoga, or dance, which involve a lot of stretching (and mild sweating). These may be available in community centers.
- Plant a garden and maintain it in the spring and summer. Mow your lawn and shovel your driveway instead of hiring someone else to do it.
- If you find it hard to be active for half an hour or an hour at a time, aim for ten-minute chunks of time, which can be just as effective. Park the car at the farthest end of the parking lot and walk to the mall. Use the stairs instead of the elevator at work. Do housework in ten- or fifteen-minute segments every day.

## Eat Less Red Meat

Eating red meat (which includes beef, pork, and lamb) even once a week increases your risk of colon cancer. The best way to eat less red meat per week is to find substitutes: chicken, fish, and vegetables. If you have to eat at a fast food restaurant, order a salad or chicken meal. Better yet, pack your own lunch at work, and bring yogurt or a vegetarian pocket sandwich instead of using lunch meat.

## Take a Daily Multivitamin with Folic Acid

Even if you are already eating plenty of fruits and vegetables, take a multivitamin that contains folic acid. Multivitamins are available in almost every grocery store and pharmacy, with many effective and inexpensive varieties available. Don't take megavitamins; aim for those that provide 100 percent of your daily needs.

## Maintain a Healthy Weight

If you gain too much weight as you grow older, you will increase your risk not only of colon cancer but also of other serious conditions. To maintain a healthy weight, increase your activity and decrease the amount of calories you consume every day. You can do this by reducing your fat intake and substituting foods like fruits and vegetables for high calorie snacks. The better your diet and exercise regimen, the easier it will be to control your weight. Although maintaining a healthy weight is not always easy, remember that you are not alone: talk to your health care provider for support and suggestions.

# CHAPTER TEN

# Lowering the Risk
# of Osteoporosis

## BACKGROUND

Osteoporosis is a disease that most women dread as they grow older. Characterized by brittle bones, this condition causes more than 1.5 million fractures a year. Although vertebral fractures (or fractures of the spine) are the most common outcome, hip fractures are the most severe. They cause not only a loss of physical functioning but also pain, anxiety, fear, and depression. Only about a third of women who have hip fractures regain the ability to function as they did prior to the fracture, and about a third are placed in nursing homes. In addition, hip fractures can lead to life-threatening complications. About 20 percent of women who have a hip fracture die of complications within a year after the fracture.

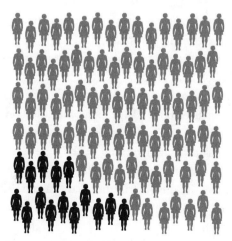

FIG. 10-1. In a group of 100 women who are fifty years old, 15 will suffer a hip fracture before they reach the age of eighty. (Source: Grady et al.)

The good news is that you can dramatically lower your risk of osteoporosis through the same healthy lifestyle that also protects you from cardiovascular disease and cancer: be physically active, eat a healthy diet, and avoid smoking. Taken collectively, these behaviors can help you maintain strong bones and a healthy body throughout your lifetime.

## Bone and Osteoporosis

Bone is a living tissue made up of three layers. At its core is bone marrow, a spongy substance that produces blood cells. Encasing the marrow is a dense, rigid layer called compact bone, which supports the weight of the body. It is made up mostly of calcium, phosphorus, and other minerals and has thousands of tiny holes and passageways. Nerves and blood vessels run through these passages, supplying the bone tissue with oxygen and nutrients. The outer layer of bone is a tough membrane called the periosteum. Packed with nerves and blood vessels, this membrane supplies the compact bone with osteoblasts, the cells that build the bone.

Bone serves two vital functions. First, it supports the weight of the body. Ounce for ounce, bone bears as much weight as reinforced concrete. Second, it acts as a storage site for calcium and phosphorus. Bone holds about 99 percent of the body's calcium, with the remaining 1 percent free to circulate in the blood. There the calcium aids in a variety of crucial bodily functions, including muscle contraction, nerve function, and blood clotting. When the level of calcium in the blood drops, the bones release a new supply. In this way, bone helps to maintain the balance of minerals in the blood and ensure that the body has enough calcium to function properly.

Throughout a woman's life, her bone is continuously broken down and replaced with new bone. This process, called remodeling, is necessary for the growth and maintenance of healthy bones. Cells called osteoclasts are responsible for the breakdown of bone. They chew into the bone tissue, releasing small amounts of calcium and other minerals into the blood. Cells called osteoblasts then rebuild the bone by filling in the holes created by osteoclasts. They do this by creating a meshwork of collagen and other proteins and then embedding themselves in the matrix they have created. Bone formation is complete when calcium, phosphorus, and other minerals from the blood are deposited into the matrix.

Although bone is continuously broken down and rebuilt during all phases of a woman's life, the two processes occur at different rates. During childhood, bone is built up much more rapidly than it is broken down, enabling the bones to become longer, denser, and heavier. Bone mass continues to increase throughout young adulthood until a woman reaches her mid-twenties. At that time, bone destruction and bone formation start to occur at about the same pace. Bone mass is neither gained nor lost. When a woman reaches her mid-thirties, however, she starts to lose bone mass, because bone is being torn down more rapidly than it is built. Between her thirties and fifties, the average woman will lose about 0.5 percent of her bone mass each year. With the arrival of menopause, and the subsequent drop in estrogen levels, the rate of bone loss accelerates. Women lose between 1 and 5 percent of their bone mass each year during the first few years of menopause. Bone loss continues at a slower rate throughout menopause, resulting in bones that are lighter, less dense, and lower in mineral content.

Osteoporosis occurs when the bones in the body lose so much mass and become so brittle that they are prone to fracture. This condition is often caused by an acceleration of the normal changes that occur with age. For example, a woman with osteoporosis may have lost bone mass more rapidly during menopause than most women, or she may not have accumulated enough bone mass during childhood to withstand the normal loss that occurs during adulthood. This suggests that there are two ways to prevent or delay the development of osteoporosis: first, promote the accumulation of bone mass during childhood and adolescence; and second, slow the rate of bone loss during adulthood.

## LESSONS FROM THE NURSES' HEALTH STUDY AND OTHER STUDIES

If you asked a group of women what you can do to lower your risk of osteoporosis, you would most likely be told to get more calcium. While this is a good means of maintaining bone mass, it is not the only way (or even the best way) to protect your bones. Scientists have identified a number of factors that are related to the risk of osteoporosis and the subsequent risk of fractures. Most of these probably influence your risk by altering the amount of bone mass that you gain or lose at different points in your life. However, most fractures are not caused solely by low bone mass.

Most fractures are precipitated by a fall, and there are many factors that can increase your likelihood of falling, including impaired vision, poor mobility, and low physical strength. In addition, your risk of fracture may depend on the ability of your bones to absorb the impact of a fall. For example, one woman's hipbones may fit together in such a way that they are less likely to fracture upon impact, while another's may not. Many factors that affect your risk of osteoporosis, such as age, physical activity, and weight, are thought to influence not only your bone mass but also your propensity to fall and your bones' ability to absorb impact.

## Factors You Cannot Control

As with many other diseases, age, family history, and race/ethnicity have an important influence on your risk of osteoporosis. Despite the fact that you cannot control these factors, you should know how they might affect your risk so that you can be even more careful about the factors you can control, such as your physical activity and diet.

### AGE

Because women naturally lose bone mass as they grow older, they become increasingly vulnerable to the effects of osteoporosis. Compounding this problem is the fact that older women are also more likely to fall and subsequently fracture a bone. In a large study of postmenopausal women, researchers found that the risk of hip fracture rose steadily with age. For every five-year increase in age after sixty-five, there was a 40 percent increase in the risk of hip fracture.

### FAMILY HISTORY

Because families tend to have similar bone structure and may share a propensity for falling, it has been suggested that hip fractures might run in families. Data from several studies support this notion, including a large-scale study conducted among postmenopausal women. In that study, having a mother who suffered a hip fracture doubled a woman's risk of suffering one herself. How old the mother was at the time of the fracture appeared to determine the extent of the daughter's risk (see Figure 10-2).

### RACE AND ETHNICITY

There are significant racial and ethnic differences in the rates of osteoporosis in women. Most notably, the rate of hip fracture is about twice as high in white women as it is in African American women. The reason for this disparity is unclear, but may have to do with differences in bone mass. Throughout their lifetimes, white women tend to have less bone mass than African American women.

Not all of the racial and ethnic differences are due to differences in bone mass, however. Compared to white women, Japanese women accumulate less bone mass during childhood and early adulthood, but still have lower rates of hip fracture. The reason for this is not yet fully understood, but may be due to

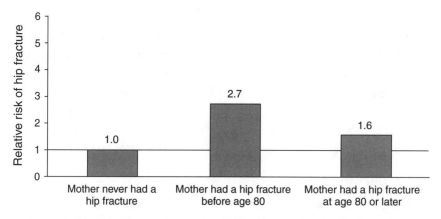

FIG. 10-2. The risk of hip fracture is increased in women whose mothers have had a hip fracture. It is particularly high if the mother had the fracture before age eighty. (Source: Cummings et al.)

differences in height, bone geometry, and participation in activities that lead to falls. Other ethnic groups have also been compared in terms of bone mass, but not fracture rates. For example, Mexican American women tend to have greater bone mass than white women, while Native American women have less.

## LIFETIME PRODUCTION OF ESTROGEN

The more estrogen that a woman produces during her lifetime, the less likely she is to develop osteoporosis. Several things determine a woman's lifetime production of estrogen, including her age at menarche, history of irregular menstrual periods, age at menopause, and weight.

*Menarche.* The onset of menstruation (menarche) marks the beginning of a woman's potential childbearing years. During these years (from menarche to menopause), the body produces substantial amounts of estrogen. Because estrogen prevents bone loss, it may be better, in terms of osteoporosis, to reach menarche earlier rather than later. Those who reach menarche early may produce more estrogen in their lifetimes and thus have greater bone mass than those who reach menarche late.

*Irregular Menstrual Cycles.* At some point in their reproductive lives, most women will experience irregular menstrual cycles. They will either skip periods occasionally or have them come earlier or later than normal. In general, these types of cycles are harmless. However, if a woman has abnormal cycles repeatedly, it can be an indication of low estrogen levels. If such low levels are sustained over time, it can lead to a loss in bone mass.

*Menopause.* Most women go through menopause between the ages of forty-five and fifty-five. During this time, the body's production of estrogen drops dramatically, to less than one-third of what it was during the childbearing years. The later a woman goes through menopause, the more estrogen she produces in her lifetime. This suggests that women with a later age at menopause may have greater bone mass than women with an early age at menopause.

*Weight.* Body weight also influences the amount of estrogen produced by the body and is discussed in greater detail below as a factor you can control.

## Factors You Can Control

Although your risk of osteoporosis is determined in part by your age and family history, your lifestyle also plays an important role. Key behaviors that can lower your risk—while also improving your overall health—include being active, eating a healthy diet, and not smoking.

### PHYSICAL ACTIVITY

Physical activity is a well-established means of protecting against osteoporosis. When a woman is physically active, it places mechanical stress on her bones, forcing the tissue to absorb calcium and become stronger. In this way, physical activity directly promotes the building up of bone. However, it also strengthens the bone tissue indirectly by stimulating the muscles that surround bone tissue. As these muscles become larger and stronger, they place increasing pressure on the bone. This pressure stimulates the bone tissue to absorb calcium and grow stronger. Remember, however, that the only bones protected by physical activity are those that are stressed during the activity. For example, walking will place stress on the bones of the spine and hips, but it will have no impact on the wrist.

Numerous studies have shown that being active early in life can have a long-term effect in preventing osteoporosis. This is because activity during childhood promotes the accumulation of bone mass—and the more bone that is accrued early in life, the lower the chance of osteoporosis later. In one study, bone mass was higher among women who had participated in youth sports than among women who had not. While this evidence is reassuring for women who exercised as children, it need not be frightening for those who did not: being active in adulthood can also prevent osteoporosis by slowing the rate of bone loss.

While most studies have shown that weight training and vigorous activity (like running) are the most effective activities for preventing osteoporosis and

subsequent fractures, recent data suggest that walking might be just as beneficial. In a large study conducted among women over age sixty-five, researchers
found a 30 percent reduction in the risk of hip fracture among those who
walked for exercise compared to those who did not (see Figure 10-3). The farther women walked, the lower their risk. Several small, randomized controlled
trials have supported these results, showing greater bone mass among women
who walked than among women who were sedentary.

Women who are active may have a lower risk of fractures not only because
of greater bone mass, but also because they are less likely to fall. Numerous

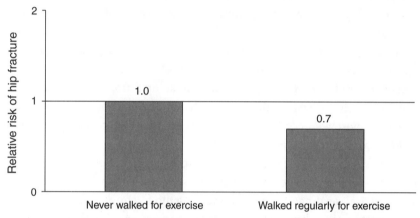

FIG. 10-3. The risk of hip fracture is moderately reduced among women who regularly walk for exercise. (Source: Cummings et al.)

randomized controlled trials have confirmed this, including a two-year study
that involved women age eighty and older. In that study, half of the women participated in a home exercise program that included walking, strength training,
and balance training, while the other half were given no specific instructions
about activity. Researchers found that the risk of falling was about 30 percent
lower among those participating in the two-year exercise program. This reduction in risk was probably due to improvements in muscle mass, muscle
strength, and overall balance.

Although physical activity has a beneficial effect on bone for most women,
engaging in too much strenuous activity can lead to dangerously low levels of
estrogen and subsequent bone loss. One indication of low estrogen levels is
the absence of menstrual periods among women who have not yet reached
menopause.

## POSTMENOPAUSAL HORMONES

One of the greatest long-term benefits of postmenopausal hormone use is that estrogen can prevent, and even partially reverse, postmenopausal bone loss. It does this by inhibiting the cells that break down bone and stimulating the cells that make new bone. For this reason, estrogen has been acknowledged by the Federal Drug Administration to help prevent and treat osteoporosis.

Women who take postmenopausal hormones tend to *gain* bone mass in the early years of menopause, when most women are losing bone at a rate of 1 to 5 percent per year. In one randomized controlled trial, postmenopausal women took estrogen and progestin daily for ten years and had a 6 percent increase in bone mass.

Estrogen's beneficial effects on the bone appear to translate into a reduced risk of hip fracture, the most serious effect of osteoporosis. Nearly a dozen epidemiologic studies have shown that women taking estrogen are about 25 percent less likely to have a hip fracture than women who have never taken estrogen. Those who begin taking estrogen early in menopause and continue to do so for at least seven to ten years may attain even greater protection. Though few studies have examined the effect of both estrogen and progestin on the risk of hip fracture, those that have suggest that the combined therapy is as effective as estrogen alone in preventing hip fracture.

Unfortunately, when a woman stops taking postmenopausal hormones, she begins to lose bone mass quickly, as if she were in the early years of menopause. The protection she gained from the hormones eventually disappears, and her risk of hip fracture returns to that of a woman who never took hormones.

While the protection offered by postmenopausal hormones is substantial in terms of osteoporosis, it must still be weighed against the other benefits and risks of hormones. Ultimately, a woman and her health care provider must balance her risk of various diseases before deciding whether hormones are right for her.

## SMOKING

Although all women lose bone mass after menopause, smokers appear to lose more than nonsmokers. In a large analysis combining the results of nearly thirty studies, researchers found that, by age eighty, smokers had lost 6 percent more of their bone mass than nonsmokers. Although the reason for this is uncertain, smoking does lower the level of estrogen in the body, and this can have a detrimental effect on bone. In addition, smoking may reduce bone's ability to absorb calcium.

The bone-weakening effects of smoking appear to translate into an increased risk of hip fracture. In the Nurses' Health Study, we found a 20 percent increase in risk among women who smoked compared to those who did not. The more cigarettes a woman smoked, the more likely she was to suffer a hip fracture (see Figure 10-4). We also found that smoking has long-lasting effects on bone. After women stopped smoking, it took at least ten years before their risk dropped to that of women who had never smoked.

Similar results were reported in a large analysis that combined the results of twenty studies. In that analysis, researchers also found that smoking had more of an impact on the risk of hip fracture among older women than among middle-aged women. This is of particular concern since older women are already at increased risk because of their age.

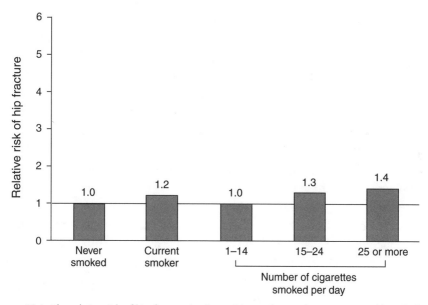

FIG. 10-4. The relative risk of hip fracture is elevated in smokers and increases steadily with the number of cigarettes smoked per day. (Source: Nurses' Health Study)

## CALCIUM

An essential building block of bone, calcium has long been touted as the perfect agent for preventing osteoporosis. This mineral not only helps build bone mass early in life but also helps slow the rate of bone loss during adulthood. Despite these positive effects, however, calcium may not be as beneficial as researchers once thought. While it does lead to stronger bones, there is no solid evidence that calcium-rich diets or calcium supplements offer long-term protection against the most serious consequence of osteoporosis: bone fractures.

Numerous observational studies have examined the long-term effects of dietary calcium (that is, calcium from foods) on fracture risk. To date, nearly all of these have shown that dietary calcium has no effect on the risk of fractures. In the Nurses' Health Study, women who drank two glasses of milk a day were just as likely as those who drank one glass a week to suffer a fracture of the hip or wrist. We found similar results when we looked at other foods rich in calcium.

What about calcium from supplements? A number of randomized controlled trials have shown that calcium supplements improve bone mass. However, most of these trials have not looked directly at fracture risk because randomized controlled trials do not generally last long enough to study such long-term effects. A nine-year trial to address the issue is currently underway in the Women's Health Initiative. In that trial, researchers assigned women to take either a daily placebo or a daily supplement containing both calcium and vitamin D. At the end of the trial, researchers will determine which group has lower fracture rates: those on the placebo or those on the supplements. Two smaller trials have shown lower rates of fracture among women on supplements compared to women on placebo, but both of these studies were short in duration.

What should a woman make of all of this? First, there is no doubt that calcium is very important for building strong bones during childhood and adolescence. Teenage girls should strive to get 1,300 milligrams of calcium a day, as recommended by the National Academy of Sciences. Second, even though a high calcium intake is not yet proven to provide additional protection against fractures, adult women are currently still advised to get sufficient amounts of this mineral either through their diets or through supplement use. The National Academy of Sciences recommends 1,000 milligrams a day for women ages nineteen to fifty and 1,200 milligrams a day for those over age fifty.

## Vitamin D

Vitamin D helps bone absorb calcium and also plays an important role in maintaining bone mass. Because of this, researchers have speculated that increasing the intake of vitamin D might lower the risk of osteoporosis. But does the evidence bear this out? To date, studies have had mixed results. The most positive findings come from studies described above that combine vitamin D with calcium.

Taken collectively, the current evidence does suggest that women can benefit from increasing their intake of vitamin D. They can do this by taking supplements (400 IU per day), eating fortified foods (like breakfast cereals, dairy products, and eggs), and spending time outdoors. When women are exposed to ultraviolet radiation from the sun for as little as fifteen minutes a day, their skin produces vitamin D from a cholesterol that is found naturally in the body.

## Vitamin K

Found mainly in green leafy vegetables, vitamin K plays an important role in maintaining healthy bones. First, it is essential for the production of osteocalcin, one of the main proteins used to build bone. Second, it inhibits the production of substances known to promote the breakdown of bone. Finally, vitamin K helps regulate the amount of calcium that is excreted in the urine. If too much calcium is excreted and the body does not have enough to perform its normal functions, it will leach calcium away from the bones. Vitamin K helps prevent this by maintaining adequate levels of calcium in the blood.

Several studies have shown that low levels of vitamin K lead to low bone mass. In the Nurses' Health Study, we found that such low levels of vitamin K might also lead to hip fractures. Women who got at least 100 micrograms of vitamin K a day were 30 percent less likely to break a hip than those who got less of this vitamin. Notably, vitamin K is easy to obtain through daily diet, with kale and other greens being the best sources: a half a cup of kale contains about 715 micrograms. Spinach, broccoli, and lettuce are also excellent sources. There are 215 micrograms of vitamin K in a cup of raw spinach, 150 micrograms in half a cup of broccoli, and 70 micrograms in a cup of lettuce.

## Caffeine

Caffeine can indirectly promote bone loss by increasing the amount of calcium that is excreted in the urine. Several studies have suggested lower bone mass among women who consume large amounts of caffeine, such as four or more cups of coffee per day, compared to those who consume little. We saw a similar relationship in the Nurses' Health Study: the more caffeine a woman consumed, the more likely she was to fracture a hip. Coffee appeared to be the main culprit, probably because it contains more caffeine than tea or cola drinks and is consumed much more frequently. These data suggest that women who consume caffeinated beverages should do so in moderation.

## PROTEIN

Eating a diet rich in protein may have detrimental effects on bone. When proteins are digested, acids are released into the bloodstream. To neutralize these acids, the body must leach calcium from the bones. This can lead to bone loss and an increased risk of fracture.

In the Nurses' Health Study, we found that the more animal protein a woman consumed, the more likely she was to suffer a wrist fracture. Those who ate at least five servings of red meat a week were 20 percent more likely to have a wrist fracture than those who ate less than one serving a week. The protein in red meat and other animal products may be worse than the protein in vegetables, because it raises acid levels more and causes more calcium to be leached from the bones. We did not find a similar relationship for protein and hip fractures.

## FLUORIDE

Fluoride has long been used as a treatment for osteoporosis because it can stimulate bone formation. However, it remains uncertain whether this mineral also helps lower the risk of osteoporosis. When bone is being rebuilt and fluoride is available in the body, it takes the place of calcium in the bones. While this may help improve overall bone mass, it also makes the bones more brittle, and this can lead to fractures.

Numerous studies have examined whether low levels of fluoride (such as those found in fluoridated tap water) might influence the risk of fracture. Although results have been inconsistent, overall they suggest that fluoridated water does not offer much risk or benefit to women's bone health. In an analysis that combined the results of nearly twenty studies on the topic, researchers found no link between low levels of fluoride and the risk of fractures.

In the Nurses' Health Study, we measured the level of fluoride in women's toenails to determine their long-term dietary intake of this mineral. We found a suggestion of a lower risk of hip fracture among those with high levels of fluoride versus those with low levels. Overall, however, the data are too inconsistent for fluoride use to be considered a means of preventing fracture.

## OTHER MINERALS

In addition to calcium and fluoride, there are a variety of other minerals that may influence bone health. For example, phosphorus and magnesium account for about half of the mineral content in bone, while potassium helps regulate calcium absorption. What is not yet clear is whether, at high intakes, these minerals can help improve bone mass and reduce the risk of osteoporosis. For phosphorus, this is not likely: most women already get so much of this mineral in their diets that they do not need additional amounts. Increasing magnesium and potassium, on the other hand, may be more beneficial. A handful of studies have suggested that a diet rich in these minerals can promote the accumulation of bone mass in early adulthood.

## CERTAIN MEDICATIONS

Certain medications can affect a woman's risk of osteoporosis and subsequent fractures. Some, such as thiazide diuretics, offer protection against osteoporosis, while others, such as corticosteroids and thyroid pills, increase the risk of osteoporosis.

*Thiazide Diuretics.* Commonly used to treat high blood pressure, thiazide diuretics help reduce the amount of calcium that is excreted in the urine. They may also inhibit the breakdown of bone. Several studies have shown greater bone mass among women who take thiazide diuretics, and a growing body of evidence suggests that these medications also offer protection against fractures. In the Nurses' Health Study, we found a 20 percent reduction in the risk of wrist fracture among women taking thiazide diuretics. When we looked at the risk of hip fracture, we found that the diuretics lowered risk only among women who had already gone through menopause. Among these women, thiazide diuretics reduced the risk of hip fractures by about 30 percent. Similar results have been reported in other studies.

*Corticosteroids.* These drugs are commonly taken for the treatment of such chronic conditions as asthma, arthritis, and psoriasis. However, numerous studies have shown that these drugs have a serious side effect: they promote the loss of bone by inhibiting calcium absorption and interfering with bone formation. This translates into a large increase in the risk of fractures, particularly among women who take doses exceeding 5 milligrams for more than two months.

*Thyroid Pills.* These drugs are prescribed when the thyroid gland does not produce enough of the hormone thyroxin. When a woman does not have enough of this hormone, it slows her body's metabolism, and when she has too much, it accelerates the turnover of bone and causes bone loss. Excess thyroid hormone can result from an overactive thyroid gland (such as Graves' disease) or from taking high dose thyroid pills for extended periods of time.

## ALCOHOL

Drinking in moderation carries a variety of risks and benefits for women. Relative to nondrinkers, women who drink up to two drinks a day are less likely to develop heart disease and ischemic stroke. However, they are also at increased risk of breast cancer and possibly colon cancer and hemorrhagic stroke. Added to this risk-benefit equation are the seemingly contradictory effects of alcohol on osteoporosis: moderate alcohol consumption helps build bone mass, but it also increases the risk of hip fracture.

In the Nurses' Health Study, we found that women who drank about one alcoholic beverage a day had greater bone mass in the spine than women who did not drink at all. This may be due to the fact that alcohol increases estrogen levels, and estrogen prevents bone loss.

Although alcohol might protect bone, it is probably more detrimental to overall bone health than it is beneficial. Drinking alcohol, even in moderate amounts, can make a person less steady and can increase the likelihood that they will fall and injure themselves. In the Nurses' Health Study, we found that women who consumed about one drink a day were twice as likely to fracture their hips as women who did not drink at all. Similar results have been reported in several other studies, including the Framingham Study.

## WEIGHT

Being overweight can help protect women from the bone-weakening effects of osteoporosis and from the subsequent risk of hip fracture. There are several reasons for this. First, women who are overweight after menopause have higher levels of estrogen than women who are lean, and estrogen helps keep bone from losing calcium. Second, overweight women have extra padding around their hips that can help cushion a fall. Finally, the more weight that women carry, the more stress it places on their bones. This stress, which is similar to that created by weight-bearing exercise, can lead to stronger bones.

In the Nurses Health Study, we found that obese women have a lower risk of hip fracture than lean women—a result confirmed by numerous other studies. But should women gain weight to protect themselves from osteoporosis and hip fractures? Given the many adverse health consequences associated with obesity and weight gain, definitely not. A healthier and more positive approach would be to increase one's level of physical activity or wear protective garments that provide padding around the hips.

## WHAT IT ALL MEANS

Osteoporosis is a common, debilitating disease, with hip fracture being the most severe consequence. Although scientists have long focused on dietary means of preventing this disease, the best way to prevent it is actually through the same combination of behaviors that will help protect you from other chronic diseases: engage in regular physical activity, eat a diet rich in vitamins and minerals, and avoid smoking. Postmenopausal hormones and certain medications also play a role in osteoporosis and should be discussed with your health care provider.

## Screening and Early Detection of Osteoporosis

Getting screened for osteoporosis means having a health care provider pass an imaging device over your bones. This device, which works like an X-ray machine, measures your bone mass and compares it to that of a healthy woman of the same age and size. Although routine screening is not necessary for all women, it may be important if you have a personal or family history of bone fractures or if you are age sixty-five or older. You may also want to have your bone mass measured if you are considering postmenopausal hormones. These hormones slow postmenopausal bone loss, but also increase the risk of several serious diseases. By having your bone mass measured, you can better decide whether you need to incur the risks of postmenopausal hormones.

## WHAT I TELL MY PATIENTS ABOUT LOWERING THEIR RISK OF OSTEOPOROSIS

DR. NANCY RIGOTTI

My patients often think about only one thing, calcium, when they ask me about how to avoid osteoporosis. Getting enough calcium is certainly important, but it is only one element of what should be a broader strategy for avoiding this disease and the debilitating bone fractures it causes. A woman should also think about exercise, other vitamins and minerals, tobacco use, and medications such as postmenopausal hormones.

Exercise is a critical element in any plan to preserve bone mass, and one that is often overlooked. Regular physical activity helps the bones absorb calcium, which makes them stronger. Exercise also strengthens the muscles that attach to the bones. Stronger muscles provide better support to the skeleton,

## Established, Probable, and Possible Factors Associated with the Risk of Hip Fractures

| Risk factor | Approximate risk* |
|---|---|
| *Established* | |
| Age (greater than 60 vs. less than 50) | ↑↑↑ |
| Ethnicity (white vs. African American) | ↑↑↑ |
| Mother had a hip fracture | ↑↑ |
| Regular physical activity (walking or other weight-bearing activity vs. no activity) | ↓↓ |
| Postmenopausal hormones (current use vs. never use) | ↓↓ |
| Use of thiazide diuretics | ↓↓ |
| Greater weight (overweight vs. lean) | ↓↓ |
| *Probable* | |
| Smoking (25 cigarettes a day vs. none) | ↑↑ |
| Alcohol (one drink a day vs. none)** | ↑↑ |
| Caffeine (4 or more cups of coffee a day vs. none) | ↑↑ |
| Vitamin D (400 IU a day) plus calcium (500 milligrams a day) vs. neither | ↓↓ |
| Vitamin K (100 micrograms a day vs. less than 100 micrograms a day) | ↓↓ |

| | |
|---|---|
| *↑ Small increase in risk | ↓ Small decrease in risk |
| ↑↑ Moderate increase in risk | ↓↓ Moderate decrease in risk |
| ↑↑↑ Large increase in risk | ↓↓↓ Large decrease in risk |
| ↑↑↑↑ Very large increase in risk | ↓↓↓↓ Very large decrease in risk |

** Consuming this amount of alcohol will improve bone mass, but since it increases the likelihood of falling, it also increases the risk of hip fracture.

and the muscle tension acting on bone stimulates bone to become denser. In childhood, exercise helps to build bone mass; in adulthood, it helps to slow bone loss. So it's never too late to start exercising even if you have lived a sedentary life. The best strategy is to start slowly and to do both resistance exercises, which build muscle by pushing against a weight or some other resistance, and weight-bearing aerobic exercises such as walking, which increase cardiovascular endurance and strengthen muscles. You don't have to go to a gym to benefit; even walking regularly can reduce your risk of hip fracture later on. See Chapter 15 for tips on how to build an exercise routine.

Many women do not realize that cigarette smoking harms bones in addition to causing cancer, heart disease, and lung disease. Smoking accelerates bone loss and significantly increases the risk of hip fracture (by about 20 percent). These effects last about ten years after a woman stops smoking. Obviously, it's best never to smoke, but if you have already started, quitting as soon as possible will still help protect your bones. (See Chapter 17 for tips on how to quit smoking.)

Medications can also affect bone strength. Taking estrogen therapy after menopause clearly reduces bone loss and can prevent fractures. Deciding whether to take postmenopausal hormones is a complex decision, and your bones are not the only consideration. This is an important issue for you to discuss thoroughly with your health care provider. He or she can help you to weigh the risks and benefits of your decision. Other medications, such as corticosteroids, can increase your risk of developing osteoporosis. If you take them regularly, you need to take special precautions to avoid osteoporosis. Be sure to talk this over with your health care provider, too.

Diet is the final, and in some ways the most complicated, component of a strategy to reduce osteoporosis risk. Certainly getting enough calcium is important, but it's also essential to eat a variety of foods that will provide a full range of vitamins and minerals so that your body can best benefit from that calcium. Here's what I recommend my patients pay attention to:

- **Calcium.** Teenagers should get 1,300 milligrams a day; women should get 1,000 milligrams a day before menopause and 1,200 milligrams a day after menopause. Very few women eat enough dairy products to reach this level of calcium intake from their diets. It's especially hard for postmenopausal women to reach their higher calcium goal. You can work with your health care provider or a dietitian to estimate the amount of calcium you are getting in your daily diet. If you're not getting enough, take supplements to make up the difference.
- **Vitamin D.** You need vitamin D in order to absorb the calcium you eat. It's pretty easy to do this. Having cereal with a glass of milk for breakfast every day will help, because milk is fortified with vitamin D. Or take vitamin D in a supplement form. The easiest way to do this is to take a daily multivitamin, which supplies 400 IU a day.

- **Eat green leafy vegetables.** Lettuce and spinach are just two examples of green leafy vegetables, which have plenty of vitamin K and may help to maintain bone mass. You can also obtain vitamin K from some cruciferous vegetables, such as broccoli.
- **Drink caffeine and alcohol in moderation.** Caffeine causes bones to lose calcium; alcohol can increase a woman's unsteadiness and may lead to falls. Obviously, these risks have to be weighed against the benefits of both types of drink. (Who hasn't needed a cup of coffee or two to get started in the morning? And drinking alcohol in moderation can reduce your risk of heart disease.) The best strategy is to try to limit caffeine and alcohol as much as possible.

# CHAPTER ELEVEN

# Lowering the Risk of Endometrial Cancer

## BACKGROUND

Although endometrial cancer is the most common reproductive cancer in American women, it does not need to be: you can lower your risk of this disease by maintaining a healthy weight throughout adulthood and making wise decisions about birth control pills and postmenopausal hormones. The other good news about endometrial cancer is that it produces noticeable symptoms (e.g., irregular bleeding) in its early stages. As a result, it can usually be found while it is still treatable. About 75 percent of women with this disease are diagnosed before the cancer spreads beyond the uterus, and most can be cured with treatment.

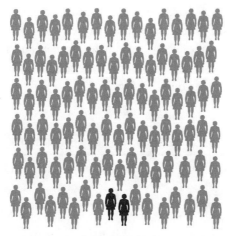

FIG. 11-1. In a group of 100 women who are fifty years old, 2 will develop endometrial cancer before they reach the age of eighty. (Source: National Cancer Institute)

## The Endometrium and Endometrial Cancer

The endometrium is the membrane that lines the inside of the uterus (or womb). During each menstrual cycle, the endometrium undergoes a series of changes, stimulated primarily by two hormones, estrogen and progesterone. At the beginning of the menstrual cycle (when a woman is having her period), the surface cells of the endometrium are shed, leaving only a thin layer of endometrial cells in the uterus. A few days later, after menstrual flow has ceased, the ovaries increase their production of estrogen. This stimulates the cells in the endometrium to divide and grow, and the endometrium gradually becomes thicker. About halfway through the cycle, in a process called ovulation, the ovaries release a mature egg for fertilization. Following this, the ovaries produce substantial amounts of both estrogen and progesterone. This stimulates the endometrium to mature in preparation for a fertilized egg. During maturation, the lining itself stops growing. Small blood vessels form and the cells begin to store nutrients that are needed to support a pregnancy. These changes are primarily an effect of progesterone; without it, the endometrium would just keep growing under the influence of estrogen. At the end of the menstrual cycle, if fertilization does not occur, estrogen and progesterone levels drop again. The endometrium deteriorates, separates from the wall of the uterus, and is shed as menstrual blood. If fertilization does occur, progesterone levels remain elevated so that the endometrium can support the pregnancy.

Endometrial cancer occurs when cells in the endometrium divide and grow uncontrollably. Although this may happen for a number of reasons, it is thought to be caused primarily by an imbalance between estrogen and progesterone, or more specifically, by too much estrogen and not enough progesterone. The excess estrogen may stimulate cell growth in the endometrium, just as it does during the menstrual cycle.

## Endometrial Cancer: The Larger Picture

- Endometrial cancer is the most common gynecologic cancer in American women.
- About 75 percent of cases are diagnosed before the cancer has spread beyond the uterus, making it highly curable.
- The symptoms of endometrial cancer include irregular vaginal bleeding, unusual spotting, and bleeding after menopause.

Although endometrial cancers can spread beyond the uterus, they are usually found before they do because the symptoms of the disease are so prominent. They include irregular vaginal bleeding, unusual spotting, and bleeding after menopause.

## LESSONS FROM THE NURSES' HEALTH STUDY AND OTHER STUDIES

Most of the factors linked to endometrial cancer probably influence risk by altering your body's production of estrogen and progesterone. Among the most important factors are ones that you can control: your weight and your use of hormones.

*In the Nurses' Own Words . . .*

There have been so many changes in my life in the past twenty or so years. The loss and gain of family members and friends, change in my place of employment, and now retirement. But through it all, my lifestyle has not changed greatly. I think the greatest benefit I've received from the study is that at each stage I've had to stop and review some aspect of my life, and I've seen what I've been doing right and where my weaknesses lay. Then I've been left with the choice of going on as I had been or improving my lifestyle. Some choices have been wise: diet, making time for my interests. Some not so wise: I am still not physically active and am paying for it with low stamina and high cholesterol despite a low fat diet. That's human nature, I guess. I feel very privileged to have been part of this study. I'm sure many will benefit from it.

—From DM

### Factors You Cannot Control

Being older or having a family history of endometrial cancer may raise your risk of this disease. Although you cannot change these things, you can be more vigilant about your weight and other factors within your control.

### AGE

Although endometrial cancer does occur in younger women, more than 95 percent of cases are diagnosed in those over age forty. The rate of endometrial cancer increases dramatically between the ages of forty and seventy and then declines around age eighty (see Figure 11-2).

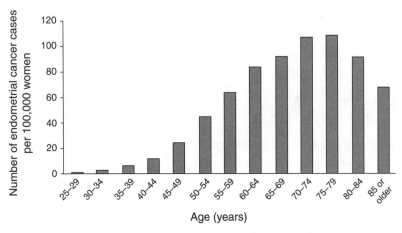

FIG. 11-2. Rates of endometrial cancer increase dramatically after age forty and continue to rise steadily until age eighty, when rates begin to decline. (Source: National Cancer Institute)

## FAMILY HISTORY

Only a handful of studies have evaluated the relationship between family history and endometrial cancer. Most have found varying degrees of increased risk among women with a family history of the disease. However, in the large Iowa Women's Health Study, researchers found no such link. Taken collectively, these studies suggest that if there is an association between endometrial cancer and family history, it is probably modest. An exception is in the case of rare genetic syndromes, which can substantially increase the risk of this disease.

## Factors You Can Control

Your risk of endometrial cancer is influenced by several factors within your control, including your weight and use of birth control pills and postmenopausal hormones. By understanding how each of these factors affects your risk, you can take appropriate steps to protect yourself from this disease.

## WEIGHT AND WEIGHT GAIN

Over the past thirty years, a large number of epidemiologic studies have examined the effect of weight on endometrial cancer. These have been remarkably consistent in demonstrating what we have also found in the Nurses' Health Study: overweight women have a substantially increased risk of endometrial cancer, as do women who gain excess weight during adulthood. This is because overweight women tend to have higher levels of estrogen and lower levels of progesterone than lean women.

Just how much of an impact does a woman's weight have on her risk of endometrial cancer? The answer appears to depend on whether or not she has gone through menopause. In the Nurses' Health Study, we found a direct relationship between weight and endometrial cancer in both premenopausal and postmenopausal women: the more a woman weighed, the higher her risk was. However, the risk was elevated to a much greater degree among postmenopausal women. This same relationship held true when we looked at the amount of weight that women had gained since age eighteen. A weight gain of more than forty pounds doubled the risk of endometrial cancer among premenopausal women but quadrupled it among postmenopausal women (see Figure 11-3). The reason for this difference is that fat tissue becomes the primary source of estrogen after menopause. The more weight a woman carries after menopause, the more estrogen her body produces.

## BIRTH CONTROL PILLS

Birth control pills can substantially lower the risk of endometrial cancer. More than a dozen epidemiologic studies have confirmed this relationship, with some of the most conclusive results to date coming from a large study conducted by

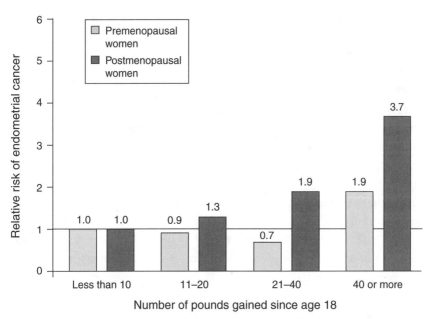

FIG. 11-3. Women who gain substantial amounts of weight during adulthood have an increased risk of endometrial cancer. Risk is particularly elevated among postmenopausal women who have gained more than forty pounds. (Source: Nurses' Health Study)

the U.S. Centers for Disease Control. In that study, women who used the pill for one year received moderate protection, while those who used it for at least two years received substantial protection (see Figure 11-4). After women stopped taking the pill, they remained at reduced risk of endometrial cancer for at least another fifteen years. When we examined this relationship in the Nurses' Health Study, we found similar results.

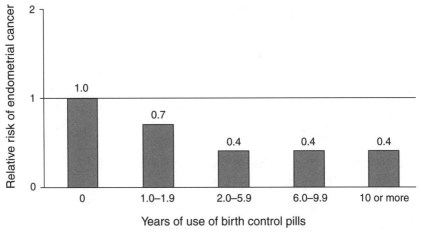

FIG. 11-4. The risk of endometrial cancer is largely reduced among women who take birth control pills for at least two years. (Source: Centers for Disease Control and Prevention)

Researchers are not yet sure why this long-term protective effect exists, but suspect that the short-term benefits are due to the fact that pills contain both estrogen and progestin (a synthetic form of the hormone progesterone). In the absence of progesterone or progestin, estrogen stimulates the growth of endometrial cells. Since birth control pills contain both hormones, they may reduce the amount of time that a woman's endometrium is exposed to estrogen alone.

While the protection offered by the pill in terms of endometrial cancer is substantial, it must still be weighed against the other risks and benefits of birth control pills. Assessing these risks and benefits and how they impact a woman's lifestyle is an important factor in determining her approach to contraception.

## POSTMENOPAUSAL HORMONES

To alleviate the symptoms of menopause—and to lower the risk of osteoporosis and possibly cardiovascular disease—many women supplement their natural supply of estrogen by taking postmenopausal hormones. These hormones have changed considerably over the past thirty years, mainly because of their potential effect on the risk of endometrial cancer.

Prior to the 1970s, women taking postmenopausal hormones took daily doses of estrogen without progesterone. By the mid-seventies, however, it became clear that in the absence of progesterone, estrogen stimulated cell growth in the endometrium and raised the risk of endometrial cancer. In an analysis that combined more than twenty studies on the topic, researchers found that taking estrogen alone doubled women's risk of endometrial cancer. The longer women took estrogen without progesterone, the greater their risk was.

Consequently, in the late 1970s, researchers developed hormone regimens that were designed to preserve the beneficial effects of estrogen while reducing the risk of endometrial cancer. On these regimens, women take both estrogen and progesterone (either natural or synthetic). They may take estrogen alone for part of each month and then take estrogen and progesterone together for the rest of the month (called cyclic therapy), or they may take both estrogen and low dose progesterone every day (called continuous therapy). Both of these regimens appear to substantially reduce the increased risk associated with estrogen alone. This is because the progesterone counterbalances the estrogen, inhibiting the growth of endometrial cells. This combination of hormones is now recommended for all women who have an intact uterus and choose to take postmenopausal hormones.

As with birth control pills, there is more to consider than endometrial cancer risk when deciding whether to use postmenopausal hormones. Ultimately, a woman and her health care provider must balance her risk of various diseases before deciding what approach is best for her.

## SMOKING

More than a dozen studies have found that smoking is associated with a lower risk of endometrial cancer. This is primarily because smokers are leaner and have lower estrogen levels. However, smoking is *not* recommended for the prevention of endometrial cancer or for any other reason. Smoking is the single most important cause of premature death among women.

## DIABETES

Several studies have shown that women with diabetes have an increased risk of endometrial cancer. However, it is not yet clear whether these women are at increased risk because of their diabetes or because of their weight. Women who have diabetes tend to be overweight, and being overweight can substantially increase the risk of endometrial cancer.

## High Blood Pressure (Hypertension)

Having high blood pressure, or hypertension, may also increase a woman's risk of endometrial cancer. However, like diabetes, hypertension is related to weight, and weight is related to endometrial cancer risk. This makes it unclear whether women with hypertension are at increased risk because of their blood pressure or because of their weight.

## Dietary Fat

High fat diets appear to have little effect, if any, on the risk of developing endometrial cancer. Although some smaller studies have shown that eating high amounts of fat might increase risk, most larger studies have found no link. However, the amount of fat consumed might not be as important as the type of fat consumed. For example, in the Nurses' Health Study, total fat did not appear to influence the risk of endometrial cancer, but saturated fat did increase risk. The more saturated fat postmenopausal women had in their diets, the more likely they were to develop the disease. These fats, which come largely from animal products, are thought to alter the body's natural production of hormones. Although not yet established, similar findings have been reported in several smaller studies.

## Fruits and Vegetables

Several small studies have shown that fruits and vegetables protect against endometrial cancer. However, this relationship is not well established. Only one large cohort study has examined it, and that study found no link. However, fruits and vegetables should still be an important part of the diet. Eating at least five servings of these foods a day can lower the risk of cardiovascular disease, other forms of cancer, and a variety of other diseases.

## Fiber

Found only in plant foods, fiber provides the bulk necessary to move waste through the large intestine and out of the body. It is thought to reduce women's risk of endometrial cancer by affecting the way estrogen is absorbed in the intestines. However, as in the case of fruits and vegetables, fiber has been linked to a reduced risk of endometrial cancer only in smaller studies. A few large cohort studies, including the Nurses' Health Study, have examined the relationship but to date have not found a link.

## Reproductive Factors

Your risk of endometrial cancer is largely influenced by the amount of estrogen your body produces during your lifetime. Estrogen plays an essential role not only during pregnancy but throughout your reproductive life. Among other things, it influences when you begin menstruating, how long your menstrual cycle lasts, and when you reach menopause. As a result, many of the events in your reproductive life affect your risk of endometrial cancer. While the timing of some of these events (like childbearing) is within your control to some extent, it is also largely influenced by your age and social circumstances. For most women making reproductive choices, concerns about endometrial cancer will likely be overshadowed by a number of other important considerations.

### AGE AT FIRST MENSTRUAL PERIOD (MENARCHE)

The onset of menstruation marks the beginning of a woman's potential childbearing years. During these years (from menarche to menopause), the body produces substantial amounts of estrogen. Because estrogen can cause excessive cell growth in the endometrium, it may be better, in terms of endometrial cancer risk, to reach menarche later in adolescence rather than earlier. Those who reach menarche late may produce less estrogen in their lifetimes and thus have a lower risk of endometrial cancer.

In the Iowa Women's Health Study, researchers found a substantial reduction in risk among women who began menstruating at age fifteen compared to those who began at age ten. Although similar findings have been observed in almost every study that has examined the relationship, some doubt still remains. The age at which a girl begins menstruating may be related to other factors that also influence her risk of endometrial cancer. For example, girls who are overweight have higher estrogen levels and thus tend to begin menstruating earlier than girls who are lean. Girls who are overweight may also carry their weight into adulthood, which increases their risk of endometrial cancer. Thus, it is not clear whether a girl reaching menarche late is at low risk because of her delayed menarche or because she is lean.

## Endometriosis

Although endometriosis originates in the same tissue as endometrial cancer, the two conditions are not related. Endometriosis occurs when tissue from the endometrium grows outside of its normal place in the uterus. For example, it may be found on the ovaries, fallopian tubes, or tissues surrounding the uterus, bladder, and rectum. This displaced tissue can cause infertility, as well as a variety of other symptoms, including severe menstrual discomfort, abdominal pain, pain during sexual intercourse, backache, rectal discomfort during bowel movements, diarrhea, and constipation. Birth control pills are often prescribed to relieve pain, but other treatments depend on the severity of the disease. Mild endometriosis typically requires no treatment, while more advanced cases may require surgery.

### IRREGULAR MENSTRUAL CYCLES: AMENORRHEA OR OLIGOMENORRHEA

At some point in their lives, most women will experience an irregular menstrual cycle. They will skip a period occasionally or have it come earlier or later than normal. In general, these types of cycles are harmless. However, there are two patterns of irregular cycles that may be of concern when it comes to endometrial cancer: amenorrhea and oligomenorrhea.

*Amenorrhea.* This condition is characterized by the absence of menstrual periods for six or more months, and it may indicate that a woman is not ovulating. While her body may continue to produce relatively high levels of estrogen, as it does at the beginning of a normal cycle, the estrogen is not balanced by high levels of progesterone. At least one study has indicated that this may lead to a substantially increased risk of endometrial cancer.

*Oligomenorrhea.* In women with oligomenorrhea, the interval between menstrual periods is longer than usual and can be different from one cycle to the next. For example, a woman may have an excessively long cycle, followed by a normal cycle, followed by a slightly prolonged cycle. When women have abnormally long and irregular menstrual cycles, their estrogen levels remain elevated for extended periods of time. As with amenorrhea, this may lead to an increased risk of endometrial cancer.

### NUMBER OF CHILDREN

There is abundant evidence to suggest that having a child reduces the risk of endometrial cancer. In fact, the more children a woman has, the lower her risk

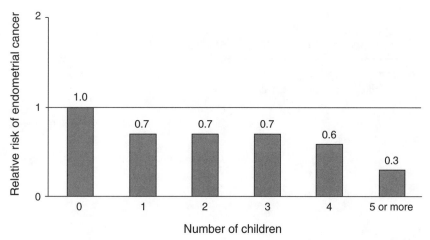

FIG. 11-5. Having children lowers a woman's risk of endometrial cancer. (Source: Nurses' Health Study)

is. In the Nurses' Health Study, we found a moderate reduction in risk among women who had one child and a large reduction in risk among those who had more than four children (see Figure 11-5).

The reason for this relationship is not yet known, but researchers are focusing on at least two possibilities. First, cells in the endometrium may divide much more slowly during pregnancy, thus reducing the chance for abnormal cell growth. Second, the many hormonal changes that occur in the body during pregnancy may offer some protection against endometrial cancer. For example, although estrogen levels are higher than normal during pregnancy, they are balanced by equally high levels of progesterone.

## AGE AT MENOPAUSE

Most women go through menopause between the ages of forty-five and fifty-five. During this time, the body's production of estrogen drops dramatically, to less than a third what it was during the childbearing years. The earlier a woman goes through menopause, the shorter her potential childbearing years are. Because of this, the total amount of estrogen that she produces during her lifetime is reduced. This suggests that those with an earlier age at menopause may have a lower risk of endometrial cancer.

A number of studies have shown a reduced risk of endometrial cancer among women who go through menopause in their forties versus those who do so in their fifties. In the Nurses' Health Study, women who reached natural menopause between the ages of forty-five and forty-nine had a moderate reduction in risk compared to those who did so between the ages of fifty and fifty-

## Endometrial Cancer: Weighing the Risks

- Being overweight greatly increases the risk of endometrial cancer. Gaining weight during adulthood also increases risk.
- Taking postmenopausal estrogen without progestin greatly increases the risk of endometrial cancer. Taking estrogen with progestin, however, has very little effect on risk.
- Taking birth control pills for at least two years offers women long-term protection against endometrial cancer.
- Having children lowers the risk of endometrial cancer.

two. Women who went through menopause before the age of forty-five had the largest reduction in risk.

## WHAT IT ALL MEANS

Endometrial cancer is the most common reproductive cancer in American women. Fortunately, though, it can be detected early through close attention to symptoms and cured through treatment. In addition, you can lower your risk of this disease by focusing on two important factors: your weight and your use of hormones. While there are other factors that also influence your risk of endometrial cancer—like having children—they are probably dictated by other concerns and priorities in your life. By maintaining a healthy weight and talking to your health care provider about whether birth control pills and postmenopausal hormones are right for you, you can lower your risk of endometrial cancer while also improving your overall health.

## WHAT I TELL MY PATIENTS ABOUT LOWERING THEIR RISK OF ENDOMETRIAL CANCER

DR. CELESTE ROBB-NICHOLSON

Even though endometrial cancer is the most common reproductive cancer in American women, most of my patients do not know much about it or express concern over it. That is not unreasonable since it is usually detected early and cured through treatment. However, it is important to report unusual patterns of vaginal bleeding to your health care provider, especially if you are past menopause.

## Established, Probable, and Possible Factors Associated with the Risk of Endometrial Cancer

| RISK FACTOR | APPROXIMATE RISK* |
|---|---|
| *Established* | |
| Age (greater than 60 vs. less than 50) | ↑↑↑ |
| Greater weight (obese vs. lean) | ↑↑↑ |
| Weight gain after age 18 (more than 40 pounds vs. less than 10 pounds) | ↑↑↑ |
| Postmenopausal use of estrogen *without* progesterone (ever vs. never) | ↑↑↑ |
| Birth control pills (more than two years of use vs. never) | ↓↓↓ |
| Number of children (one vs. none) | ↓↓ |
| *Probable* | |
| Age at first menstrual period (greater than 14 vs. less than 11) | ↓↓ |
| Smoking (current vs. never) | ↓↓ |
| Age at menopause (less than 45 vs. greater than 50) | ↓↓ |
| *Possible* | |
| Personal history of diabetes | ↑↑↑ |
| Personal history of absent or irregular menstrual cycles | ↑↑↑ |
| Personal history of hypertension | ↑↑ |
| Immediate family member with endometrial cancer | ↑ |
| High saturated fat intake | ↑ |
| High fruit and vegetable consumption | ↓↓ |
| High fiber intake | ↓ |

| | |
|---|---|
| *↑ Small increase in risk | ↓ Small decrease in risk |
| ↑↑ Moderate increase in risk | ↓↓ Moderate decrease in risk |
| ↑↑↑ Large increase in risk | ↓↓↓ Large decrease in risk |
| ↑↑↑↑ Very large increase in risk | ↓↓↓↓ Very large decrease in risk |

Endometrial cancer develops when your uterus is exposed to too much estrogen and not enough progesterone. A number of factors increase your risk of this disease. Although you cannot change some of these factors, you can alter others. Here are my recommendations for lowering your risk of endometrial cancer:

1. If you have reached menopause, have not had a hysterectomy, and are considering taking postmenopausal hormones, make sure your prescription contains both estrogen and progesterone.

2. If you have gained weight since you were eighteen (particularly if you have gained forty pounds or more, are diabetic, have hypertension, or are postmenopausal), try to lose weight by exercising more and eating a sensible diet. Weight gain significantly increases your risk of endometrial cancer as well as heart disease and certain other cancers. Eat a diet low in fat and high in fruits, vegetables, and fiber. Try to do at least thirty minutes of moderate exercise a day (a vigorous walk, a bicycle ride, gardening), even if you have to build up slowly or do it in ten-minute increments.

3. If you are still of childbearing age, you can also talk with your health care provider about whether you should take birth control pills. You don't have to take them forever; a large study by the U.S. Centers for Disease Control found that taking the pills for at least two years provides significant protection. The benefit remains for as many as fifteen years after you stop taking the pills.

You should also be alert to the early warning signs of endometrial cancer: irregular vaginal bleeding, unusual spotting between periods, and bleeding after menopause. Contact your health care provider if you notice any of these symptoms.

# CHAPTER TWELVE

# Lowering the Risk of Ovarian Cancer

## BACKGROUND

Ovarian cancer is often referred to as a silent killer: it rarely produces symptoms before progressing to an untreatable stage, and even then, the symptoms are difficult to distinguish from those of other conditions. Each year, about 25,000 American women are diagnosed with this disease. Nearly three-quarters of them have late-stage cancer at the time of their diagnosis, and only about half survive beyond five years.

Clearly, we still have a lot to learn about this disease. Scientists continue to focus not only on improving treatments and finding screening tests, but also on identifying factors that might lower women's risk.

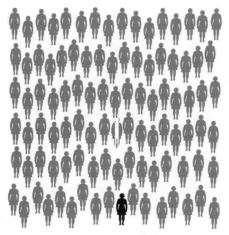

FIG. 12-1. In a group of 100 women who are fifty years old, 1 will develop ovarian cancer before she reaches the age of eighty. (Source: National Cancer Institute)

## The Ovaries and Ovarian Cancer

Located on either side of the uterus (see Figure 12-2), the ovaries serve two vital functions throughout the reproductive years. They produce estrogen and progesterone (the hormones that regulate the menstrual cycle), and they release mature eggs for fertilization.

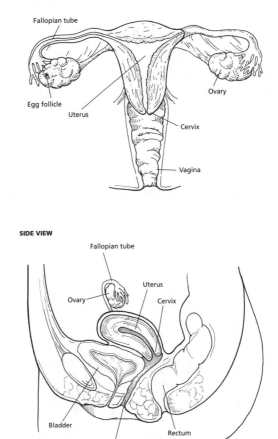

**FRONT VIEW**

Fallopian tube

Egg follicle

Uterus

Ovary

Cervix

Vagina

**SIDE VIEW**

Fallopian tube

Ovary

Uterus

Cervix

Bladder

Rectum

Vagina

FIG. 12-2. Internal Female Reproductive System. The female reproductive system consists of two ovaries (where eggs are stored), two fallopian tubes, the uterus, cervix, vagina, and outer genitals. Each month during menstruation, an egg is released from the ovaries. If fertilized by a sperm cell, the egg begins its journey to the uterus for implantation.

At a girl's birth, her ovaries contain a lifetime supply of eggs—over 1 million per ovary. Each egg is enclosed in a small pocket of cells (called a follicle) that sits in the ovary. During the menstrual cycle, a hormonal signal is sent to one of the ovaries, stimulating the egg follicles to expand and secrete estrogen. In a process called ovulation, one of the follicles eventually enlarges to the point that the ovary wall is ruptured, and a mature egg is released. The egg is then swept into the fallopian tube, where it may or may not be fertilized. More often than not, fertilization does not occur, and the egg is excreted as part of the normal menstrual flow. If fertilization does occur, the egg may implant itself in the uterus.

Ovarian cancer develops when the cells in the ovary divide and grow at an abnormal rate. About 90 percent of ovarian cancers arise from the cells that cover the ovary surface (or epithelium), while about 10 percent start in the egg follicles or the tissue that holds the ovary together. Cancerous tumors in the ovary tend to metastasize (or spread) only within the pelvis or abdomen. In rare cases, the cancer will metastasize to other parts of the body via the lymphatic system, ultimately causing more widespread illness.

There are often no symptoms of ovarian cancer until the tumor has spread to other organs. Even then, the symptoms—persistent nausea or vomiting, frequent urination, constipation, abdominal bloating, and a sense of fullness—can be easily confused with those caused by less serious problems. Consequently, most women with ovarian cancer are not diagnosed until their disease has progressed to a stage that is difficult to treat.

## LESSONS FROM THE NURSES' HEALTH STUDY AND OTHER STUDIES

Most of the factors linked to ovarian cancer probably influence risk by altering certain hormone levels or suppressing ovulation. Women who have intermittent breaks from ovulation (such as those afforded by pregnancy, birth control pills, and breast-feeding) are thought to be at lower risk of ovarian cancer than

## Ovarian Cancer: The Larger Picture

- Ovarian cancer often goes undetected until it has reached an advanced stage that is difficult to treat.
- Symptoms of ovarian cancer can be easily confused with those caused by less serious problems. They include persistent nausea, vomiting, frequent urination, constipation, abdominal swelling, and a sense of fullness.

women who ovulate continually throughout their reproductive years. This is because the ovary wall is ruptured each time ovulation occurs, and the cells must divide rapidly to repair it. This repeated trauma to the surface of the ovaries—coupled with the rate of cellular division necessary for repair—may contribute to the development of ovarian tumors.

### Factors You Cannot Control

Your risk of ovarian cancer is influenced by factors that are beyond your control, such as your family history. If you have a family history of either breast cancer or ovarian cancer, you should talk to your health care provider about it. You may wish to discuss screening or consider being more vigilant about things you can control, like your contraceptive choices.

### AGE

Age is a well-established factor linked to ovarian cancer. In general, the older a woman is, the more likely she is to develop the disease. National data show that rates of ovarian cancer begin to increase dramatically after age fifty and are highest in women over sixty-five (see Figure 12-3). Only after age eighty does the risk stop increasing with age.

### FAMILY HISTORY AND GENETICS

A woman's risk of ovarian cancer is influenced by her family history of ovarian cancer, and to a lesser extent, by her family history of breast cancer. In the Iowa Women's Health Study, having a mother, sister, or daughter with ovarian can-

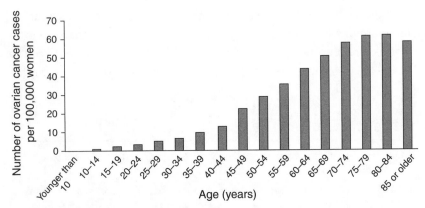

FIG. 12-3. Rates of ovarian cancer are low in women under age forty, begin to increase dramatically after fifty, and are highest in women over sixty-five. Only after age eighty do rates of ovarian cancer stop increasing. (Source: National Cancer Institute)

cer more than doubled a woman's risk of the disease (see Figure 12-4). Although this particular study did not observe a similar relationship between ovarian cancer and a family history of breast cancer, another large cohort study did. In the American Cancer Society's Cancer Prevention Study II, researchers found a moderate increase in the risk of fatal ovarian cancer among women whose mother or sister had breast cancer.

*Genetics.* In *rare* instances, families share an inherited genetic mutation and, as a result, experience an excess of breast cancer and ovarian cancer. This mutation occurs in the BRCA 1 gene and, less frequently, the BRCA 2 gene. These genes have received much attention in the media for their role in breast cancer, but they also appear to influence the risk of ovarian cancer. Studies have found that women with the BRCA 1 mutation have about a 50 percent chance of developing ovarian cancer in their lifetimes, and women with BRCA 2 about a 15 percent chance.

Because of the very high risk of cancer associated with BRCA 1, women with a strong family history of breast cancer or ovarian cancer (that is to say, with multiple immediate family members with the disease) may want to consider genetic testing to determine whether or not they have the mutation.

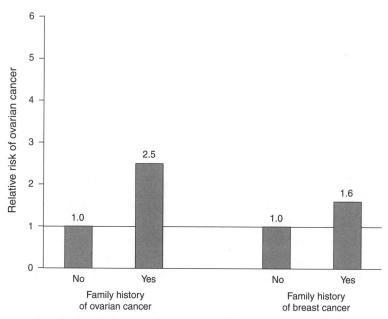

FIG. 12-4. The risk of ovarian cancer is substantially increased in women with a family history of ovarian cancer and moderately increased in those with a family history of breast cancer. (Source: Mink and Poole)

## Ovarian Cysts

Having an ovarian cyst does not increase the risk of ovarian cancer. Even though they can be quite painful, ovarian cysts are usually harmless. Some may push on surrounding organs, twist the ovary, or rupture suddenly, causing severe nausea, bleeding, pain, and fever. These cysts are sometimes removed because of the intolerable symptoms. However, most cysts cause no symptoms and are found during routine pelvic examinations. They are usually monitored by ultrasound and tend to shrink or disappear without treatment.

BRCA 1 mutations seem to be particularly prevalent among certain Jewish women (those of Ashkenazi descent), making it especially important for them to know their family history and seek genetic testing when appropriate. Many hospitals and medical centers now have on-staff genetics counselors who can talk through the risks and benefits of being tested for the BRCA 1 mutation. Women found to have a gene mutation have certain options that may help lower their risk of getting ovarian cancer, or at least increase their chances of identifying the disease early when it is most treatable.

### Factors You Can Control

Some factors that influence the risk of ovarian cancer are within your control. Among the most important are two forms of contraception, birth control pills and tubal ligation, both of which can lower your risk of this disease.

### BIRTH CONTROL PILLS

Birth control pills are thought to influence the risk of ovarian cancer in one or more ways. First, the pill suppresses ovulation, and the number of times a woman experiences ovulation in her lifetime may affect her risk of ovarian cancer. In addition, the pill lowers the level of hormones that may stimulate cell growth in the ovaries.

We examined the relationship between birth control pills and ovarian cancer by combining the results of more than twenty epidemiologic studies on the topic. We found that birth control pills substantially lower the risk of ovarian cancer, particularly if used for at least five years (see Figure 12-5). This reduction in risk has been observed in almost all of the studies that have assessed this relationship. We also found that after women stop taking the pill, they remain protected against ovarian cancer for at least another decade, if not longer.

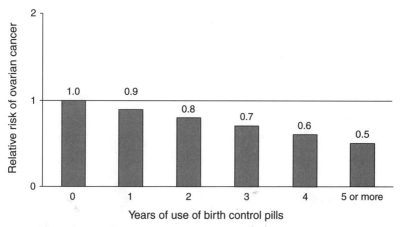

FIG. 12-5. The longer women use the pill, the lower the risk of ovarian cancer. (Source: Nurses' Health Study)

Although this evidence pertains to the older, high dose pills, recent study findings suggest that the modern, low dose pills offer a similar pattern of protection against ovarian cancer.

## TUBAL LIGATION AND HYSTERECTOMY

Tubal ligation and hysterectomy are among the most commonly performed surgeries in the United States. Tubal ligation involves having the fallopian tubes cut, tied, or clamped. Hysterectomy involves having the uterus removed, either by itself (called a simple hysterectomy) or in addition to the fallopian tubes and ovaries (called a complete hysterectomy).

Both tubal ligation and simple hysterectomy are thought to offer long-term protection against ovarian cancer, though tubal ligation appears to have more of an effect than hysterectomy. In the Nurses' Health Study, we observed a large reduction in risk among women who had a tubal ligation and a moderate reduction among women who had a simple hysterectomy (see Figure 12-6). Reductions in risk have been observed in most other studies as well.

Researchers have proposed several explanations for the protective effects of tubal ligation and hysterectomy. First, high levels of circulating hormones in the blood may increase the risk of ovarian cancer. After a tubal ligation or hysterectomy, there may be less blood flowing to the ovaries and thus less exposure to circulating hormones. Second, having a tubal ligation or hysterectomy might alter the length of a woman's ovulatory cycle, so that she experiences ovulation less frequently. Finally, researchers have speculated that some ovarian cancers might be caused by carcinogens that have been introduced into the

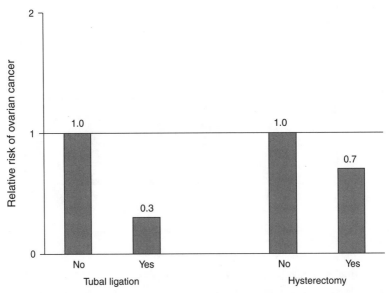

FIG. 12-6. Having a tubal ligation or hysterectomy may lower the risk of ovarian cancer. Tubal ligation appears to offer about twice as much protection as hysterectomy. (Source: Nurses' Health Study)

vagina and have then traveled to the ovary via the uterus and fallopian tubes. After a tubal ligation or hysterectomy, the pathway between the fallopian tubes and ovaries is blocked, preventing the possible passage of carcinogens.

## POSTMENOPAUSAL HORMONES

While postmenopausal hormones do lower the risk of osteoporosis and possibly coronary heart disease, they also increase the risk of breast cancer, blood clots, and gallbladder disease. Several studies have suggested that these hormones may also increase the risk of ovarian cancer.

In the only large cohort study to examine this relationship to date, the American Cancer Society's Cancer Prevention Study II, researchers found a small increase in the risk of fatal ovarian cancer among women who had ever used postmenopausal hormones. The risk increased with duration of use and was greatest among those who were currently on hormones and had been for at least ten years. These women had a twofold increase in risk compared to women who had never used postmenopausal hormones. Smaller studies have corroborated these findings but have not been entirely consistent. Taken collectively, the current evidence suggests that the long-term use of postmenopausal hormones has at least a moderate effect on the risk of ovarian cancer.

## WEIGHT

Being overweight can have a dramatic influence on hormone levels and the monthly menstrual cycle. This may in turn affect the risk of ovarian cancer, though researchers are still determining the exact nature of the relationship. To date, results have been inconsistent. In the Nurses' Health Study, we observed that women who were obese in early adulthood had a moderately increased risk of premenopausal ovarian cancer. This finding will need to be confirmed with additional study. Overall, a woman's current weight probably does not have a large effect on her risk of ovarian cancer.

In the Iowa Women's Health Study, there was no difference in the risk of ovarian cancer between heavy women and lean women. However, waist size did appear to influence risk. Women who carried their excess weight around their waists were twice as likely to develop ovarian cancer as women who carried their excess weight in their hips, buttocks, or thighs. These results suggest that where a woman carries her weight might have more impact on her risk of ovarian cancer than the amount of weight she carries. The reason for this is unknown, but may be due to the hormonal effects of fat accumulating around the organs. However, much more research is needed before waist size can be conclusively linked to ovarian cancer.

## LACTOSE

Lactose is the primary sugar found in milk and other dairy products. When consumed and digested, lactose is broken down into two components, galactose and glucose, which are then broken down even further. If galactose is not metabolized properly, it can accumulate in the ovaries, affecting ovarian function and hormone levels. This may in turn contribute to the development of ovarian tumors.

Two large cohort studies, the Nurses' Health Study and the Iowa Women's Health Study, have examined the impact of lactose consumption on ovarian cancer. Both studies found a slight to moderate increase in risk among women with a high intake of lactose.

## VEGETABLES

Eating vegetables may lower a woman's risk of ovarian cancer, although few studies have addressed the issue and results have not been consistent. In the Iowa Women's Health Study, vegetables in general were not related to ovarian cancer, but green leafy vegetables were. Women who ate at least six servings a

## Ovarian Cancer: Weighing the Risks

- Having a family history of ovarian cancer increases a woman's risk of the disease.
- Having children lowers the risk of ovarian cancer, as does breast-feeding.
- Taking birth control pills substantially lowers the risk of ovarian cancer.
- Having a tubal ligation or simple hysterectomy can significantly lower the risk of ovarian cancer.

week were half as likely to develop ovarian cancer as women who ate two servings a week. One smaller study reported similar findings, although others, including the Nurses' Health Study, observed no relationship.

It is not yet clear why eating vegetables might reduce the risk of ovarian cancer. Some researchers have suggested that vegetables contain a cocktail of potential cancer-fighting substances, including antioxidant vitamins. Others have attempted to identify a specific nutrient or vitamin that possibly protects against ovarian cancer. Some studies point to vitamin A, others to carotenoids, and still others to vitamins C and E. Despite the inconsistency of these studies, fruits and vegetables should be an important part of the diet. Eating at least five servings of these foods a day can lower the risk of cardiovascular disease, other forms of cancer, and a variety of other diseases.

### TALCUM POWDER

Several studies have suggested that using talcum powder on the genitals may increase the risk of ovarian cancer. Talcum powder can be absorbed by the vagina and carried up into the fallopian tubes and ovaries, where it can cause inflammation.

In the Nurses' Health Study, we found that women using talcum powder on their genitals or on sanitary napkins had a slight increase in their risk of one specific type of ovarian cancer. A number of studies have reported similar findings, though results have not been entirely consistent. Taken collectively, these findings suggest that talcum powder has only a modest effect, if any, on the risk of ovarian cancer.

### Reproductive Factors

Several reproductive factors, including childbearing and breast-feeding, have been linked to the risk of ovarian cancer. While these factors are within your control to some extent, they are also largely influenced by your age and your social circumstances. For most women making reproductive decisions, concerns about ovarian cancer will likely be overshadowed by a number of other important considerations.

## NUMBER OF CHILDREN

The number of children a woman has can greatly influence her risk of ovarian cancer. More than twenty epidemiologic studies have examined this relationship, and nearly all of them have shown what we found in the Nurses' Health Study: that women who have at least two children are at lower risk of ovarian cancer than women who do not. In general, the more children a woman has, the less likely she is to develop the disease (see Figure 12-7).

The protection afforded by having children may be due to some of the many hormonal changes that occur in the body during pregnancy. Alternatively, it may be due to the suppression of ovulation during pregnancy.

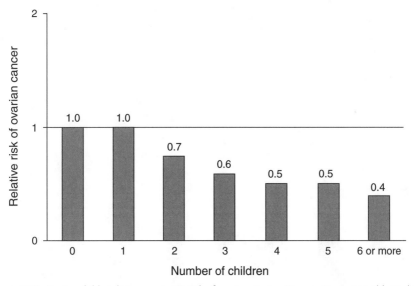

FIG. 12-7. Having children lowers women's risk of ovarian cancer. (Source: Nurses' Health Study)

## BREAST-FEEDING

After a woman gives birth, her body slowly returns to its pre-pregnancy state. The ovaries begin to produce and release eggs again, and hormone levels resume their normal balance. However, if a woman breast-feeds, these changes are delayed. She continues not to ovulate, and her hormone levels remain altered. Thus, breast-feeding is thought to lower the risk of ovarian cancer in the same ways that pregnancy does.

Most studies have shown that breast-feeding lowers the risk of ovarian cancer. When researchers combined the results of twelve different studies, they found that the risk of ovarian cancer was modestly reduced among women who breast-fed for at least six months (see Figure 12-8).

## INFERTILITY AND THE USE OF FERTILITY DRUGS

Infertility is caused by a variety of disorders, which makes it difficult to determine its impact on the risk of ovarian cancer. For example, some disorders may increase the number of times a woman ovulates in her reproductive years, thereby increasing the risk of ovarian cancer. Others may suppress ovulation, leading to a lower risk. Many disorders probably influence the levels of certain hormones, which in turn influence the development of the disease. Given the complexity of this relationship, it is not surprising that studies on infertility and ovarian cancer have had largely inconsistent results.

Slightly more consistent, but still not definitive, is the relationship between fertility drugs and ovarian cancer. Several large studies conducted among infertile women have suggested that fertility drugs may increase the risk of ovarian cancer, but more research is needed.

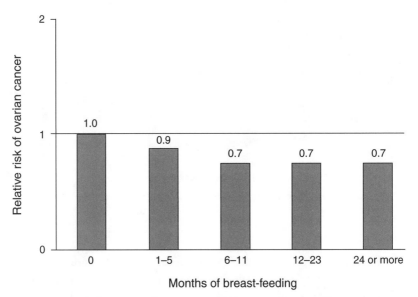

FIG. 12-8. Women who breast-feed for at least six months have a moderately reduced risk of ovarian cancer. (Source: Whittemore et al.)

## WHAT IT ALL MEANS

Ovarian cancer is a relatively rare but deadly disease. Many of the factors that influence your risk, such as having children, taking the pill, and breast-feeding, are probably dictated by other concerns and priorities in your life. However, one factor in particular—your family history—warrants careful attention if it affects you. If your mother, sister, or daughter has been diagnosed with either breast cancer or ovarian cancer, you need to discuss this with your health care provider.

### Established, Probable, and Possible Factors Associated with the Risk of Ovarian Cancer

| RISK FACTOR | APPROXIMATE RISK* |
|---|---|
| *Established* | |
| Immediate family member diagnosed with ovarian cancer | ↑↑↑ |
| Confirmed genetic test for BRCA 1 or 2 | ↑↑↑ |
| Age (greater than 60 vs. less than 50) | ↑↑ |
| Tubal ligation | ↓↓↓ |
| Birth control pills (more than 5 years of use vs. never) | ↓↓ |
| Number of children (2 or more vs. less than 2) | ↓↓ |
| *Probable* | |
| Use of postmenopausal hormones | ↑ |
| Breast-feeding (6 or more months vs. less than 6 months) | ↓↓ |
| Hysterectomy | ↓↓ |
| *Possible* | |
| Immediate family member diagnosed with breast cancer | ↑↑ |
| Larger waist | ↑↑ |
| Use of fertility drugs | ↑↑ |
| High lactose (dairy) intake | ↑ |
| Use of talcum powder on the genitals | ↑ |
| High vegetable intake | ↓ |

| | |
|---|---|
| *↑ Small increase in risk | ↓ Small decrease in risk |
| ↑↑ Moderate increase in risk | ↓↓ Moderate decrease in risk |
| ↑↑↑ Large increase in risk | ↓↓↓ Large decrease in risk |
| ↑↑↑↑ Very large increase in risk | ↓↓↓↓ Very large decrease in risk |

# WHAT I TELL MY PATIENTS ABOUT LOWERING THEIR RISK OF OVARIAN CANCER

DR. CELESTE ROBB-NICHOLSON

Ovarian cancer is relatively uncommon, but it is frightening because it can develop and even spread without causing noticeable symptoms. As a result, my patients often ask me what they can do to reduce their risk of developing this cancer. My advice depends on whether they are at high risk or not. Some factors that put you at high risk are beyond your control, whereas others you can control.

You are considered high risk if:

1. Your mother, sister, or daughter has been diagnosed with either breast cancer or ovarian cancer.
2. You test positive for BRCA 1, a genetic mutation that increases your chances of developing ovarian cancer as well as breast cancer.
3. You are over age sixty-five.

If you are at high risk, I'd recommend the following steps to reduce your chances of developing ovarian cancer:

1. If you are still menstruating, consider using birth control pills in addition to or instead of other contraceptives. Birth control pills can substantially reduce your risk of developing ovarian cancer, especially if used for at least five years. The protective effect remains for at least a decade after stopping the pills.
2. If more than one of your family members has been diagnosed with ovarian or breast cancer, you should also undergo regular screening. Although the two screening tests used—transvaginal ultrasound and the CA125 blood test—are not perfect, they are our best methods for detecting the disease early, when it can be most successfully treated.

    Transvaginal ultrasound involves having a small tampon-shaped probe placed in the vagina so that an image of your uterus and ovaries is projected by ultrasound. This test can sometimes show ovarian cancer at an early stage, but often does not. It also frequently identifies suspicious areas that turn out to be nothing serious, particularly in women who have not yet gone through menopause.

False positive test results can lead to fear and unnecessary surgical procedures.

The CA125 blood test detects the amount of CA125 protein in your blood. CA125 is sometimes shed by ovarian cancer cells and thus is present at elevated levels in women with ovarian cancer. However, this test is not highly accurate: CA125 levels can be normal in women with ovarian cancer and can be elevated in those with noncancerous conditions. Recent studies indicate that having CA125 levels measured periodically and looking for changes over time may provide more accurate results than having only a single measurement taken.

Most women are only at average risk for developing ovarian cancer. If you are one of them, there are few clear guidelines for reducing your risk of this disease. Because the risk increases the more you ovulate, we do know that your risk is reduced if you use birth control pills for at least five years, have multiple children, and breast-feed your children. But most women decide to have children or breast-feed based on other considerations. And none of us can grow younger or control when we enter menopause, so there is really not much you can do to change the reproductive factors implicated in ovarian cancer.

Postmenopausal hormones, lactose (dairy) intake, and talcum powder have all been linked to a slight to moderate increase in the risk of ovarian cancer, although the data are not as consistent and well confirmed as for other factors such as birth control pills. These are all factors that you can control, and limiting your exposure to them would be reasonable if you are concerned about ovarian cancer risk. However, discuss these issues with your health care provider, as postmenopausal hormones have other potential health effects, too. There is also a possible link between ovarian cancer and a large waist size— the so-called apple shape—so watching your caloric intake may also be helpful, especially as you grow older. Your weight and waist size can influence your risk of a variety of conditions other than ovarian cancer, so it is particularly important to keep these in check.

The yearly pelvic exam and Pap smear, which are valuable for detecting cervical and endometrial cancer, may also be used to detect ovarian cancer, since your ovaries can often be felt during that examination. However, this exam is not as sensitive at detecting ovarian cancer as the transvaginal ultrasound. Remember that ovarian cancer is relatively rare. If you are at high risk or have additional concerns about this disease, make sure to discuss the issue with your health care provider.

# CHAPTER THIRTEEN

# Lowering the Risk of Skin Cancer

## BACKGROUND

Skin cancer is a disease about which we know much but seem to do little. Scientists knew as early as 1896 that skin cancer was caused by harmful ultraviolet radiation from the sun. Yet more than a hundred years later, rates of skin cancer are rising more rapidly than ever, due largely to America's obsession with the perfect tan. More than a million people are diagnosed with skin cancer each year, and while the disease is usually not fatal, it can be severely disfiguring.

It is never too late in life—or too early—to protect yourself from the sun's harmful rays. By incorporating sun protection habits into your everyday life, you can protect yourself from skin cancer, as well as from wrinkles and other blemishes caused by sun damage.

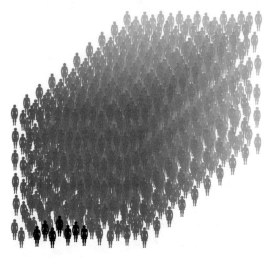

FIG. 13-1. In a group of 1,000 women who are fifty years old, 7 will develop melanoma before they reach the age of eighty. (Source: National Cancer Institute)

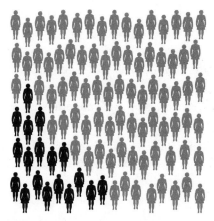

FIG. 13-2. In a group of 100 women who are fifty years old, 18 will develop basal cell cancer before they reach the age of eighty. (Source: Miller et al.)

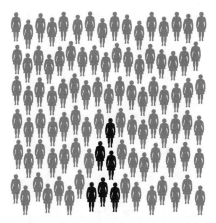

FIG. 13-3. In a group of 100 women who are fifty years old, 6 will develop squamous cell cancer before they reach the age of eighty. (Source: Miller et al.)

## The Skin and Skin Cancer

The skin is the largest organ in the body, serving a variety of essential functions. The most obvious are that it keeps the body together and protects internal organs from injury, sunlight, and infection. It also aids in storing water and fat, helps to regulate body temperature, and serves as a sensory organ for temperature, touch, and pain.

The skin is composed primarily of three layers: the subcutis, the dermis, and the epidermis (see Figure 13-4). The subcutis is the deepest layer and attaches the skin to underlying tissue and organs. The dermis is the thick middle layer that contains blood vessels, hair follicles, nerves, and glands. Together, the subcutis and dermis form a network that helps to absorb shock and protect the internal organs from injury. The thin outer layer of the skin is called the epidermis and contains several different types of cells, including keratinocytes and melanocytes. Keratinocytes produce the protein that helps waterproof the skin and give it its resilience. Melanocytes produce melanin, the brown-black pigment that gives skin its color and protects it from ultraviolet radiation.

Skin cancer tends to develop in the epidermis, usually as a result of excessive exposure to ultraviolet radiation. There are three primary types of skin cancer: basal cell cancer, squamous cell cancer, and malignant melanoma. Basal cell cancer and squamous cell cancer are the most common forms, affecting nearly as many women each year as all other cancers combined. Both originate from the keratinocytes and are often referred to collectively as nonmelanoma skin cancer. Almost all nonmelanomas develop on areas of the skin that are

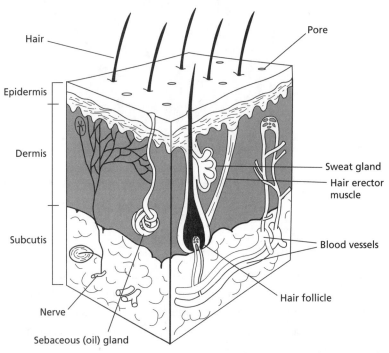

FIG. 13-4. Cross Section of Skin and Hair. The skin consists of the epidermis (the thin outer layer made up mostly of dead cells) and the dermis (the thicker layer containing blood vessels, nerves, oil glands, and hair follicles). A subcutaneous (literally "under the skin") layer forms the base.

consistently exposed to the sun; more than 80 percent of basal cell cancers and at least 60 percent of squamous cell cancers are found on the face, neck, and head. These cancers rarely spread to other parts of the body and are almost always curable. However, they can be severely disfiguring if they are not diagnosed and treated early.

Malignant melanoma is considerably less common, but it is far more deadly. It originates from the melanocytes and can spread rapidly to other parts of the body, causing death within months of diagnosis. Though it can occur anywhere on a woman's body, including areas like the soles of the feet that are not exposed to the sun, malignant melanoma is most often found on the arms and legs.

## LESSONS FROM THE NURSES' HEALTH STUDY AND OTHER STUDIES

Most diseases are influenced by a variety of factors. Skin cancer, however, is primarily caused by one factor: sun exposure. Although there are several inherited factors that can increase your risk of this disease, such as family history and natural coloring, they are important to understand mainly because of the way that they interact with sun exposure. For example, if you have fair skin, you might be particularly vulnerable to the harmful effects of the sun and should take special precautions to protect yourself.

### Factors You Cannot Control

Having a particular skin tone or a family history of skin cancer can increase your susceptibility to skin cancer. Although you cannot change these things,

## Squamous Cell Cancer and Basal Cell Cancer: The Larger Picture

- Squamous cell cancer and basal cancer are often referred to collectively as non-melanoma skin cancer.
- Nonmelanoma skin cancer can be severely disfiguring if it is not diagnosed and treated early.
- Most nonmelanoma skin cancers develop on the face, neck, and head.
- Almost all nonmelanoma skin cancers are caused by ultraviolet radiation from the sun.
- The best way to prevent this disease is to practice safe sun habits.

## Malignant Melanoma: The Larger Picture

- Malignant melanoma is the least common but most deadly form of skin cancer.
- Though it can occur anywhere on a woman's body, it is most often found on the arms and legs.
- Melanoma affects women at much earlier ages than most cancers do. It is the most common cancer found in women ages twenty-five to twenty-nine.
- Almost all malignant melanomas are caused by ultraviolet radiation from the sun.
- The best way to prevent this disease is to practice safe sun habits.

being aware of their impact may lead you to be more vigilant about things you can control, especially your sun exposure.

## AGE

Skin cancer affects women at much earlier ages than most cancers do. Malignant melanoma is the most common cancer found in women ages twenty-five to twenty-nine and is second only to breast cancer among those ages thirty to thirty-four. The older a woman gets, the more likely she is to develop both malignant melanoma (see Figure 13-5) and nonmelanoma skin cancer.

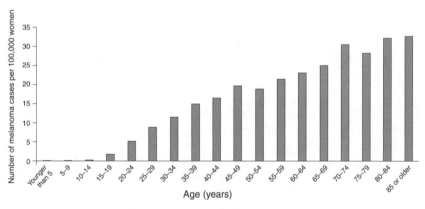

FIG. 13-5. The risk of malignant melanoma increases with age. Unlike most cancers, melanoma occurs frequently in women under age fifty. (Source: National Cancer Institute)

## FAMILY HISTORY

A number of studies have confirmed that malignant melanoma runs in families, though nonmelanoma skin cancer probably does not. Having a relative

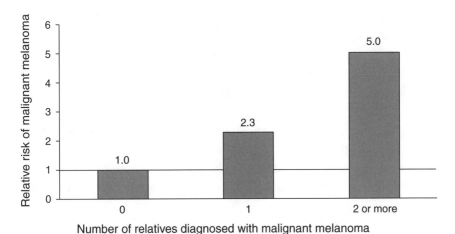

FIG. 13-6. The risk of malignant melanoma is greatly increased among women with a family history of melanoma, particularly for those who have more than one affected relative. (Source: D'Arcy et al.)

with melanoma more than doubles a woman's risk of the disease. The more relatives a woman has with melanoma, the more likely she is to develop it herself (see Figure 13-6). This may be because family members have similar sun exposure habits, or because they share genetic traits and physical features that predispose them to skin cancer.

## NATURAL HAIR AND SKIN COLOR

A woman's natural coloring is determined primarily by the amount of melanin produced by her melanocytes: the more melanin she has, the darker her skin and hair. Melanin shields the genetic material in skin cells from ultraviolet radiation, the predominant cause of skin cancer. Women who produce large amounts of melanin receive greater protection against ultraviolet light and thus have a lower risk of skin cancer.

White women are at least 10 times more likely to develop skin cancer than African American women, and the risk of skin cancer varies substantially with skin tone even among white women. In the Nurses' Health Study, we found that women with fair skin were 70 percent more likely to develop malignant melanoma than women with medium- or olive-colored skin. Other studies have shown that fair-skinned women may also be at increased risk of nonmelanoma skin cancer.

Natural hair color is also determined by melanin, such that women with light-colored hair are more susceptible to skin cancer than women with dark-colored hair. In the Nurses' Health Study, we found an elevated risk of both melanoma and nonmelanoma skin cancer among women whose hair was naturally blond, red, or auburn. The lighter a woman's hair was, the more likely she was to develop skin cancer (see Figure 13-7).

Women with fair skin and light-colored hair are often sensitive to the sun, and this sensitivity further increases their risk of skin cancer. When a woman's skin is exposed to ultraviolet light, her melanocytes compensate by increasing the production of melanin. The extra melanin provides enhanced protection against ultraviolet light and causes the skin to darken, or tan. Women who tan poorly, burn easily, or freckle heavily are not producing enough melanin to protect their skin and are at increased risk of both melanoma and nonmelanoma skin cancer.

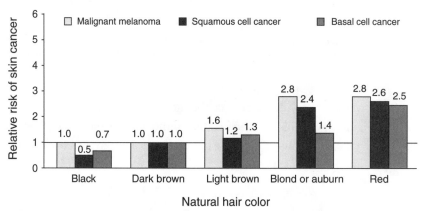

FIG. 13-7. Having blond or red hair greatly increases a woman's risk of developing malignant melanoma, squamous cell cancer, and basal cell cancer. (Source: Nurses' Health Study)

## MOLES

Like melanoma, moles develop when melanocytes cluster on the surface of the skin. Although moles are noncancerous, there is substantial evidence that people who develop them are at increased risk of developing melanoma. In the Nurses' Health Study, having at least one mole on the arms or legs doubles a woman's risk of melanoma. The more moles she has, the more likely she is to develop the disease (see Figure 13-8).

Some researchers have argued that moles might actually develop into melanomas. If this were the case, having a mole on one part of the body would increase the risk of having melanoma on the same part of the body. Evidence from numerous studies suggests otherwise. In the Nurses' Health Study, we found that a woman with a mole on her arm was more likely to develop melanoma but not necessarily on the arm with the mole. This suggests that moles and melanomas might not be as directly linked as was once thought. It may be that having a mole simply indicates that a woman was exposed in childhood to the ultraviolet radiation that causes melanoma. Several studies have shown that the number of moles an adult has is related to the amount of time they spent in the sun as children.

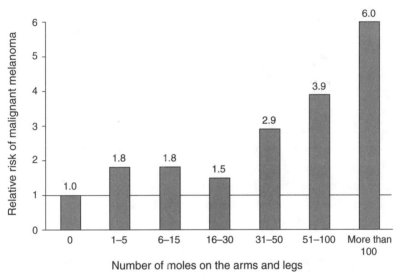

FIG. 13-8. The more moles a woman has, the higher her risk of malignant melanoma. (Source: Nurses' Health Study)

## SOLAR KERATOSES

Solar keratoses, also called actinic keratoses, are blemishes that appear as rough, flat, pink spots on sun-exposed areas of the skin. These blemishes are indicators of sun damage and substantially increase a woman's risk of both melanoma and nonmelanoma skin cancer. The more solar keratoses a woman has, the more likely she is to develop skin cancer.

### Factors You Can Control

Although there are other factors that can increase your risk of skin cancer, your sun exposure has the most impact and is also the most modifiable.

## SUN EXPOSURE

Almost all malignant melanomas and nonmelanoma skin cancers are caused by ultraviolet radiation from the sun, and there is substantial evidence to support this. First, skin cancer rates are about twice as high in southern states as in northern states, and the rates increase with proximity to the equator, where sunlight is most intense. Second, nonmelanoma skin cancer is most common in people who work outdoors and in people with sun-damaged skin. Finally, almost all nonmelanoma skin cancers occur on areas of the skin that are regularly exposed to the sun, like the face, neck, and head. Scientists have confirmed the relationship between sunlight and skin cancer on a molecular level: upon examining cancerous skin cells, they found genetic mutations that had been caused by ultraviolet light.

The effects of ultraviolet radiation on the skin appear to be cumulative. That is, the more sun exposure a woman gets during her lifetime, the more likely she is to develop skin cancer. But how can researchers or even women themselves tell how much sun a woman has been exposed to in her lifetime? One way is to look at the number of sunburns accumulated since childhood. In the Nurses' Health Study, we found that the more sunburns a woman had in her lifetime, the more likely she was to develop basal cell cancer and squamous cell cancer. This was true for women of all skin types, though the risk was highest among those with sun-sensitive skin and light-colored hair. Notably, cumulative exposure to the sun, even in the absence of sunburns, can increase the risk of nonmelanoma skin cancer.

Having a history of severe sunburns may also increase a woman's risk of malignant melanoma, though the relationship appears to be more complex. While cumulative sun exposure may increase risk, what appears to be even more harmful is occasional intense exposure. For example, people who work indoors seem to have a higher risk of melanoma than people who work outdoors. This may be because they are shielded from the sun most days of the week and are then exposed to intense sunlight on the weekends and during vacations. It is this type of intermittent exposure to strong sunlight that often leads to sunburns—and perhaps melanoma.

When a woman is exposed to ultraviolet light daily, her body is able to partially protect itself by developing a store of melanin. When she is exposed to the sun only occasionally, her body has to produce melanin each time. Without the protective store, her skin is much more sensitive to sunlight, and the exposure is therefore more dangerous. This does not mean, however, that a woman should spend excessive amounts of time in the sun trying to develop a protective tan. The amount and intensity of sun exposure necessary to develop a tan can still damage the skin cells and increase the risk of skin cancer.

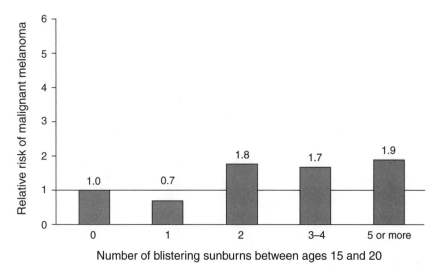

FIG. 13-9. Women who experienced multiple sunburns between the ages of fifteen and twenty have an increased risk of developing malignant melanoma in adulthood. (Source: Nurses' Health Study)

While it is never too late to reduce sun exposure, the majority of most women's lifetime exposure will have occurred during childhood and adolescence, when there was more leisure time to play outdoors and sunbathe. This childhood sun exposure may have a large impact on the risk of skin cancer. In the Nurses' Health Study, we found that having multiple severe sunburns before the age of twenty nearly doubled a woman's risk of malignant melanoma (see Figure 13-9). We also found that women who lived in the southern United States during adolescence had an elevated risk of melanoma compared to women who lived in northern states. Other studies have confirmed these results by showing childhood residence to be an important risk factor for melanoma.

Overall, excessive sun exposure at any age can increase the risk of both malignant melanoma and nonmelanoma skin cancer. Women need to protect their skin against sunburn at all ages, and those with sun-sensitive skin may need to take extra precautions.

## Tanning Beds and Skin Cancer

Given the strong relationship between natural ultraviolet light and skin cancer, it would seem logical that artificial sources of ultraviolet light, like tanning beds and sun lamps, might also increase the risk of skin cancer. Though many studies have examined this, the results have been somewhat inconsistent. To date, there has not been a single study showing a protective effect for tanning beds. Some studies have reported no link, while others have suggested that tanning beds might increase the risk of melanoma. Despite the inconsistency of these results, one thing seems certain: the ultraviolet light emitted from tanning beds and sun lamps is not any safer than that emitted from the sun. In fact, it is two to three times stronger and may intensify the skin's response to subsequent ultraviolet exposure.

## BIRTH CONTROL PILLS

Researchers have long suspected that the estrogen in birth control pills might influence a woman's risk of melanoma. Estrogen is known to stimulate the growth of melanocytes and to increase the amount of melanin in the cells. In addition, women taking birth control pills sometimes notice that their skin darkens, which is direct evidence of estrogen's effect on the melanocytes.

Although not all studies have been consistent, birth control pills do appear to increase a woman's risk of melanoma but only while she is taking them. In the Nurses' Health Study, we found that women who were on the pill were twice as likely to develop melanoma as women who had never used the pill. Once women stopped taking the pill, however, their risk returned to that of women who had never used the pill.

Of course, there is more to consider than melanoma risk when deciding whether to take birth control pills. Taking the pill can lower the risk of ovarian cancer, endometrial cancer, and probably colon cancer, in addition to protecting against unwanted pregnancies. However, it may also increase the risk of breast cancer and cardiovascular disease in some women. Women who are considering the use of birth control pills should talk to their health care provider about the various risks and benefits.

## SMOKING

Several studies have suggested that smoking may increase a woman's risk of squamous cell cancer, particularly on the lips. Researchers are not yet sure why this relationship might exist, and additional studies are needed to confirm it.

## Malignant Melanoma: Weighing the Risks

A woman's risk of malignant melanoma is increased if she:

- Has family members with the disease
- Has fair skin or light-colored hair
- Tends to tan poorly, burn easily, or freckle heavily
- Has moles or solar keratoses on her skin
- Has a history of blistering sunburns, particularly during adolescence
- Takes birth control pills

## Squamous Cell Cancer and Basal Cell Cancer: Weighing the Risks

A woman's risk of nonmelanoma skin cancer is increased if she:

- Has fair skin or light-colored hair
- Tends to tan poorly, burn easily, or freckle heavily
- Has solar keratoses on her skin
- Has a history of severe sunburns

## WHAT IT ALL MEANS

A number of factors can influence your risk of skin cancer, but your sun exposure is by far the most important. Although there are three types of skin cancer, each influenced somewhat differently by sun exposure, the message for prevention remains the same: avoid unnecessary and excessive exposure to sunlight. This does not mean that you cannot enjoy the outdoors. You simply need to take precautions: avoid the sun during peak midday hours, wear protective clothing, and use sunscreen.

## Established, Probable, and Possible Factors Associated with the Risk of Malignant Melanoma

| RISK FACTOR | APPROXIMATE RISK* |
|---|---|
| *Established* | |
| Family member diagnosed with malignant melanoma | ↑↑↑ |
| Natural hair color (blond, red, or auburn vs. brown or black) | ↑↑↑ |
| Moles on the arms or legs | ↑↑↑ |
| Solar keratoses | ↑↑↑ |
| History of blistering sunburns during adolescence (2 or more vs. none) | ↑↑ |
| Skin color (fair skin vs. medium- or olive-colored skin) | ↑↑ |
| Age (greater than 60 vs. less than 50) | ↑ |
| *Probable* | |
| Use of birth control pills | ↑↑↑ |
| *Possible* | |
| Smoking (current vs. never) | ↑↑↑ |

| | |
|---|---|
| *↑ Small increase in risk | ↓ Small decrease in risk |
| ↑↑ Moderate increase in risk | ↓↓ Moderate decrease in risk |
| ↑↑↑ Large increase in risk | ↓↓↓ Large decrease in risk |
| ↑↑↑↑ Very large increase in risk | ↓↓↓↓ Very large decrease in risk |

## WHAT I TELL MY PATIENTS ABOUT LOWERING THEIR RISK OF SKIN CANCER

DR. CAROL BATES

There are just three general rules for lowering your risk of skin cancer: protect yourself from the sun; keep an eye on your skin and point out any changes to

### DECIPHERING THE LABELS ON YOUR SUNSCREEN BOTTLES

You are no doubt familiar with SPF (sun protection factor), the rating system for sunscreens. But what exactly does it mean to use SPF 15 as opposed to SPF

30? The number of the SPF corresponds to the number of minutes you can spend outdoors before experiencing the equivalent of one minute of harmful ultraviolet (UV) radiation. For example, SPF 4 blocks only 75 percent of the UV light that causes sunburn. This means that for every four minutes you spend in the sun, your skin will receive approximately one minute of radiation exposure. The higher the SPF, the more protection you receive. For example, SPF 15 blocks out 93 percent of harmful UV light, and your skin will receive one minute of radiation exposure for every fifteen minutes that you're in the sun. Experts recommend that you use sunscreen with a minimum SPF of 15, though any protection is better than none.

You may also have read about UVA and UVB on your sunscreen bottle. These are the two types of radiation from the sun that reach the Earth's surface and thus have the potential to damage your skin. Though UVB causes most sunburns, UVA is much more intense and can penetrate to underlying tissues of the skin, causing long-term skin damage. UVB is also the component of sunlight that stimulates melanin production, which protects your skin from further UV radiation. Although most sunscreens block only UVB, some provide protection against UVA as well. To tell if your sunscreen blocks both, look for the label "broad-spectrum sunscreen" or check the ingredient list for micronized zinc oxide, titanium oxide, or avobenzene.

Some sunscreens are also labeled as water-resistant or waterproof. Water-resistant sunscreens protect for only forty minutes when you're swimming or sweating, while waterproof protect you for at least eighty minutes. Whenever there's a chance that your sunscreen might be washed off by water or sweat, opt for a sunscreen that is clearly labeled waterproof.

your health care provider; and let your health care provider check your skin regularly as part of your general checkup.

I tell my patients that skin damage from the sun probably is involved in causing all three kinds of skin cancer, including the deadly malignant melanoma. The problem is that most of us like the sun: we like the feel of warmth on our bodies, and we generally like the way we look with a suntan. Also, the sun helps us make vitamin D, which can protect against osteoporosis. So the trick is to enjoy the sun while minimizing the risks. There are three general approaches: avoid the sun altogether during the peak midday hours when it is most intense, wear protective clothing, and use sunscreen. Here are some practical hints:

1. Avoid significant sun exposure during the peak hours of 10 AM to 4 PM.
   - Mow your lawn and do other types of gardening early in the morning or toward dusk.
   - When you do go outdoors, make sure that you wear sunscreen or protective clothing.
2. Find or create shade.
   - Bring an umbrella to the beach.
   - Sit under trees in a park while reading or picnicking.
3. Wear sunscreen with an SPF of at least 15 (the higher the SPF, the more protection you receive).
   - It may be simplest to routinely use waterproof sunscreen with SPF 30 or more for all outdoor activities.
   - If you wish to vary SPF for different activity levels, you may choose to wear a sunscreen with SPF 15 for routine outdoor activities. If you intend to spend some time at the beach or plan hours of yard work, consider an SPF of 30 or more.
   - Reapply several times a day, especially if you've been outside and sweating, using at least one ounce of sunscreen to cover your arms, legs, neck, and face.
   - Look for skin care products that include SPF protection. Many lotions, lip balms, and cosmetics now include this.
   - For optimal protection, apply the sunscreen twenty to thirty minutes before you go out into the sun. Sunscreen must be absorbed by your skin in order to be effective.
   - UV light can reflect off of snow and pass through water, so remember, whether you're skiing in the mountains or wading in the lake, use sunscreen for all outdoor activities.
   - UV exposure is more intense in summer, near the equator, and at high altitude. Protect yourself accordingly.
   - Don't relax healthy habits on cloudy days, as UV light can penetrate clouds.
   - Know your skin type. UV protection is important for everyone, but be extra vigilant if you have fair skin or light hair.

4. Wear protective clothing, including hats.

- Most nonmelanoma skin cancers, and some malignant melanomas, develop on the head, even under the hair (where they are hard to see). So wear a broad-brimmed hat while running errands and a shade cap (similar to a baseball cap with material that hangs over the ears toward the shoulders) while at the beach or doing gardening, to protect your neck and ears as well as your face and scalp.
- Wear long-sleeved shirts while gardening.
- Slip on some long pants or wear a caftan at the beach or while outside for prolonged periods.
- Dark and tightly woven fabrics offer the most protection, but if these are too heavy in the sun, choose light-colored fabric that breathes and wear sunscreen underneath.
- Wear gloves while doing yard work; your hands can get overexposed too.

## Screening and Early Detection of Skin Cancer

Getting screened for skin cancer means having your doctor examine your entire body for early-stage cancers. Whenever I do a complete checkup, I examine the skin carefully. If I see something suspicious, I will send my patient to a skin specialist for further examination. If a cancerous growth is found, it can usually be removed to treat the disease before it spreads further.

There is some controversy, however, about whether early detection actually improves a woman's chance of survival. The National Cancer Institute and the United States Preventive Services Task Force have concluded that there is not enough scientific evidence to warrant a recommendation on screening for skin cancer. The American Cancer Society, however, recommends that all women be screened yearly for this disease.

Overall, it is best to talk to your health care provider about whether you need to be screened for skin cancer. If my patients have any of the following risk factors for malignant melanoma, I am vigilant about checking their skin carefully on a regular basis:

- A family history of malignant melanoma
- A personal history of malignant melanoma or nonmelanoma skin cancer

## THE ABCD RULE

People with melanoma often report that their cancer developed at the exact site of a preexisting mole. However, what appeared to be a mole may in fact have been a melanoma in its earliest stages. Normal moles are evenly colored and do not change in size, shape, or appearance. The ABCD rule can help you distinguish between a normal mole and a melanoma. Look for the following characteristics to see if your mole might be an early-stage melanoma:

**A**symmetry: One half of the mole does not look like the other half.

**B**order: The edges of the mole are not even but instead appear ragged or notched.

**C**olor: The mole is not evenly colored. It has different shades of tan, black, or brown and may have patches of red, blue, or white.

**D**iameter: The mole is at least a quarter of an inch wide (the size of a pencil eraser).

If you notice a mole that has any of these characteristics—or if you notice a sudden change in the size, shape, or color of a mole—you should see your health care provider immediately. He or she will most likely want to remove the mole and make sure it is not an early melanoma.

- An unusually high number of moles on the skin
- Solar keratoses or other suspicious blemishes on the skin
- Fair skin or light hair

If my patients have any of these risk factors for melanoma, I teach them how to examine their own skin and how to have a family member help look at the places that are hard for them to see (the back or scalp, for example). I also teach them the ABCD rule (see box).

## Protecting Your Children and Grandchildren

Most children spend a fair amount of time in the sun. In fact, more than 80 percent of a person's lifetime sun exposure is accumulated during childhood and adolescence. Unfortunately, skin cells may be particularly vulnerable to damage this early in life. With a few simple steps, you can help protect your children and grandchildren from the sun's harmful rays.

- Hats, clothing, and shade work best for protecting babies younger than six months. If these are not available, however, dab a little sunscreen on the baby's exposed skin.
- Use sunscreen for all of your child's outdoor activities. Choose one with SPF 15 or higher and UVA/UVB protection.
- Don't forget to send sunscreen with your child to camp or school each day. It's important to reapply sunscreen regularly, especially if your child swims or exercises.
- Encourage your child to wear a hat that covers the face, scalp, ears, and neck. If your child prefers a baseball cap, be sure to cover the ears and neck with sunscreen.
- Try to plan your child's outdoor activities before or after peak sunlight hours (between 10 A.M. and 4 P.M.).
- Although it's good for children to play outdoors, encourage them to spend part of the middle of the day indoors to limit their sun exposure.
- Be creative about choosing shady play spaces. Build a tree fort, bring a pop-up tent to the beach, or picnic under an umbrella.
- Pitch a tent for children in the backyard so they can play in the shade.

Remember to protect yourself, too: you are an important role model.

# CHAPTER FOURTEEN

# Lowering the Risk of Asthma, Arthritis, Age-Related Eye Disease, and Alzheimer's Disease

I N THE NURSES' HEALTH STUDY, we have focused on the diseases that are most common and most deadly among middle-aged women—mainly cancer and cardiovascular disease. While the diseases presented in this chapter are certainly common, they tend to affect a woman's *quality* of life rather than her *quantity* of life. As the participants in our study have grown older and have begun to develop age-related diseases in greater numbers, we have been able to gather the information we need to look at diseases like arthritis, cataracts, and Alzheimer's disease. In fact, a number of substudies are either under way or in the planning stages on a variety of age-related diseases, as well as on diseases such as asthma that affect a growing number of adults.

## ASTHMA

### Background

If an epidemic is defined as a disease that rapidly spreads to affect a large number of people, then the United States is in the midst of an asthma epidemic. In just twenty years, the number of Americans affected by this potentially disabling lung disease has nearly tripled and now stands at more than 17 million. While asthma rates have increased most among those who live in large inner cities, suburban adults and children have also experienced substantial increases.

To date, scientists do not know exactly what causes asthma. However, they do have a firm understanding of *how* the condition occurs. People with asthma are said to have hyperreactive (or "twitchy") airways that are exceptionally sensitive

## Medical Care and the Risk of Asthma

Early detection is particularly important because it can help prevent permanent damage to the airways. Unfortunately, such early detection is not easy, particularly for those who do not have regular medical care. Asthma is often misdiagnosed as another condition, such as a nighttime cough or wheezy bronchitis, and its symptoms tend to come and go unpredictably. Thus, if people do not have a regular health care provider, their asthma may not be managed correctly, and they may be more likely to experience repeated attacks of severe asthma.

For patients without medical insurance, asthma management often occurs in the emergency room when an asthma attack leaves them struggling for breath. While the medical attention provided may resolve the crisis, they often receive little follow-up care to prevent future attacks. Many people have difficulty with access to proper medical care, and this is especially true for young children. If you think that you or your child has asthma, and a chronic cough or wheeze is persistently attributed to chronic bronchitis or twitchy airways, you may need to insist on seeing an asthma specialist. This is an important first step to controlling the disease.

to irritants like cigarette smoke, cold air, pollen, and pollution. When the airways are exposed to these irritants (or triggers), the walls thicken with inflammation and the muscles begin to contract, narrowing the airways. At the same time, the airways also fill with mucus, further interrupting the flow of air. As airflow continues to deteriorate, wheezing and coughing usually develop. Some asthma attacks are mild, while others can be severe and even life-threatening. Although asthma is generally not considered to be a curable disease, it can usually be controlled through education, lifestyle changes, and medication.

### Factors You Cannot Control

#### ETHNICITY

Although asthma rates are similar across racial and ethnic groups, African Americans and Hispanic Americans are more likely than whites to suffer from severe asthma attacks that require emergency room visits or hospitalization. Whether this difference represents an increased susceptibility to severe asthma or a gap in access to regular health care is under investigation.

#### FAMILY HISTORY

Asthma tends to run in families: a third of those who suffer from asthma share the condition with an immediate family member. In one large study of newborns, half of those with an asthmatic parent developed the disease within ten years. This suggests that one or more genes may either cause asthma directly or make the people that inherit the genes more susceptible to asthma's environmental triggers. Additional support for a link between asthma and genetics comes from the fact that people with asthma often have allergies or the skin disorder known as eczema. Both of these conditions have been shown to be genetically linked, suggesting that asthma may be caused by a combination of a person's genetic makeup and her environmental exposures.

## Low Birth Weight

An intriguing hypothesis suggests that poor nutrition in utero (in the womb) sets the stage for a host of medical problems later in life. These include not only diabetes, high blood pressure, and heart disease but also asthma. Several studies have shown that the less people weigh at birth, the more likely they are to develop asthma later.

### Factors You Can Control

## The Surrounding Environment

For most people, home is a safe haven from the hazards of the world. For people susceptible to asthma, however, home may harbor many asthma triggers. The most common ones are molds that grow indoors, dander (flakes of skin from dogs, cats, birds, or other people), dust mites (tiny insects that thrive on dust), cockroach particles, and combustion products (from passive cigarette smoke, fireplaces, woodstoves, natural gas, etc.). Triggers also abound outdoors (pollen, air pollution, and cold, dry air) and in the workplace (fumes, dusts, and vapors).

There is no evidence that avoiding these pervasive triggers will protect a woman from developing asthma. However, for women who have already been diagnosed, it is important to identify what triggers their condition and then either eliminate those triggers entirely or at least limit exposure to them.

## Weight

The Nurses' Health Study has identified a number of health hazards linked to excess weight, and asthma can be added to the list. In the Nurses' Health Study II, women who were overweight were more likely to develop asthma over a four-year period than women who were lean. This was especially true for obese women, who had a threefold increase in the risk of asthma.

Although it is unclear how excess weight can lead to asthma, there are several possible explanations. First, people who are overweight tend to exercise less and spend more time indoors. As a result, they may be exposed to indoor allergens for longer periods of time. Second, the combination of less physical activity and excess weight may mean fewer deep breaths and more obstructed airways. Together these may lead to airway inflammation and asthma. Finally, carrying excess weight increases a woman's risk of developing gastroesophageal reflux, a condition in which acidic stomach juices get into the airways, causing irritation and potentially leading to asthma.

## POSTMENOPAUSAL HORMONES

Several observations have led researchers to speculate that hormones might play a role in the development of asthma. First, the rate of asthma becomes higher among girls than boys with the onset of puberty and remains higher throughout the reproductive years. Second, women tend to be hospitalized with asthma for longer periods than men are, suggesting that asthma may be more severe among women. Finally, the severity of asthma symptoms appears to vary with the menstrual cycle. Several studies have reported that nearly a third of all women with asthma have exacerbated symptoms before and/or during menstruation.

Although there is little direct evidence to support a relationship between hormones and asthma, our findings in the Nurses' Health Study are consistent with the idea that higher levels of estrogen are linked with higher rates of asthma. We found that premenopausal women had higher rates of asthma than postmenopausal women. However, among postmenopausal women, the rate of asthma was elevated for those taking postmenopausal hormones. Women who were currently using estrogen, as well as those who had used it in the past, were 50 percent more likely to develop asthma than women who had never used estrogen. The longer women used the hormone and the higher the dose, the more likely they were to develop the condition.

## PHYSICAL ACTIVITY

Low levels of physical activity appear to be related to an increased risk of asthma. This may be because people who do not exercise spend more time indoors exposed to asthma triggers. Alternatively, it may be that regular physical activity strengthens the muscles around the airways and makes them less responsive to triggers.

For some people, exercise actually provokes asthma. An asthma management plan that includes adequate warmup and cooldown sessions and use of medications before exercising can help prevent these attacks.

## Cigarette Smoke

Although the link between smoking and asthma has been examined in several studies, the results to date have been inconsistent. What is clear, however, is that parents' use of cigarettes raises their child's risk of asthma. When a child is exposed to smoke from another person's cigarette—known as passive smoke—it can increase the risk of asthma.

## Lowering Your Child's Risk of Asthma

Asthma prevention truly begins before birth. A growing body of evidence suggests that early-life exposure to cigarette smoke and poor nutrition predisposes children to asthma. If you are pregnant or plan to become pregnant, give your child a healthy start: do not smoke, avoid passive smoke, eat well, and breastfeed your child if you can. These things will improve both your child's health and your own.

## Controlling Your Asthma

If you have asthma, you can play a very active role in minimizing the severity of your condition and preventing asthma flares. Here are some key steps:

*Quit smoking.*
- Ask your health care provider for help in quitting.
- Don't get discouraged. It may take you more than one try before you are able to quit for good.

*Minimize your exposure to passive smoke.*
- Encourage others to quit.
- Ask that family and friends not smoke in your home or car.
- Advocate for a smoke-free workplace.
- Avoid smoky bars and restaurants.

*Take charge of your asthma.*
- Learn how to monitor your asthma with peak flow measurements.
- Develop an asthma action plan with your health care provider in order to aggressively treat asthma flares at the outset.

- When your airways are exposed to irritants, they may respond in two ways: the walls of the airway may become swollen, and the bronchial muscles may contract. In any given individual, one response may be more dominant than the other, and this can be tested by a health care provider. Make sure that your treatment plan controls both responses adequately if necessary.

*Avoid allergen triggers.*

- Consider allergy testing, especially if your asthma is difficult to control.
- Learn how to minimize exposure to your triggers.

*Control gastroesophageal reflux (heartburn), which can trigger asthma attacks.*

- Avoid eating before bedtime.
- Avoid tobacco, alcohol, and chocolate.

*Prevent exercise-induced asthma.*

- Talk to your health care provider about using a preventive inhaler before you exercise.

## Asthma: What It All Means

The three most effective things you can do to lower your risk of asthma are to not smoke, get (or keep) your weight in the healthy range, and be physically active. If you think that you or your child has asthma, talk with your health care provider about what you can do at home. With early diagnosis and adequate control, people with asthma can live full, unlimited lives.

## ARTHRITIS

### Background

When most people think of arthritis, they conjure up achy fingers, creaky knees, and stiff hips. That's usually osteoarthritis, the slow erosion of the cushioning cartilage inside the joints. While this is the most common form of arthritis—it affects one of every five women in the Nurses' Health Study—there are actually more than 100 other varieties. These include a variety of autoimmune disorders such as rheumatoid arthritis, systemic lupus erythematosus, and scleroderma. The autoimmune forms of arthritis are caused by an immune system that, for unknown reasons, attacks the body's own tissues and joints as if they were foreign invaders.

## Osteoarthritis

Osteoarthritis, also called degenerative joint disease, is the painful and gradual deterioration of the joint cartilage, without much inflammation. It is the most common form of arthritis, affecting more than 16 million Americans. Symptoms typically emerge in women after age fifty-five, affecting the hips, knees, hands, and spine. Women with osteoarthritis also sometimes develop Heberden's nodes, which are small bony growths on the joint nearest the fingertip.

In osteoarthritis, the cartilage that protects the joint surfaces from rubbing together changes and starts to wear away. Without this cushioning, bone surfaces rub directly against each other. The body responds by trying to repair the damage, but instead of generating normal bone, the body forms bony protrusions called osteophytes or bone spurs. These spurs can irritate surrounding soft tissues and cause inflammation. People whose joints are severely damaged sometimes have periods of joint swelling.

## Rheumatoid Arthritis

Rheumatoid arthritis is an inflammatory disease that damages the tissue connecting bones and joints. One of the most crippling forms of arthritis, it affects more than 2.5 million Americans. It is not known what triggers the immune system to produce the substances that cause the inflammation, which can destroy all components of the joint. The membrane covering the joints, normally smooth, develops into a rough and grainy tissue called pannus that invades the joint cavity. The pannus then releases enzymes that eat into the cartilage, bone, and soft tissues. Inflamed tendons can shorten, immobilizing the joint and causing the bones to fuse. If tendons rupture, the result can be loose, floppy joints. Rheumatoid arthritis can occur at any age but usually develops between twenty and forty-five.

Given that osteoarthritis and rheumatoid arthritis can be controlled but not cured, preventing them is critically important. While there is no single magic strategy, we have learned enough from the Nurses' Health Study and other studies to suggest a few important steps you can take.

### Factors You Cannot Control

#### Age

The longer a woman lives, the more likely she is to develop some form of arthritis. According to a national survey, arthritis affects approximately 3 percent of women under age twenty-five and more than half of those over age sixty-five.

## GENES

Although the root cause of osteoarthritis has not yet been determined, scientists suspect that only a small proportion of osteoarthritis can be attributed directly to heredity. Most cases are probably caused by factors like smoking, excess weight, and occupational hazards. When it comes to rheumatoid arthritis, a gene called HLA-DR4 appears to play an important role. People who carry this gene tend to more susceptible to this particular form of arthritis.

## Factors You Can Control

### WEIGHT

Carrying excess weight is one of the most common predisposing factors that predicts osteoarthritis in the knees and hips. This has been clearly demonstrated in numerous studies, including the Nurses' Health Study and the Framingham Heart Study. The more weight that a woman carries, the more force she puts on her joints. More force means more mechanical stress, and this can lead to the erosion of protective cartilage.

### INJURY

A sudden injury like a twisted knee or sprained finger can cause long-term damage that leads to osteoarthritis. So can the buildup of infinitesimally small injuries that are caused by repeatedly performing the same motion. While sudden injuries are not usually preventable, the small daily ones may be.

### SMOKING

Several studies, including the Nurses' Health Study, have shown that smoking increases the risk of rheumatoid arthritis. However, this relationship is not well established, given that other studies have found no link. Despite the inconsistency of the evidence, it is still extremely important to avoid smoking, as it is the single most important cause of premature death among women.

### BIRTH CONTROL PILLS AND POSTMENOPAUSAL HORMONES

The painful symptoms of rheumatoid arthritis often disappear during pregnancy, when levels of estrogen and progesterone are high, only to flare up again three to four months after delivery, when estrogen levels plummet. Breast-feeding seems to make symptoms worse, possibly because of the high levels of the hormone prolactin, which promotes inflammation. Observations such as these have prompted researchers to look at estrogen and other hormones as risk factors for arthritis.

In the Nurses' Health Study, we have seen a small increase in the risk of systemic lupus erythematosus among women who used birth control pills and those who use postmenopausal hormones. Because lupus is a relatively uncommon condition, affecting fewer than 2 women per 1,000, and the increased risk associated with hormones is small, this disease should not be a dominant factor in deciding whether to use hormones. Neither osteoarthritis nor rheumatoid arthritis appear to be more common among women who use (or have used) birth control pills or postmenopausal hormones.

## Arthritis: What It All Means

Excess weight is the number one preventable cause of osteoarthritis. If your weight is in the healthy range, keeping it there will help lower your risk of arthritis. If you are overweight, losing weight will reduce your chances of developing arthritis.

Taking care of your knees and hips during work or play is also a good way to prevent arthritis. This means trying to avoid repetitive kneeling and squatting. If you regularly run, jog, or walk, try to wear shoes that cushion your step, and whenever possible, exercise on surfaces that have a little "give."

# AGE-RELATED EYE DISEASE

## Background

One of every two women who read this book will experience some sort of age-related vision loss, most likely a cataract or macular degeneration. Together, these two conditions are the leading cause of vision loss and blindness in the United States. Although we tend to treat cataracts as something that can be fixed with relatively simple surgery, they account for about half of the 30 million to 50 million cases of blindness worldwide.

A cataract is the gradual clouding of the eye's lens. This rigid disc of protein sits near the front of the eye, right behind the pupil (see Figure 14-1). Its job is to focus light onto the retina, the light-sensitive tissue that lines the back of the eye. In a child, the lens is crystal clear. Unfortunately, decades of use and abuse can change that. Sunlight, cigarette smoke, and other noxious agents can damage the proteins in the lens, often by generating free radicals. These are highly reactive particles that damage many of our tissues.

Free radical attacks can make the lens proteins clump together. These clumped proteins scatter light in all directions. Light coming out of a clouded

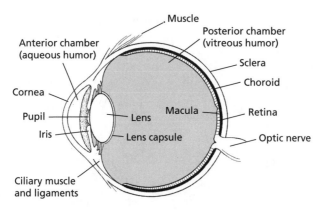

FIG. 14-1. Cross Section of the Eye. Rays of light are bent as they pass through the cornea, lens, and vitreous humor, ultimately coming to focus on or near the retina. The retina has light-sensitive cells that capture light energy and send it as electric impulses via the optic nerve to the brain. You experience this as sight.

lens spreads out, hitting parts of the eye that cannot translate the signals, instead of streaming straight down in a tightly focused beam onto the retina. This dispersion of light can cause blurred or clouded vision. Other symptoms include halos around lights, poor night vision, and less vibrant colors. When a cataract interferes with vision, it can usually be fixed by surgically removing the lens and replacing it with an artificial one.

Macular degeneration affects a different part of the eye. The macula is a spot about the size of this O that sits at the very center of the retina. Millions of tiny photoreceptors in the macula turn light into electrical signals that are then transmitted to the brain, where they are turned into mental pictures. The macula, in other words, is responsible for central vision. In the most common form of macular degeneration, photoreceptors in the macula begin to break down, usually in one eye. The other eye may or may not follow suit. The earliest symptom of macular degeneration is usually blurred or distorted vision (see Figure 14-2). So far, there is not an effective treatment for this form of macular degeneration.

Until recently, these two eye diseases were seen as inevitable consequences of aging. However, some exciting research in the Nurses' Health Study and other ongoing projects indicates that healthy habits are an excellent strategy for keeping your eyesight intact.

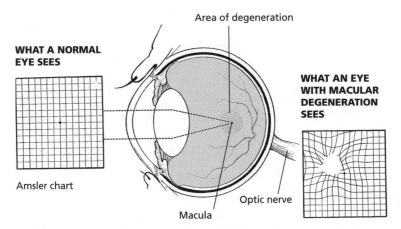

FIG. 14-2. Age-related macular degeneration (ARMD) results from deterioration of the light-sensitive cells of the central retina (macula). To demonstrate ARMD effects, you will be asked to look at a dot on an Amsler chart (*far left*). If lines near dot appear wavy (*far right*), ARMD may be the cause. In people with ARMD, the lines may appear wavy or broken, colors may fade, objects may look larger or smaller than they should, and letters within a word or sentence may seem distorted or may seem to disappear.

## Factors You Cannot Control

### AGE

Clearly, the risk of age-related eye disease increases as a woman grows older. Less than 1 percent of Americans under age fifty-five have cataracts, while nearly 40 percent of those aged seventy-five and older have it. Macular degeneration follows a similar pattern, affecting less than 1 percent of adults under age sixty-four and 7 percent of those aged seventy-five and older.

### GENES

The limited information available on age-related eye disease suggests that genes may play a modest role in both cataracts and macular degeneration. Having a parent or sibling with macular degeneration slightly increases a woman's chance of developing the disease. Just how large that increase is remains to be determined. Habits during youth and adulthood probably cause the majority of age-related vision problems.

## Factors You Can Control

### SUNLIGHT

The radiant energy that the eyes and brain transform into images of the world can also damage the delicate proteins in the eye. One of the main culprits is ultraviolet light, the same slice of the spectrum that is responsible for sunburns. Pigment in the iris and the white of the eye can filter out some of this extra-energetic light. However, too much ultraviolet light for too long can cloud the lens and damage the macula, either directly or by generating free radicals.

Sunglasses offer a simple, portable, and unfortunately often overlooked or forgotten tool for protecting the eyes. A good pair of sunglasses can filter out most of the ultraviolet light and reduce the total amount of energy that enters the eye, while still allowing for clear, sharp vision. Wearing a wide-brimmed hat or visor is another easy way to protect the eyes.

## SMOKING

Smoking has been proposed as a possible cause of both cataracts and macular degeneration. Although not entirely consistent, most studies have found a link between smoking and each of these diseases. In the Nurses' Health Study, when we assessed the link between cataracts and smoking, we found that the heaviest smokers—those who had smoked the most cigarettes throughout their lives—had a 60 percent greater risk of the disease than nonsmokers. Although it is unclear exactly how smoking might cause cataracts, it may be that substances in tobacco smoke cause oxidation in the lens. Stopping smoking helps, but any healing takes a long time. Women in the Nurses' Health Study who stopped smoking had a 20 percent lower risk of developing cataracts than current smokers, but their risk was still higher than those who had never smoked, even twenty-five years after quitting.

When we assessed macular degeneration, we found that smoking was related to a moderate to large increase in risk for both current and past smokers. The more a woman smokes, the greater the increase in risk. Whether the increased risk declines after quitting is uncertain; what is clear is that if any decline in risk does occur, it takes many years.

## WEIGHT

Cataracts and macular degeneration are among the many adverse consequences of being overweight. Carrying excess weight can substantially increase the risk of having high blood sugar and insulin levels. When too much sugar is supplied to the eye, it can literally sugarcoat the proteins of the lens, making them opaque. In the Nurses' Health Study, we found that women who were overweight were more likely to develop cataracts than those who were lean.

A similar link has been observed in several studies of age-related macular degeneration. Excess weight often causes cholesterol levels to head in unhealthy directions, a trend that can lead to clogged arteries in the heart and elsewhere. Cholesterol-clogged arteries in the eye or leading to it may increase the risk of macular degeneration.

## ANTIOXIDANTS

Eating a diet rich in antioxidants may lower the risk of cataracts and macular degeneration. Antioxidants are a special group of vitamins and minerals that counter damage done to the cells by free radicals. Common antioxidants include vitamin C, vitamin E, and beta-carotene (the substance that gives carrots and pumpkins their orange color).

Two antioxidants that accumulate in the eye, lutein and zeaxanthin, seem to provide protection against age-related eye diseases. In the Nurses' Heath Study, women who got the most lutein and zeaxanthin in their diets were 20 percent less likely to need a cataract removed than those who got the least. These particular antioxidants can be found abundantly in dark green leafy vegetables such as spinach and kale. At least one study has suggested that lutein and zeaxanthin may also provide protection against macular degeneration; however, additional research is needed to confirm this. Because of remaining uncertainty about these relationships, and because other antioxidants may also protect against free radical damage in the eye, a woman's best insurance is to eat a variety of fruits and vegetables.

Although it may seem easier to take a vitamin pill instead of eating more fruits and vegetables, the vitamin pill will not necessarily provide the same benefits. Studies, including the Nurses' Health Study, that have examined the use of specific vitamin supplements and risk of age-related eye diseases have not consistently found a link between the two.

## MEAT AND FISH

In the Nurses' Health Study, we found that eating less animal fat and more fish might lower the risk of macular degeneration. This is the first report of a possible link between meat, fish, and macular degeneration and thus needs to be confirmed in other studies.

## Age-Related Eye Diseases: What It All Means

Protecting your eyesight from age-related conditions such as cataracts and macular degeneration is relatively easy. Wear sunglasses and a visor or hat when you are outside. If you smoke, try to quit as soon as possible. Keep your weight in the healthy range, and eat plenty of fruits and vegetables.

## ALZHEIMER'S DISEASE

### Background

When our grandmothers were young, few women lived long enough to experience the frightening condition known as Alzheimer's disease. Thanks to safer childbirth, the development of antibiotics and vaccines, and a host of improvements in public health and clinical medicine, the average sixty-five-year-old woman can now expect to live another twenty years. During those added years, however, the risk of Alzheimer's disease steadily increases.

Mental function doesn't invariably decline with age. In fact, things like numerical skills and spatial orientation actually improve with age, peaking around age sixty. Short-term memory does tend to taper off beginning in middle age. Occasional forgetfulness—losing your keys, blanking on a name or phone number—is *not* Alzheimer's disease. It may be aggravating, but it shouldn't be a concern unless it becomes routine and is sometimes accompanied by sudden mood swings, irritability, depression, or other behavioral changes.

There are several types of dementia, with Alzheimer's disease being one of the most common. The other common type of dementia is caused by multiple small strokes and has different characteristics from Alzheimer's. True Alzheimer's disease erases memory progressively and irreversibly, changes behavior and personality, destroys language skills, and in its terminal stage may eradicate the ability to walk or chew. The pace and intensity of Alzheimer's varies from person to person, progressing rapidly in some and slowly in others. It may wipe out memory completely, or it may lead to only modest memory loss after several years, with little loss of old skills or memories.

While researchers haven't yet pinned down exactly what causes Alzheimer's disease, we know that it occurs in the part of the brain known as the basal forebrain. It has its greatest impact on the hippocampus, a seahorse-shaped region of the brain that is active in converting information into long-term memory (see Figure 14-3). The disease also involves other regions of the brain, especially the outer cerebral cortex, the seat of language and reasoning. The biological hallmarks of Alzheimer's disease are dense protein deposits called plaques, which cluster between nerve cells in the brain, and twisted strands of fiber called tangles, which can be found inside brain cells.

Today, an estimated 4 million Americans have Alzheimer's disease, and two-thirds of them are women. Current projections show that each year in the United States, 360,000 people are newly diagnosed with Alzheimer's disease.

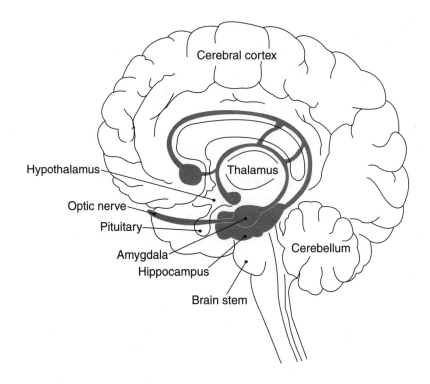

FIG. 14-3. In Alzheimer's disease, brain cells die and neuronal connections wither in all parts of the brain but especially in the hippocampus and the amygdala, important parts of the limbic system that coordinate memory storage and recall, and the cerebral cortex, the seat of higher-level thinking, memory, and language.

While some drugs have shown promise for slowing the spread of Alzheimer's disease, there's currently no cure for it. Is prevention an option? Maybe. There are indications that a healthy lifestyle may help. In addition, a number of tactics, including postmenopausal hormones, aspirin, antioxidant vitamins, and a variety of "use it or lose it" strategies are being tested as possible preventive strategies.

## Factors You Cannot Control

### AGE

The most important factor linked to Alzheimer's disease is unquestionably age. Only a small percentage of Alzheimer's cases occur among people in their fifties, and most of these people are genetically predisposed to the disease. The large majority of cases occur in those over age sixty. Alzheimer's disease affects

5 to 10 percent of people over age sixty-five and up to half of those over age eighty-five. These percentages are for men and women combined and are even higher for women alone.

## GENES

As is true for most diseases, genes play a complex role in the development of Alzheimer's disease. Specific mutations have been linked with familial Alzheimer's disease, a relatively rare form that affects people at younger ages and accounts for less than 10 percent of Alzheimer's cases. Other genes are involved in the more common form of Alzheimer's disease, which generally affects those over age sixty. One top contender is a gene that codes for a protein called amyloid precursor protein. Fragments of this protein, which are called beta-amyloid, make up the clumps of plaque that appear in the brains of people with Alzheimer's disease. Another leading candidate is a family of genes called APOE. Inheriting different forms of APOE can raise or lower a woman's risk of developing Alzheimer's disease.

People whose parents or siblings have Alzheimer's disease often wonder if they should be tested for these Alzheimer's-linked genes. Most experts do not recommend testing, in large part because there are not yet effective strategies for preventing Alzheimer's disease. If ongoing research eventually points to ways that people with a genetic predisposition can prevent Alzheimer's disease, or at least slow its progression, then testing would make sense.

### Factors You Can Control

## DIABETES

There is some evidence that poorly controlled diabetes increases the risk of developing Alzheimer's disease and other types of dementia. Diabetes has long been known to cause poor circulation to the hands and feet. If the same thing happens to the brain, the reduced blood flow could hinder brain function and cause mental decline. The high levels of blood sugar that are a characteristic of diabetes could also promote the onset or progression of Alzheimer's disease in two ways: by speeding the deposition of beta-amyloid around brain cells and by stabilizing the protein fibers that make up tangles inside brain cells.

## POSTMENOPAUSAL HORMONES

As we have described throughout this book, estrogen plays many nonreproductive roles in the body. While we are not yet certain exactly what estrogen does in the brain, it's apparent from animal studies that it has some task in mental function. Estrogen receptors are present in many kinds of brain cells, including those in the hippocampus and cerebral cortex. It improves blood flow in diseased blood vessels, including those in the brain, and also stimulates the growth of nerve-to-nerve connections.

These biological observations suggest that taking estrogen could prevent Alzheimer's disease or slow its progression. Data from epidemiologic studies, however, do not show a consistent pattern. A number of preliminary studies show that women who use postmenopausal hormones gain protection against Alzheimer's disease.

To look at the possible effects of estrogen on the memories of healthy women, we telephoned more than 2,000 women in the Nurses' Health Study between the ages of seventy and seventy-eight and asked them if they would be willing to take four simple memory and mental function tests by phone. As ever, the response was overwhelmingly positive. Overall, women who were using postmenopausal hormones or had done so in the past did not score any better on these tests than women who had never used hormones. The only difference was that women on hormones had slightly better verbal skills. In the future, we plan to further evaluate the influence of estrogen on Alzheimer's disease.

More information on estrogen and the brain is also on the horizon from other studies. For example, one very large trial is the ongoing Women's Health Initiative. The memory study of this trial includes 8,000 women, half of whom are taking estrogen pills and half of whom are taking placebo pills. Results from this trial are expected in 2006. Similar trials of antioxidant vitamins, folic acid, and aspirin in the prevention of cognitive decline are in progress.

## Mental Exercise

A popular myth is that each of us is born with a certain number of brain cells and that we lose about 10,000 to 100,000 of them a day. However, this is not true. New technology shows that even older adults make new brain cells and new connections between existing cells.

Just as women can strengthen their muscles through regular exercise, they can also "strengthen" their brains. Exactly what kinds of mental gymnastics will accomplish this is still an open question. But studies of older people who stay mentally active—by reading, pursuing hobbies or activities, playing an instrument, doing crossword puzzles, or learning a new skill—show that they are less likely to develop Alzheimer's disease than those whose activities are more mentally passive. Several studies have shown that higher education appears to offer protection, although it is not yet known whether this is merely a marker for continued use of the mind throughout life.

## PHYSICAL ACTIVITY

Despite its diminutive size, the brain uses about one-fifth of the oxygen that a woman breathes. Some studies suggest that a diminished blood supply to the brain is part of the cause of Alzheimer's disease. Giving one's body a daily workout strengthens the heart, lungs, and circulatory system and makes them more efficient at oxygenating and pumping blood. It helps prevent, or at least slow, the formation of cholesterol-laden, artery-narrowing plaque. It also helps control blood sugar and blood pressure. By keeping blood flow steady and strong, physical activity may also keep the brain healthy and the memory intact.

### Alzheimer's Disease: What It All Means

Since the mid-1980s, the MacArthur Foundation Studies of Successful Aging have been redefining the aging process. These studies show that an interplay of physical and mental factors determine who will maintain memory and mental function. The four most important factors are regular physical activity, higher or ongoing education, good lung function (and an improved supply of oxygen to the brain), and feelings of control over what life has to offer. Other strategies may emerge down the road, as researchers test the impact of antioxidants like vitamin E, anti-inflammatory drugs like aspirin and ibuprofen, postmenopausal hormones, and dietary factors like the amounts and types of dietary fat.

For right now, though, no one knows exactly how to lower the risk of Alzheimer's disease. The best bet is to adopt or stick with a healthy lifestyle. That strategy clearly helps prevent cardiovascular disease, a variety of cancers, and other chronic diseases.

## WHAT I TELL MY PATIENTS ABOUT ASTHMA, ARTHRITIS, AGE-RELATED EYE DISEASE, AND ALZHEIMER'S DISEASE

DR. CAROL BATES

Many of my patients are concerned about their quality of life as they get older, and when we talk about this, topics such as arthritis, cataracts, and Alzheimer's disease invariably come up in the conversation. Although these conditions have long been seen as an inevitable part of aging, research now suggests that they don't have to be: you can lower your risk to some extent through the same healthy behaviors you use to lower your risk of cancer, heart disease, and osteoporosis.

- **Stop smoking.** If you currently smoke, this is the single most important step you can take to improve your overall health. In addition to its many important health benefits, quitting smoking can lower your child's risk of asthma and possibly your own risk of rheumatoid arthritis, cataracts, and macular degeneration.
- **Maintain a healthy weight.** Asthma, osteoarthritis, and age-related eye disease are among the many possible consequences of being overweight. The best way to maintain a healthy weight—or lose weight if you are currently overweight—is to exercise regularly and eat a healthy diet.
- **Be physically active.** I recommend that all of my patients be active on a daily basis, even if it just means going for a few short walks throughout the day. Among the many mental and physical benefits of daily activity is a decreased risk of asthma, arthritis, and possibly Alzheimer's disease.
- **Eat a healthy diet.** When my patients ask me about the latest diet, I tell them to stick with what we know: eat a variety of grains, fruits, and vegetables every day, and cut down on saturated fat.
- **Protect yourself from the sun.** When you're in the sun, you need to protect not only your skin, but also your eyes. Too much sunlight can raise your risk of macular degeneration, and you can lower this risk by simply wearing sunglasses and a hat.
- **Make an informed decision about whether to use hormones.** Birth control pills and postmenopausal hormones can have a variety of effects on your health, some good and some not. Talk to your health care provider about these effects, so that you can make the decision that is right for you.

Many of my patients ask me whether postmenopausal hormones will affect their risk of Alzheimer's disease. I tell them that the current data are too inconsistent for me to answer that. I'm waiting for information from ongoing studies before I recommend estrogen specifically for the treatment or prevention of dementia.

# PART THREE

# Changing Behaviors

# CHAPTER FIFTEEN

# Physical Activity

---

## Key Lifestyle Message

- Being physically active is one of the best ways to improve your overall health and quality of life.

---

## BACKGROUND

"No pain, no gain" is a phrase you hear frequently. But is it true that you can lose weight or improve health only by putting yourself through grueling workouts? Current federal guidelines suggest otherwise: weary bodies and sore muscles are not prerequisites for achieving the many health-related benefits of physical activity. All it takes is a minimum of thirty minutes of brisk walking a day (or the equivalent). This level of moderate activity is recommended for all women and has been shown to lower the risk of cardiovascular disease, diabetes, and some types of cancer. If you choose to do more than this minimum amount, you will most likely gain even greater benefit.

### What Is Physical Activity?

Physical activity consists of any movement that substantially increases the amount of calories you burn in a day (also called energy expenditure). Walking, gardening, washing the car, dancing, raking, swimming, and jogging are all types of physical activity. However, as most people know, not all activities burn the same amount of calories. Activities that require modest energy expenditure and therefore burn fewer calories per hour are considered light or moderate, while those that burn more calories per hour are considered to be vigorous. Examples of each type are listed on page 276.

You can burn the same amount of calories doing moderate activity for an extended period of time as you can doing vigorous activity for a shorter duration. For example, you can burn 150 calories by either running hard for fifteen

| Light activity | Moderate activity | Vigorous activity |
| --- | --- | --- |
| Walking at less than 3 mph | Walking briskly at 3 to 5 mph | Race walking |
| Golf, using a cart | Golf, carrying clubs | Stair climbing |
| Cycling at less than 6 mph | Cycling 6 to 9 mph | Cycling 10 or more mph |
| Pruning or weeding | Raking the lawn | Pushing a nonmotorized lawn mower |
| Dusting or sweeping | Scrubbing floors or vacuuming | Carrying heavy loads |
| Shuffleboard | Competitive volleyball | Jogging or running |
| Bowling | Badminton | Backpacking |
| Boating | Canoeing | Competitive rowing |
| Playing catch | Weight training | Calisthenics (pushups, situps) |
| Table tennis | Doubles tennis | Singles tennis |
| Yoga | Ballroom dancing | Aerobic or fast dancing |
| Tai chi | Skiing downhill, light effort | Karate or judo |
| Coaching | Recreational swimming | Lap swimming |

minutes, raking leaves for thirty minutes, or playing recreational volleyball for forty-five minutes (see Figure 15-1)

## What Is Exercise?

Physical activity that is planned, structured, and done specifically to improve your physical fitness is considered exercise. There are three basic types: aerobic exercise, flexibility exercise, and strength training. Aerobic exercise, such as jogging, brisk walking, or swimming, improves cardiovascular fitness by con-

## Physical Activity: The Larger Picture

- Less strenuous activities, when performed for longer periods of time, are just as beneficial as vigorous activities.
- All women should get at least thirty minutes of moderate activity a day.
- Brisk walking, recreational swimming, canoeing, vacuuming, and weight training are all good examples of moderate-intensity activity.

## Minutes of Activity Required to Burn 150 Calories

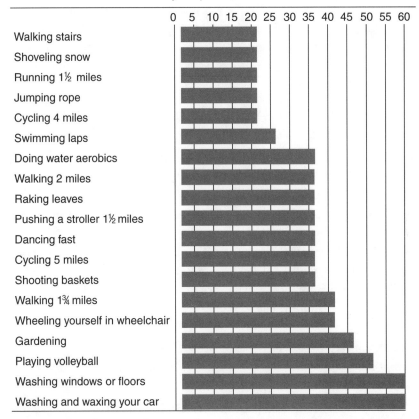

FIG. 15-1. Number of Minutes of Activity to Burn 150 Calories. (Source: U.S. Dept. of Health and Human Services)

ditioning your heart and lungs to provide oxygen to your muscles. Flexibility exercises stretch your muscles, thereby improving your ability to recover from exercise. Often incorporated into warmup and cooldown routines, these exercises help prevent muscle strain. Finally, strength training involves working your muscles against some form of resistance, which can help preserve bone mass, improve strength and balance, and increase muscle mass. Strength training may also improve insulin metabolism, since it increases the proportion of muscle in your body relative to the proportion of fat.

Despite America's supposed obsession with muscle tone and exercise, sedentary lifestyles have become the norm. Less than 20 percent of all women participate in physical activity for at least thirty minutes five times a week, as recommended by the Surgeon General, and only a quarter of all women report that they are active in their leisure time. Due to technological advances, it is no longer necessary to be active on the job, and people rely increasingly on their cars, even if their destinations are within walking or bicycling distance. This shift toward inactivity contributes substantially to society's overall burden of disease and may increase your own personal risk of illness, disability, and premature death.

## LESSONS FROM THE NURSES' HEALTH STUDY AND OTHER STUDIES

The relationship between health and physical activity was noted as early as the fifth century B.C.E., when Hippocrates wrote, "Eating alone will not keep a man well; he must also take exercise. For food and exercise, while possessing opposite qualities, yet work together to produce health." Although achieving the delicate balance between physical activity and diet continues to elude many people, it is now clear that activity alone has a vast impact on women's health. This means that regardless of your diet or weight, you can benefit greatly from engaging in regular physical activity. Strive for a minimum of thirty minutes of brisk walking a day (or the equivalent).

---

*In the Nurses' Own Words . . .*

At first, when I was enrolled in the study, I didn't appreciate its value. The form was just something I filled out once every two years, often working very hard to estimate with any degree of honesty just how many carrots I ate weekly! As I have matured in my professional life, I appreciate more and more the importance of this work. Too often women have been excluded from studies. We are very complex. It makes such sense to study a large population and see what happens to us. I am now happy to be part of the study and look forward to reading the results. The study becomes very important when I fill out the form. Then I wish I had eaten more carrots! Filling out the form is now an introspective act, where I pause and reflect on my life habits and wonder where they will lead me as I age. And I think that being part of the study is one more thing I do that keeps me conscious about my life habits and, hopefully, on track for a long and healthy life.

—From ASL

## The Benefits of Physical Activity
### WEIGHT CONTROL

Most women gain about one pound a year between the ages of thirty-seven to sixty-four. Though this may seem inconsequential, the accumulation of small weight gains over time can lead to excess body weight, which has serious health consequences. By engaging in regular physical activity, women can prevent such cumulative weight gains and possibly even lose weight.

In the Nurses' Health Study, we looked at how changes in physical activity over a two-year period affected changes in weight. We found that, among nonsmokers, women who became more active during the study period lost or maintained their weight, while those who became less active gained weight. Women who added at least twenty minutes of moderate activity to their daily schedules (or thirty minutes of walking) lost an average of 2.25 pounds over two years, depending on their weight at the beginning of the study. Lean women lost an average of 0.2 pounds, overweight women 1.4 pounds, and obese women 2.3 pounds. These results suggest that changes in physical activity have an immediate though fairly small impact on body weight.

Physical activity may also minimize the weight gain that typically occurs when people stop smoking. In a two-year period of the Nurses' Health Study, women who quit smoking gained about 5 pounds more than those who continued smoking. However, women who became more active when they stopped smoking gained less weight than those who quit smoking but did not change their activity level. The more active women became, the less weight they gained after quitting smoking.

Physical activity can also play an important role in maintaining weight loss. In a study of women who had previously lost weight, regular physical activity was reported by 90 percent of those who maintained their weight loss and by only 34 percent of those who did not.

### IMPROVED MENTAL HEALTH

For centuries, people have speculated that physical activity might improve mental health, but only in the past thirty years has there been scientific evidence to support this. Numerous studies have shown that physical activity can be as effective as psychotherapy, relaxation, and meditation at helping women cope with stress and depression. In one study, researchers found that women responded better to stressful tasks after being active than after resting quietly. Though this particular study demonstrated the immediate benefits of activity, several others have shown there to be long-term benefits as well. For example, in a small randomized controlled trial, adults suffering from depression were asked to adhere to a twelve-week program of either psychotherapy or running. One year after the completion of the program, those who had been assigned to running had lower levels of depression than those who had been assigned to psychotherapy.

Although the release of endorphins is often cited as the reason that activity improves mental health, there are a variety of other possibilities. First, physical activity provides a time-out from the stresses of everyday life, and this can obviously lead women to feel more relaxed and less anxious. Second, being active has been shown to enhance self-efficacy (or confidence in one's ability to do things), which can counter feelings of depression and anxiety. Finally, women are often active in social settings, such as health clubs or walking groups, and social interaction is known to promote psychological well-being.

## Physical Activity and Mental Well-Being

Physical activity does much to lower the risk of chronic disease, but many women engage in activity for a more obvious reason: it makes them feel good. Being active:

- Leads to greater satisfaction with weight and overall appearance
- Improves energy levels
- Helps women sleep more soundly
- Enhances mood
- Helps women cope with stress, anxiety, and depression

### LOWER BLOOD PRESSURE

Physical activity can help lower blood pressure in several ways. First, the blood vessels dilate (or enlarge) during physical activity, allowing blood to flow through the arteries more readily. Second, activity helps remove low density lipoproteins ("bad cholesterol") from the artery walls, thus widening them. Finally, activity can help with weight loss, which can in turn lower blood pressure.

Several controlled trials have demonstrated the efficacy of physical activity in lowering blood pressure. In one trial, high blood pressure, or hypertension, was successfully lowered among women who participated in moderate physical activity for twelve weeks. In a similar study, women with hypertension were assigned to a twelve-week program of either moderate aerobic activity or tai chi. At the end of the program, both groups of women had substantially lower blood pressure, which suggests that even low-intensity activity may be beneficial.

## IMPROVED CHOLESTEROL LEVELS

Regular physical activity may influence the amount of high density lipoprotein (HDL) cholesterol that a woman has in her blood. HDL cholesterol, the "good cholesterol," keeps low density lipoproteins, "bad cholesterol," from building up in the arteries and causing atherosclerosis.

Several studies have shown that active women tend to have higher levels of HDL than sedentary women. In one such study, conducted among female recreational runners, researchers found that HDL levels increased steadily with the number of miles women ran per week. Similar results have been reported for low intensity activity. In a randomized controlled trial, sedentary women were assigned to participate in one of three walking programs. Each program lasted for twenty-four weeks and had a slightly different walking pace. By the end of the trial, women in all three programs had substantially higher HDL levels than women who had remained sedentary.

## LOWER RISK OF CARDIOVASCULAR DISEASE

Cardiovascular disease is the leading cause of death among women, killing twice as many women each year as all cancers combined. Characterized by the buildup of cholesterol and fat in the arteries, cardiovascular disease occurs when the arteries become too narrow, blocking the flow of blood. This group of diseases includes coronary heart disease and stroke and is often preceded by hypertension and high blood cholesterol. By lowering blood pressure and increasing the level of HDL cholesterol in the blood, physical activity can substantially lower the risk of cardiovascular disease.

*Lower Risk of Coronary Heart Disease.* Coronary heart disease is the most common form of cardiovascular disease, occurring when blood flow is interrupted in the arteries that feed the heart. Although more than forty epidemiologic studies have examined the benefits of physical activity on heart disease, only about a quarter have included women. These few studies have been remarkably consistent in demonstrating that physical activity is as protective in women as it is in men, reducing the risk of heart disease by as much as 50 percent.

The Nurses' Health Study has made several important contributions to this area of research. We have shown that women need not train for marathons or spend hours at a health club in order to lower their risk of heart disease.

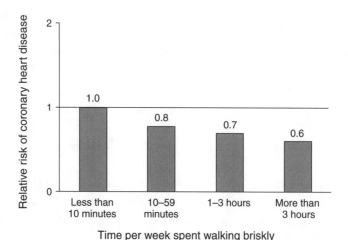

FIG. 15-2. Women who walk at a brisk pace (more than 3 miles per hour) for at least one hour a week receive moderate protection against coronary heart disease. (Source: Nurses' Health Study)

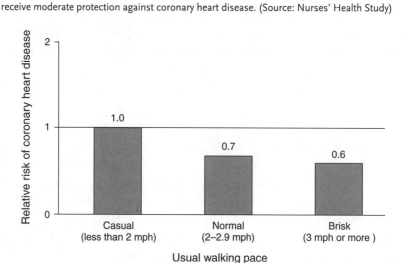

FIG. 15-3. Women who usually walk at a brisk pace are about half as likely to develop heart disease as women who usually walk at a more casual pace. (Source: Nurses' Health Study)

They can accomplish this simply by walking more often and at a faster pace (Figures 15-2 and 15-3). Women who walk briskly for at least three hours a week receive the same amount of protection against heart disease as women who exercise vigorously for an hour and a half a week. Both groups are 30 to 40 percent less likely to develop heart disease than women who are sedentary. Our study has also demonstrated that it is never too late to reap the benefits of a physically active lifestyle. Sedentary women who become active have a lower

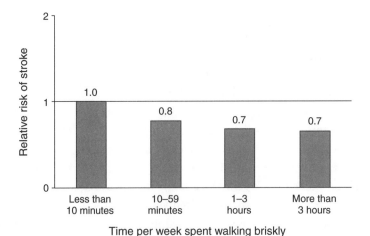

FIG. 15-4. Women who walk at a brisk pace (more than 3 miles per hour) for at least one hour a week receive moderate protection against stroke. (Source: Nurses' Health Study)

risk of heart disease than those who remain sedentary. The more active the women become, the lower their risk.

*Lower Risk of Stroke.* Characterized by the blockage of blood flow to the brain, stroke is one of the leading causes of death and permanent disability in the United States. Though only a few studies have assessed the impact of physical activity on women's risk of stroke, these studies have consistently shown that even modest amounts of activity can be beneficial. In the Nurses' Health Study, we found that walking briskly for at least one hour a week offered moderate protection against stroke (see Figure 15-4). Women who walked at even quicker paces had further reductions in risk.

## LOWER RISK OF DIABETES

Physical activity may lower the risk of adult-onset diabetes (type 2 diabetes) in two ways. First, overweight women are more likely to develop adult-onset diabetes than women at a healthy weight, and activity is an effective means of weight control and weight reduction. Second, adult-onset diabetes occurs when the pancreas does not produce enough insulin or when the body does not effectively use the insulin that is produced. Physical activity can improve the body's response to insulin and thereby lower the risk of diabetes.

The Nurses' Health Study has helped confirm what many other studies have previously found—that physical activity provides moderate protection against adult-onset diabetes. We have examined this relationship in great detail and have made several important findings. First, regardless of how much a woman weighs, she can reduce her risk of diabetes by being physically active. This is extremely important for overweight women, who have a greatly increased risk of diabetes and can thus benefit most from the protection offered by activity. Second, women who are sedentary can lower their risk of diabetes by becoming more active. Although a large increase in activity provides the most protection, even a very modest increase will offer some protection. Finally, if it is done for an extended period of time each week, walking can be as protective against diabetes as vigorous activity. In the Nurses' Health Study, women who walked briskly for three hours a week reduced their risk of diabetes as much as women who exercised vigorously for an hour and a half a week. The more time women spent walking, and the faster they walked, the less likely they were to develop the disease (see Figure 15-5). Taken collectively, these findings are encouraging. They suggest that, regardless of a woman's current weight or activity level, she can lower her risk of adult-onset diabetes by walking more frequently—or more quickly.

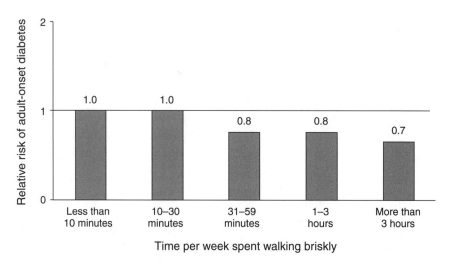

FIG. 15-5. Women who walk at a brisk pace (more than 3 miles per hour) for at least three hours a week receive moderate protection against adult-onset (type 2) diabetes. (Source: Nurses' Health Study)

## Lower Risk of Colon Cancer

Colon cancer (or cancer of the large bowel) is one of the most preventable forms of cancer, yet it is also one of the most common, affecting nearly 52,000 American women each year. In the past two decades, scientists have identified many factors linked to colon cancer and have found physical activity to be

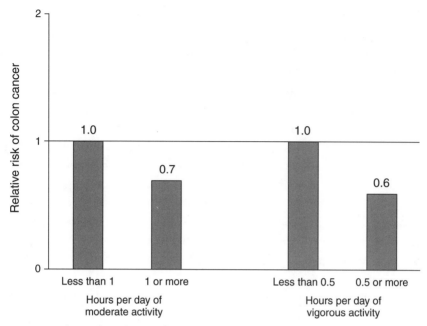

FIG. 15-6. Moderate physical activity for an hour a day provides about the same protection against colon cancer as vigorous activity for half an hour a day. (Source: Nurses' Health Study)

among the most important. There are at least two possible reasons for this. First, when a woman is physically active, waste moves through her bowels more quickly; this may reduce the exposure of the colon wall to any carcinogens in the waste. Second, physical activity may lower the level of blood insulin, which in high amounts may stimulate abnormal cell growth in the colon.

In the Nurses' Health Study, we found that physical activity cut women's risk of colon cancer in half. We also found that walking can be as effective in preventing colon cancer as vigorous activity. Walking at a normal to brisk pace for an hour a day provides the same amount of protection as doing more vigorous activity, like jogging, cycling, or swimming, for half an hour a day (see Figure 15-6).

## LOWER RISK OF OSTEOPOROSIS

Osteoporosis occurs when the bones in the body lose mass and become so brittle that they are prone to fracture. Physical activity is a well-established means of protecting against this condition. When a woman is physically active, it places mechanical stress on her bones, forcing the tissue to absorb calcium and become stronger. In this way, physical activity directly promotes the building of bone. However, it also strengthens the bone tissue indirectly by stimulating the muscles that surround bone tissue. As these muscles become larger and stronger, they place increasing pressure on the bone. This pressure stimulates the bone tissue to absorb calcium and grow in strength. Remember, however, that the only bones protected by physical activity are those that are stressed during the activity. For example, walking will place stress on the bones of the spine and hips but not the wrists.

Numerous studies have shown that being active early in life can have a long-term effect in preventing osteoporosis. This is because activity during childhood promotes the accumulation of bone mass—and the more bone that is accrued early, the lower the chance of osteoporosis later. In one study, bone mass was higher among women who had participated in sports during their childhood than among women who had not. While this evidence is reassuring for women who exercised as children, it need not be frightening for those who did not: being active in adulthood can also prevent osteoporosis by slowing the rate of bone loss.

While most studies have shown that weight training and vigorous activity (like running) are the most effective activities for preventing osteoporosis and subsequent fractures, recent data suggest that walking might be just as beneficial. In a large study conducted among women over age sixty-five, researchers found a 30 percent reduction in the risk of hip fracture among those who walked for exercise compared to those who did not. The farther women walked, the lower their risk. Several small, randomized controlled trials have supported these results, showing greater bone mass among women who walked than among women who were sedentary.

Although physical activity has a beneficial effect on bone for most women, engaging in too much strenuous activity can lead to dangerously low levels of estrogen and subsequent bone loss. Such low levels of estrogen are indicated by the absence of menstrual periods in women who have not yet reached menopause.

## PROBABLE LOWER RISK OF BREAST CANCER

A woman's risk of breast cancer depends largely on the amount of estrogen circulating in her body. Because active women tend to have lower estrogen levels than sedentary women, researchers have long speculated that physical activity might lower the risk of breast cancer. However, numerous studies have examined this possibility, and the results to date have been somewhat inconsistent.

In the Nurses' Health Study, the effect of physical activity varied, depending on whether women had gone through menopause. For postmenopausal women, activity appeared to offer modest protection: those who were active for at least one hour a day had a 15 to 20 percent reduction in the risk of breast cancer. For premenopausal women, however, there was no link between physical activity and the risk of breast cancer. This is in contrast to a number of other studies, which have shown that activity lowers the risk of breast cancer in both pre- and postmenopausal women.

## POSSIBLE LOWER RISK OF ASTHMA

Low levels of physical activity appear to be related to an increased risk of asthma, though the reason for this is not yet clear. One possibility is that sedentary people spend more time indoors and are thus exposed to things that trigger asthma, like molds, dander, and dust. Alternatively, regular activity may strengthen the muscles around the airways, making them less responsive to these triggers.

For some people, being active actually provokes asthma. An asthma management plan that includes warmup and cooldown sessions and the use of medications before exercising can help prevent these attacks.

## POSSIBLE LOWER RISK OF ALZHEIMER'S DISEASE

Physical activity may lower the risk of Alzheimer's disease by improving the flow of blood and oxygen to the brain. Additional studies are needed to confirm this.

## The Risks of Physical Activity

Although the benefits of physical activity are well established, there are risks to consider as well. A variety of adverse health effects have been associated with physical activity, including injuries, irregular menstrual cycles, and sudden cardiac events.

## INCREASED RISK OF INJURY

The risk of injury depends largely on the type of activity being done and how often and intensely it is performed. Women who participate in activities that require repetitive motion often suffer from overuse injuries. For example, women who engage in overhead sports, like swimming, tennis, and baseball, may suffer from shoulder problems, whereas runners tend to have foot, ankle, and knee injuries. The risk of these types of injuries can be reduced by stretching the muscles sufficiently before and after exercising.

Activity-related injuries can also be caused by roadway accidents. Women who walk, run, bike, or skate may be injured in collisions with motor vehicles or in falls that result from uneven road surfaces.

## IRREGULAR MENSTRUAL CYCLES

At some point in their lives, most women will experience an irregular menstrual cycle. However, women who are extremely active (e.g., marathon runners) may experience such irregularities more frequently. Several studies have shown that female athletes have higher rates of amenorrhea, a disorder characterized by the absence of menstrual periods for six or more months in a woman who has not yet gone through menopause. When a woman misses her menstrual periods for such an extended period of time, it means that she is not ovulating and has low levels of circulating estrogen. This can impair fertility and may lead to a decrease in bone mass. Notably, we found in the Nurses' Health Study that moderate (rather than strenuous) activity may actually lower the risk of infertility, perhaps in part by helping women to maintain a healthy weight.

## INCREASED RISK OF SUDDEN CARDIAC EVENTS

Though rare, heavy physical exertion can trigger chest pain and heart attacks, particularly in people who are habitually sedentary and sporadically engage in vigorous activity. Women who maintain a regular exercise program are much less likely to experience sudden cardiac events and, as noted above, have a much lower risk of coronary heart disease and stroke. The risk of exercise-induced cardiac events can be reduced by not undertaking physical activities that are well beyond one's normal level of exertion.

## How Physical Activity Affects Length and Quality of Life

Women who participate in regular physical activity tend to live longer than women who are sedentary. This has been confirmed in three of the largest ongoing studies of women's health: the Nurses' Health Study, the Iowa Women's Health Study, and the Framingham Heart Study. Regardless of their weight, active women were less likely than sedentary women to die during a sixteen-year period of the Nurses' Health Study. Those who participated in moderate activity for at least one hour a week had a slight reduction in mortality risk, while those who participated for more than seven hours a week had a moderate reduction in risk (see Figure 15-7). We observed a protective effect even among women whose only activity was walking for one hour a week.

Of course, there is more to long life than simply added years. Quality of life during those years is also important, and physical activity has been shown to

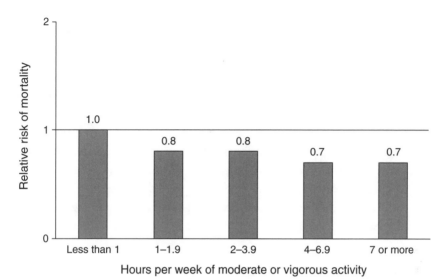

FIG. 15-7. Women who were active at least four hours a week were 30 percent less likely to die during a sixteen-year period of the Nurses' Health Study. (Source: Nurses' Health Study)

## Physical Activity: Weighing the Risks and Benefits

Women who are active tend to live longer than women who are sedentary. This is because they have a lower risk of:

- Weight gain
- Coronary heart disease
- Stroke
- Diabetes
- Colon cancer
- Osteoporosis
- Probably breast cancer

Although physical activity occasionally has its risks (namely injuries, menstrual irregularities, and cardiac events), overall it is far more beneficial than it is dangerous.

play a positive role. Active women tend to have higher self-esteem and a greater sense of well-being than sedentary women. They are also better able to perform the tasks that make up their daily lives, which is essential to maintaining independence, particularly as they get older.

## WHAT IT ALL MEANS

Being physically active is one of the best ways to improve your overall health and quality of life. Although there are risks associated with activity, they are far outweighed by the long-term health benefits. Physical activity can prolong life and lower your risk of heart disease, stroke, diabetes, colon cancer, and osteoporosis. To achieve these benefits, you need only to engage in moderate activity, like brisk walking, for at least thirty minutes a day. Walking is already the most common form of exercise among American women and appears to be as protective against disease as more vigorous activities, like jogging and tennis. While all women could benefit from becoming more active than they currently are, the greatest gain to be had is by those who are currently sedentary.

## WHAT I TELL MY PATIENTS ABOUT PHYSICAL ACTIVITY

DR. CELESTE ROBB-NICHOLSON

Most of my patients know that they should exercise more. They've read articles about the benefits of physical activity, or they've heard the advice before: try to do at least thirty minutes of moderate exercise a day. But they don't have the time. Or they've tried taking up exercise, only to get sore and discouraged. Or their children need their attention. Or they're so rushed at the beginning of the day—or so tired at the end of it—that they can't possibly think of doing anything more. Perhaps you have faced similar challenges. If so, this is the advice I give my patients, and it may help you as well.

1. **Think of activity as something you incorporate into your everyday routine.** Time is a precious commodity for most women. Many of us work, take care of children, run households, and have relationships. Who has time to exercise?

The Surgeon General recommends that we do a moderate physical activity for at least thirty minutes a day on most days. If you can create this block of time in your schedule, do it. But when it's just impossible, don't give up on physical activity. Try exercising for short periods of time over the course of the day. If you can be active for ten minutes at a time, three times a day, you will enjoy some of the same health benefits that come with the more extended workouts.

How do you integrate physical activity into your busy day? Here are some strategies that have worked for my patients:

- Park your car at the farthest end of the parking lot at work or at the grocery store, and walk.
- Use the stairs rather than the elevator at work.
- Take your dog for a walk.
- The next time you go to a mall, walk briskly around the perimeters. (You can window-shop at the same time.)
- Instead of doing all the housecleaning on one day, break it up into segments that you can do every day.
- Spend ten or fifteen minutes a day out in the garden.
- Rake leaves in the fall.
- Take a walk during your lunch break.
- Rent an exercise tape the next time you're in the video store, and do some exercises while you're getting ready in the morning or un-winding at night.
- Make the time you spend with your children or grandchildren active time. Shoot some baskets, ride bikes, go hiking, or throw a ball.
- Get together with a friend to walk and talk, instead of sitting down for a cup of coffee.

2. **Remember that being active will actually give you energy.** After an ex-hausting day, it can be hard to get yourself up and moving. But believe it or not, activity will actually increase your energy level—and help you get a better night's sleep.

- Schedule your activity when you feel most energetic. For example, if you know you'll be too tired at the end of the day, walk the dog in the morning or take a stroll at lunchtime.
- Convince yourself that if you give it a chance, being active will make you more energetic. Then try it!
- Invite a friend or family member to join you. Having fun or chatting can make you forget how tired you felt earlier.

3. **Remember that you don't have to be good at sports to enjoy being active.** For many of us, the idea of being physically active is closely tied to childhood memories of gym class or neighborhood games. If you weren't par-ticularly athletic then, you might not feel comfortable walking into a weight room or joining an aerobics class now. Fortunately, there are so many ways to get your daily dose of activity—such as those mentioned above—that it's al-most impossible not to find one that you feel good about doing.

**4. Take the appropriate steps to avoid injuring yourself.** If you have been relatively inactive until now, or if you've suffered an injury in the past, you may be hesitant to engage in activity. This is a normal fear, but keep in mind that you can prevent most injuries by using common sense and listening to your body.

- Nearly everyone can safely begin a moderate walking program. If you have not been active for a while and you would like to engage in more strenuous exercise, talk to your health care provider before you embark on a more active lifestyle. Begin slowly, with just enough exercise to get your muscles and joints used to the increased activity. Then slowly increase the length and intensity of the activity over time.
- No matter how physically fit you are, prepare your body for exercise by warming up your muscles and joints for at least five to ten minutes. When you are finished exercising, cool your body down by performing the same movements. Never stop suddenly; taper your intensity level gradually, and walk until your breathing rate returns to nearly normal. Cooling down after exercise helps prevent muscle cramps.
- If you have any of the following symptoms while you're exercising (or at any other time), stop and get help: chest pain or pressure; pain in the arms, neck, or jaw; light-headedness or dizziness; palpitations; nausea; blurred vision; breathlessness; or faintness.

**5. Do something you like.** Physical activity should be enjoyable. If it isn't, let's face it, you won't keep doing it. Sometimes the best way to get started and to ensure that you will build exercise into your everyday routine is to do things you look forward to. Here are some tips my patients have shared with me:

- Exercise with a friend. It takes your mind off the activity and makes the time go faster.
- Try a new form of exercise, such as tai chi (a series of gentle movements that originated in China), or go dancing with your partner.
- Listen to your favorite music while exercising. This will help you keep up the pace and will help the time pass.
- Close the door to your office for ten or fifteen minutes during the workday and do some stretching exercises. This will help keep you limber and may bring you a short period of uninterrupted peace.

**6. Reward yourself.** As you begin increasing your activity level, give yourself a treat. If you walked to the grocery store, for instance, buy yourself some flowers once you're there. As you become more active, the strength and sense of well-being that come with exercise will be your greatest rewards.

# CHAPTER SIXTEEN

# Weight Control

## Key Lifestyle Message

- Maintaining a healthy weight is one of the best things you can do for your overall health and quality of life.

## BACKGROUND

Achieving and maintaining a healthy weight should be a goal for everyone. As with many worthwhile goals, however, it poses a difficult challenge. Half of all adult women in the United States are currently overweight, and trends show that with each successive generation we are becoming an increasingly overweight society.

Such trends are disturbing, given the many health problems and societal issues associated with being overweight. Overweight individuals not only experience higher rates of chronic disorders such as heart disease, stroke, diabetes, and colon cancer, but also appear to be subject to social stigma and discrimination. One study found that, compared to women of average weight, overweight women were more likely to be single, to have a lower household income, and to experience higher rates of poverty.

But the picture is far from all bad. A great deal of evidence shows that some achievable goals can have significant health benefits. Most important, you don't need to look like a triathlete to improve your health. Both modest weight loss (as little as five pounds) and even maintaining your current weight (whether it is in the healthy range or not) can help combat the many bad effects associated with being overweight and gaining weight.

### Healthy Weight, Overweight, and Obesity

These terms are frequently used in health recommendations made to the public. But what is a healthy weight exactly, and what does it mean to be overweight or obese? As most people know, it is not weight per se that is a health concern, but the amount of body fat you carry (also known as adiposity). Studies have shown that above a certain amount, the accumulation of body fat begins to have adverse effects on health. A *healthy weight,* therefore, can be defined as one that corresponds to an amount of body fat linked with general good health; *overweight,* as a weight that corresponds to an amount of body fat linked to increasing health problems; and *obesity,* as a weight that corresponds to an amount of body fat linked to serious health problems.

Although these distinct categories are important tools for education, note that the risk of illness linked to weight usually increases on a continuum, not just when someone crosses from one category into another. As weight increases—even within the same category—the risk of health problems increases. With some disorders, such as diabetes, high blood pressure (hypertension), and high blood cholesterol, risk begins to increase substantially in the middle and upper part of the healthy weight range.

So how do you know to which category you belong? The main standards used today are cut points based on a person's body mass index, or BMI (see Appendix C, Table 2 for Body Mass Index chart). BMI is a simple calculation based on a person's weight and height. Specifically, it is one's weight (in pounds) divided by one's height (in inches) squared, with this result multiplied by 704.5. For many reasons, such as ease of measurement and its good estimate of body fat, BMI is the measure most often used in studies looking at weight and health. For these same reasons, it is also the measure used as the basis of most national weight recommendations.

The Nurses' Health Study has played an important role in helping to develop the federal weight guidelines in recent years. In 1995, and again in 1998, our data helped the federal government refine its definitions of healthy weight, overweight, and obesity. Under the 1998 federal guidelines, which differ only slightly from those of 1995, a healthy weight is a BMI between 18.5 and 24.9. Overweight is a BMI between 25 and 29.9, and obesity is 30 and over. A BMI of 25, the average for an adult American woman, is equivalent to weighing 145 pounds at five feet four or 164 pounds at five feet eight. A BMI of 30 is equivalent to weighing 174 pounds at five feet four and 197 pounds at five feet eight.

BMI is a good but not perfect estimate of how much body fat an average person carries. Certain individuals may have a high BMI but actually be fairly lean. Many muscular athletes, such as male football players or female ski racers and cyclists, fall into this category. For most of the population, however, BMI works well at classification in terms of adiposity.

## Weight Gain: Stemming the Tide

Independent of the weight category a person falls into, avoiding significant weight gain during adulthood is itself an important predictor of health. Simply avoiding significant weight gain as an adult (unless underweight in early adulthood) can have a large, positive impact on health. A useful way for most people to determine how much weight they have lost or gained as an adult is to compare their current weight with how much they weighed when they graduated from high school.

People tend to gain weight particularly during the holiday period, from mid-November to early or mid-January: a recent study found the gain to average just less than one pound. However, that pound is often not lost during the subsequent spring or summer months. Year after year, holiday time after holiday time, it adds up.

## Pear vs. Apple: The Issue of Central Adiposity

Outside of weight and weight gain, an increasing amount of research has looked into the health consequences of where people put on their extra weight. People who are apple shaped, who put on extra fat around the middle (known as central adiposity), are more likely to experience certain health problems compared to people who are pear shaped and put their extra weight in their hips and thighs.

The two measures most commonly used to assess central adiposity are waist size (waist circumference) and the ratio of waist size to hip size, known as the waist-to-hip ratio. Although waist-to-hip ratio is often used in scientific studies, waist circumference alone is becoming the preferred choice. Not only is it simpler to measure, it also seems to be just as accurate as waist-to-hip ratio in estimating central adiposity. The 1998 federal guidelines state that women with a BMI of 25 or higher who have a waist size of 35 inches or larger are at particularly high risk for health problems related to obesity.

Because the bathroom scale does not always reflect changes in body shape, women should keep track of their actual waist size over the years. The best way to do this is to stand up straight, hold one end of a tape measure at about the navel, and measure all the way around the waist (see Figure 16-1). By doing this regularly, women can accurately chart positive and negative changes to their waist size over time. This is important because women can stay the same weight, or even lose weight, and still add inches around the waist. Likewise, they can lose inches around the waist but actually put on weight—something that often happens when starting a regular exercise program.

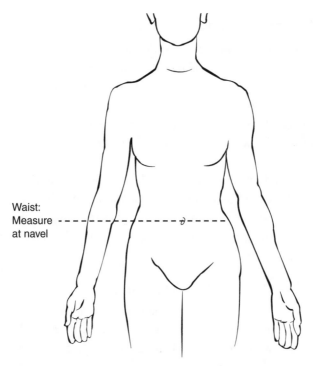

Waist:
Measure
at navel

FIG. 16-1. Accurately measuring waist size is easy. The best approach: don't wear bulky clothes, stand up straight, then hold one end of a tape measure at about the navel and measure all the way around the waist.

As the scientific evidence assessing weight and health continues to develop, the current weight and waist size guidelines may change. The results of ongoing studies like the Nurses' Health Study contribute important information to the national weight recommendations. As more knowledge is amassed on the issue, and the techniques for studying weight and health become more refined, the recommendations are revised to keep up-to-date with the science.

## LESSONS FROM THE NURSES' HEALTH STUDY AND OTHER STUDIES

The relationship between body weight and health has long been an important area of study in the scientific community. The Nurses' Health Study alone since 1976 has published over forty articles related to the topic. Overall, these studies have come to a similar conclusion: that gaining weight and being overweight are largely bad for health. The likelihood of developing coronary heart disease, stroke, diabetes, hypertension, and certain cancers is greater in over-

---

## Weight Control: The Larger Picture

- Weight has an important effect on health. Overweight individuals experience higher rates of heart disease, stroke, diabetes, and certain cancers and are also more likely to die prematurely than lean women.

- Achievable goals, such as avoiding weight gain with age and losing even ten to fifteen pounds (if overweight), can improve health significantly.

- Weight loss can also improve the quality of life of those who are overweight, increasing their ability to perform daily tasks and decreasing the amount of pain they experience.

- Body fat is a better indicator of potential health problems than weight. Therefore, body mass index (BMI), which is a good indicator of body fat, is the measure most often used in studies looking at weight and health.

- Waist size and body shape are also important indicators. Women with large waists (35 inches or more) and women who are apple shaped are more prone to health problems than those who have smaller waists or are pear shaped.

---

weight women compared to lean women. Only in the case of osteoporosis does being overweight seem to provide some protection, with rates of hip fracture in overweight women lower than in their leaner counterparts.

## The Risks of Being Overweight and Gaining Weight

### INCREASED RISK OF HYPERTENSION

Hypertension is a major risk factor for coronary heart disease and stroke. It is also exceptionally common in the United States. More than 30 million Americans have hypertension, nearly half of whom are on medication to control the disorder.

The Nurses' Health Study has confirmed what many other studies have found—that as a woman's BMI increases, so does her risk of developing hypertension. Over a sixteen-year period, we found that obese women had an extremely high risk of developing hypertension compared to women with a BMI below 20. Most notably, the risk began to increase (although very slightly) in women whose BMIs were between 20 and 21 and rose steadily as BMIs increased (see Figure 16-2).

We found a similar relationship when assessing weight gain and the risk of hypertension. Those women who had gained even small amounts as an adult (five to ten pounds) had an increased risk compared to those whose weight remained relatively stable (gained or lost less than five pounds). The

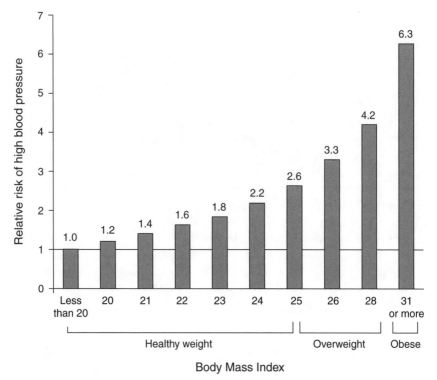

FIG. 16-2. The risk of high blood pressure (hypertension) increases as weight increases. Even women in the healthy weight range show increased risk. (Source: Nurses' Health Study)

more weight gained, the larger the risk. Those who gained fifty-five pounds or more had almost three times the risk of developing the disorder.

What the NHS has also found is that long-term weight loss can lower a woman's risk of hypertension. When we looked at this issue, we found that women who weighed ten to twenty pounds less than they did at the beginning of the study had a slightly lower risk compared to women whose weight remained steady over the same period. Women who lost more than twenty pounds were at even lower risk (see Figure 16-3).

Excessive weight may increase a woman's risk of hypertension by influencing a number of factors that can affect how the heart and blood vessels function. For example, it can promote the buildup of fluid in the circulatory system or cause certain blood vessels throughout the body to constrict, both of which can increase blood pressure. Weight loss likely reverses such conditions.

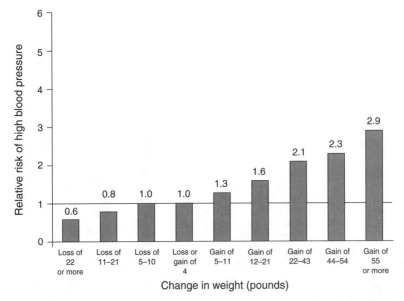

FIG. 16-3. Even a small amount of weight gain in adulthood can increase the risk of high blood pressure. Weight loss can lower the risk of the disorder. (Source: Nurses' Health Study)

## INCREASED RISK OF ADULT-ONSET DIABETES

Diabetes can contribute to a number of health problems, including coronary heart disease, stroke, blindness, skin ulcers, nerve disorders, and kidney dysfunction. The most common type of diabetes, adult-onset or type 2 diabetes, develops most often in adults and especially in people who are overweight.

What we and other cohort studies have found is that weight has a particularly striking effect on the risk of developing adult-onset diabetes. In the Nurses' Health Study, obese women had an extremely high risk for developing the disorder compared to lean women, but even women in the upper part of the healthy range had a large increase in risk (see Figure 16-4). The relationship was similar when we used measures of a woman's waist size. The risk of diabetes began to increase with waist sizes alone well within what is considered the healthy range in the 1998 federal report and rose steadily as waist size increased (see Figure 16-5).

We also found that modest weight gain or weight loss during adulthood could have a major influence on the risk of adult-onset diabetes. In the Nurses' Health Study, the women who put on twelve or more pounds from the time they were eighteen to the beginning of the study were much more likely to develop diabetes than the women whose weight remained steady. The more

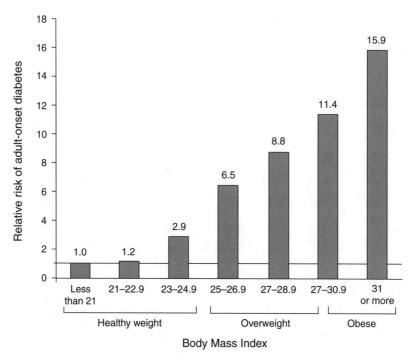

FIG. 16-4. The risk of developing adult-onset diabetes increases with weight. The increase in risk is large even for women in the upper part of the healthy range and is exceptionally high in overweight and obese women. (Source: Nurses' Health Study)

weight gained, the higher a woman's risk. Women who gained more than forty-five pounds during that time had an exceptionally high risk of the disorder. Weight loss during that same time period, however, had the opposite effect. Women who took off twelve to eighteen pounds had an almost 50 percent drop in their risk of diabetes compared to women whose weight remained steady. Women who lost more than eighteen pounds benefited even more.

An important finding from our study is that a woman's current weight seems to have a much greater influence on her risk of diabetes than what she weighed in the past, suggesting that both weight loss and weight gain have a fairly immediate influence on the risk of developing diabetes. This means that a woman who loses weight and keeps it off will likely see a fairly quick drop in her risk of the disorder.

## INCREASED RISK OF HIGH BLOOD CHOLESTEROL

Along with adult-onset diabetes and hypertension, high blood cholesterol (hypercholesterolemia) is an important contributor to the development of coronary heart disease and stroke. Numerous observational studies have found that

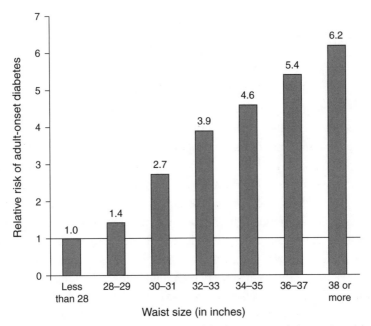

FIG. 16-5. As waist size increases, so does the risk of developing type 2 diabetes. The risk begins to increase even for women within the upper part of the healthy range and is very high in women with large waists. (Source: Nurses' Health Study)

both high BMI and large waist measures elevate women's risk of developing high blood cholesterol. Each can also adversely affect the different types of cholesterol, raising levels of LDL ("bad") cholesterol and lowering levels of HDL ("good") cholesterol.

Although the Nurses' Health Study has not assessed the association between weight and high blood cholesterol in great detail, we have generally found what most other studies have—that obese women are about twice as likely to experience the condition as lean women.

## INCREASED RISK OF CARDIOVASCULAR DISEASE

Characterized by the buildup of cholesterol and fat in the arteries, cardiovascular disease occurs when the arteries become too narrow, blocking the flow of blood. Although many studies have found that being overweight seems to increase the risk of cardiovascular disease on its own, its primary influence on the disease is likely through increasing the risk of hypertension, diabetes, and high blood cholesterol—so-called intermediate risk factors. These intermediate risk factors have a direct link to the injury of artery walls that can lead to the dangerous build up of fat and cholesterol.

*Coronary Heart Disease.* Coronary heart disease occurs when the arteries that supply oxygen and nutrients to the heart (the coronary arteries) become blocked. A number of large cohort studies, including the Nurses' Health Study, the Iowa Women's Health Study, and the Framingham Heart Study, have found that the risk of coronary heart disease increases as BMI increases. In the Nurses' Health Study, we specifically found that the risk of coronary heart disease was slightly elevated among women whose BMIs fell within the upper end of the healthy range and rose to be very large in obese women (see Figure 16-6). Those women carrying the most weight around their middles had a higher risk of heart disease compared to those women carrying the least (see Figure 16-7). Weight gain in adulthood also increased risk. Women who gained twelve to eighteen pounds since age eighteen had a slightly greater chance of developing heart disease than women whose weight remained nearly the same through adulthood. The more weight gained, the greater the risk. Women who gained forty-four pounds or more had more than double the risk of the disease.

*Ischemic Stroke.* An ischemic stroke occurs when the arteries that supply blood to the brain become blocked. Outside of the Nurses' Health Study, only

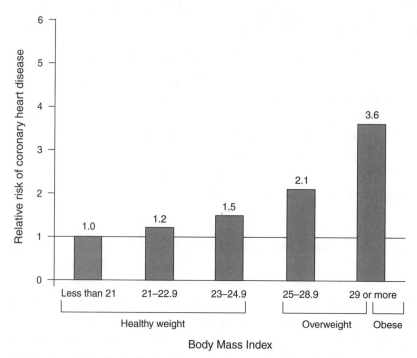

FIG. 16-6. The risk of coronary heart disease increases with weight, even for women within the healthy range. (Source: Nurses' Health Study)

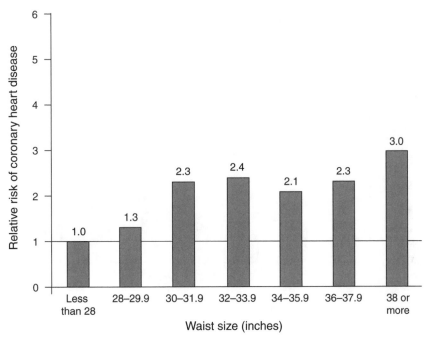

FIG. 16-7. The risk of heart disease increases with waist size. (Source: Nurses' Health Study)

one other cohort study—the Framingham Heart Study—has found that excessive weight increases the risk of ischemic stroke in women. What we have specifically found in the Nurses' Health Study is that overweight women have a moderate increase in risk compared to lean women, while those who are obese have a more than twofold increase in risk (see Figure 16-8). We also found that weight *gain* elevated the risk of ischemic stroke. Those women who put on twenty-two to forty-four pounds since age eighteen had a 70 percent increase in risk compared to women with a stable adult weight. For those who put on more than forty-four pounds, the risk increased 2.5 times.

When we looked at risk of hemorrhagic stroke—strokes caused by a bleeding blood vessel in the brain—we did not find any relationship with weight.

## INCREASED RISK OF PULMONARY EMBOLISM

Pulmonary embolism is a serious condition that results when a blood clot, usually in one of the large veins in the legs, breaks off, travels through part of the circulatory system, and becomes lodged in one or more of the blood vessels that take oxygen to the lungs. In the Nurses' Health Study, we found that the risk of pulmonary embolism was 2 to 3 times higher among overweight and

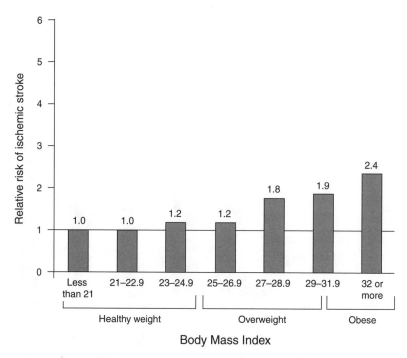

FIG. 16-8. Being overweight increases the risk of ischemic stroke. (Source: Nurses' Health Study)

obese women than lean women. This finding corroborates those from the Framingham Heart Study, where researchers found that very overweight women were more likely than women of average weight to have developed and died from pulmonary embolism.

## INCREASED RISK OF BREAST CANCER IN POSTMENOPAUSAL WOMEN

Breast cancer is the leading killer of women in midlife. Studies assessing the effect of weight on the risk of breast cancer have found that it affects women differently at different stages in life.

In the Nurses' Health Study, when we assessed the effect of weight on breast cancer risk in premenopausal women (women who still had regular menstrual periods), we found that as BMI increased, the risk of breast cancer decreased. Despite this drop in the risk of developing the disease, we also found that being overweight does not provide any substantial protection against dying from the disease. This may be due in part to the fact that over-weight women are often diagnosed with breast cancer at a more advanced stage than leaner women, making treatment less effective.

In postmenopausal women, weight gain was linked to an increase in the risk of breast cancer. Those women who had gained more than forty-five pounds since age eighteen had a small increase in the risk of developing the disease. However, because postmenopausal hormones can mask the effect of weight on breast cancer risk, we also looked specifically at women who had gained more than forty-five pounds but had never used postmenopausal hormones. When we did this, we found that there was a substantial doubling of risk linked to weight gain (see Figure 16-9). Obesity also moderately increased risk in this same group of nonhormone users.

Being overweight and gaining weight is thought to increase the risk of breast cancer after menopause by increasing levels of the hormone estrogen. Increased levels of estrogen are linked to breast cancer development. Although a woman's ovaries stop producing estrogen after menopause, fat tissue continues to produce hormones that are converted to estrogen. The more weight a woman puts on after menopause, the more estrogen she produces—a point the Nurses' Health Study helped confirm.

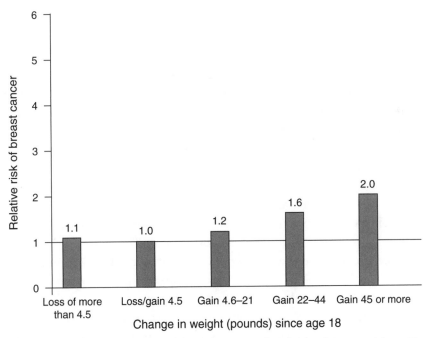

FIG. 16-9. The risk of breast cancer increases with the amount of weight gained since age eighteen. The increase in risk is even more apparent in women who have never used postmenopausal hormones. (Source: Nurses' Health Study)

## INCREASED RISK OF COLON CANCER

Colon cancer is the third leading cause of cancer death in U.S. women, despite the fact that it is a very preventable cancer. And being overweight has been consistently linked to an increased risk of developing colon cancer in women. In the Nurses' Health Study, we found that obese women had an approximately 50 percent greater risk of developing colon cancer compared to the leanest women in the cohort. We also found that, compared to lean women and women with small waists, obese women and women with very large waists had about a 50 percent greater risk of developing adenomatous polyps—precancerous growths on the lining of the colon from which almost all colon cancers arise.

The reason why being overweight or obese raises the risk of colon cancer is not well understood. Some researchers feel that it may have to do with increased insulin levels in the blood that result from obesity. The higher levels of insulin may alter cell growth in the colon, which can lead to polyp formation and the subsequent development of colon cancer.

## INCREASED RISK OF ENDOMETRIAL CANCER

Endometrial cancer occurs in the lining of the uterus (called the endometrium). Multiple studies have shown that obesity, significant weight gain, and perhaps central adiposity can substantially increase risk of the disease. As with breast cancer, obesity is thought to influence the risk of endometrial cancer by increasing a woman's estrogen levels.

In the Nurses' Health Study, when we evaluated overall weight, we found that premenopausal and postmenopausal women were affected differently. While the risk of endometrial cancer increased in both pre- and postmenopausal women as weight increased, the risk was elevated to a much greater degree in postmenopausal women (see Figure 16-10)—an effect that could be seen most clearly in women who were not on postmenopausal hormones. This same relationship held true when we looked at the amount of weight women had gained since the age of eighteen. We found that premenopausal women who had gained more than forty pounds had a risk of endometrial cancer almost two times that of women whose weight had remained steady. In postmenopausal women who had gained more than forty pounds, their risk rose to almost 4 times that of women who maintained a steady weight.

The likely reason that risk appears greatest in those postmenopausal women who are not currently using hormones relates to estrogen levels. The

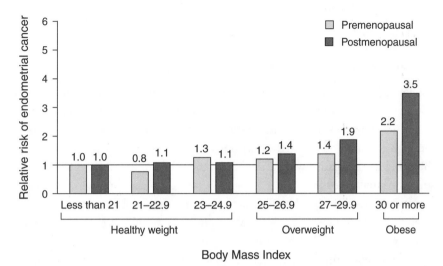

FIG. 16-10. The more a woman weighs, the greater her risk of endometrial cancer. The risk is particularly high among obese postmenopausal women. (Source: Nurses' Health Study)

amount of estrogen provided through postmenopausal hormones far outweighs that produced by a woman's fat tissue. Therefore, the full effect of weight on endometrial cancer risk becomes masked by hormone use. It is not that taking postmenopausal hormones eliminates the risk of endometrial cancer associated with being overweight (because it doesn't); it is that using hormones likely hides the effect that weight has on risk.

## POSSIBLE INCREASED RISK OF OVARIAN CANCER

Weight and body shape may be related to the risk of cancer of the ovaries (ovarian cancer). In the Nurses' Health Study, we found that women who were obese in early adulthood had a moderately increased risk of premenopausal ovarian cancer. This finding will need to be confirmed with additional study. Overall, a woman's current weight probably does not have a large effect on her risk of ovarian cancer.

In the Iowa Women's Health Study, there was no difference in the risk of ovarian cancer between heavy women and lean women. However, waist size did appear to influence risk. Women who carried their excess weight around their waists were twice as likely to develop ovarian cancer as women who carried their excess weight in their hips, buttocks, or thighs. These results suggest that where a woman carries her weight might have more impact on her risk of ovarian cancer than the amount of weight she carries. The reason for this is unknown, but may be due to the hormonal effects of fat accumulating around the organs. Additional research is needed before waist size can be linked conclusively to ovarian cancer risk.

## INCREASED RISK OF GALLSTONES

Gallstones occur more frequently in women and men who are overweight or obese than in those of lower weight. Gallstones form when bile (a liquid that helps in the digestion of fats) hardens into a rock-like substance. If large enough or numerous enough, gallstones can cause serious health problems by blocking certain pathways that lead from the liver through the gallbladder and into the small intestine.

When we looked at the effect of weight on risk of gallstones in the Nurses' Health Study, we found that as BMI increased, so did the risk of gallstones. Even women who fell within the upper part of the healthy range for weight experienced slight increases in risk compared to the leanest women, and obese women in the heaviest categories had a very large increase in risk for the disease (see Figure 16-11).

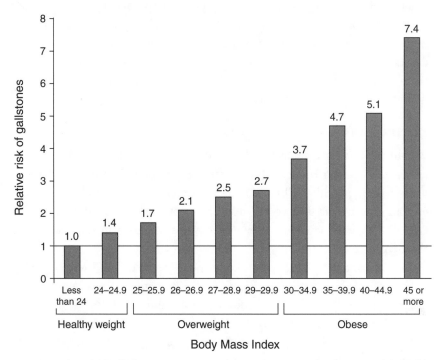

FIG. 16-11. The risk of gallstones increases as weight increases even in the upper part of the healthy weight range. (Source: Nurses' Health Study)

Contrary to what might be expected, we also found that weight loss slightly increased the risk of gallstones in the nurses. Other, smaller studies have had similar findings. This seems to occur because during weight loss the body burns fat for energy, which releases extra amounts of cholesterol into the bile. The more cholesterol present in the bile, the more likely it is that gallstones will form. It can be difficult, though, to separate out the effect of a weight-loss program from the effect that weight in general has on gallstone formation, since the people who usually go on such programs are already at increased risk because they are overweight. However, given the size of the Nurses' Health Study cohort and the large number of gallstone cases that occurred over the years we followed the nurses, we have been able to demonstrate that women who lost more than eight pounds in the previous two years increased their risk for the disorder by more than 40 percent compared to women whose weight had remained steady.

In addition to the Nurses' Health Study, only a few other cohort studies have tried to assess the link between weight and gallstone formation in women. In general, they have found similar result to ours. The Framingham Heart Study, for example, found that women with weights substantially above the average of study participants had about an 80 percent increased risk of gallstones.

## INCREASED RISK OF KIDNEY STONES

Kidney stones are a very common occurrence in the United States. Approximately 10 percent of all Americans will be afflicted by the disorder in their lifetime—men nearly three times as often as women. And even though kidney stones rarely have serious complications, they can be exceptionally painful, debilitating short-term events.

The large majority of studies that have assessed the link between body size and risk of kidney stone formation have been relatively small case-control studies, and none of them has found a link between weight and kidney stones in women. When we looked at the issue in the Nurses' Health Study, however, we discovered that as BMI increased, so did risk of developing kidney stones. Overall, the elevations in risk were not dramatic, but women did not have to be obese to be at increased risk. Nurses with BMIs in the upper part of the healthy range (23–24.9) had small elevations in their risk compared to women with BMIs between 21 and 22.9. Women with the highest BMIs (32 or greater) had a moderate increase in risk compared to the leanest women.

## Increased Risk of Arthritis

Being overweight increases the risk of the most common type of arthritis—osteoarthritis. Caused by the gradual deterioration of the protective cartilage inside joints, osteoarthritis affects over 16 million Americans. Carrying excess weight is one of the top predictors of osteoarthritis in the knee and hip. This has been clearly demonstrated in numerous studies, including the Nurses' Health Study and the Framingham Heart Study. The more weight that a woman carries, the more force she puts on her joints. More force means more mechanical stress, and this can lead to the erosion of protective cartilage.

## Increased Risk of Lower Quality of Life

The ability to perform tasks that are part of daily life is essential to remaining an independent person with a good quality of life. Difficulty doing tasks such as running errands, walking up a few steps, or getting in and out of a chair can have a greater and more immediate impact on normal living than disorders such as diabetes and hypertension.

In the Nurses' Health Study, we evaluated at the effect of a woman's weight on her ability to perform a number of daily activities. What we found was what other studies, like the Framingham Heart Study, have also found—that being overweight or obese substantially hampers the ability of women to perform normal activities on a daily basis. The more overweight a woman was, the less able she was to function normally. Overall, obese women experienced a degree of pain and a reduction in the ability to perform daily tasks that were equivalent to those experienced by a person with significant arthritis.

We also found that weight gain and weight loss had a large impact on quality of life. All women—even those starting out with a healthy weight—who gained five pounds or more in a four-year period had more problems performing normal daily activities, had less energy, and experienced more pain than women whose weight had remained relatively stable. Not surprisingly, we found that weight loss could improve certain aspects of quality of life. In the heaviest women, those with a BMI of 30 or more, weight loss improved the ability to perform daily tasks and reduced the amount of pain they experienced.

## Possible Increased Risk of Asthma

Weight has been linked in some studies to asthma. In the Nurses' Health Study II, we found that women who were overweight were more likely to develop asthma over a four-year period than women who were lean. This was especially true for obese women, who had a threefold increase in the risk of asthma.

## POSSIBLE INCREASED RISK OF CATARACTS

Being overweight may also increase the risk of cataracts. Why? Possibly because the high blood sugar levels that often result from being overweight can literally sugarcoat the lens of the eye, turning them cloudy. In the Nurses' Health Study, we found that women who were overweight were more likely to develop cataracts than those who were lean.

## The Few Benefits of Being Overweight and Gaining Weight

### LOWER RISK OF OSTEOPOROSIS AND HIP FRACTURE

Breaking a hip can be a life-threatening event in the elderly and is usually associated with the bone-weakening effects of osteoporosis. Being overweight can help protect a woman from both of these problems. First, the higher levels of estrogen in the body after menopause that result from carrying extra fat can help keep bones from losing calcium, a mineral that is essential for strong bones. Second, the padding created by the extra fat tissue can protect against a break by cushioning a fall on the hip.

In the Nurses Health Study, we have found that obese women have a much lower risk of hip fracture compared to leaner women—a result confirmed by numerous other studies. But should women gain weight to protect themselves from osteoporosis and hip fractures? Given the many adverse health consequences associated with obesity and weight gain, the answer is no. A healthier and more positive approach would be to increase one's physical activity.

Although physical activity is associated with being lean, it has also been shown to protect against osteoporosis. Physical activity places stress on the bones, which in turn stimulates the bones to absorb calcium. One study in particular found that women who had been physically active their entire lives had much stronger bones compared to women who were relatively inactive throughout life.

### HOW DOES WEIGHT AFFECT LENGTH OF LIFE?

Although it's important to know how weight affects all aspects of health, many women may be most interested in the simple bottom-line question: how does my weight affect my overall risk of dying prematurely? Even though some of the details of the relationship between weight and premature death are still be-

## Weight: Weighing the Risks

### WEIGHT

Compared to lean women, obese women have a:

- *Very high excess risk* of diabetes and hypertension
- *High excess risk* of coronary heart disease, stroke, endometrial cancer, gallstones, pulmonary embolism, and reduced quality of life
- *Moderately excess risk* of premature death, breast cancer (postmenopause), colon cancer, kidney stones, and high blood cholesterol

### WEIGHT GAIN

Compared to women whose weight has remained relatively stable in adulthood, those who have gained thirty pounds or more have a:

- *Very high excess risk* of diabetes
- *High excess risk* of stroke, hypertension, and endometrial cancer
- *Moderately excess risk* of coronary heart disease
- *Small excess risk* of breast cancer (postmenopause)

### WAIST SIZE

Compared to women with small waists, women with waist sizes of thirty-five inches or more have a:

- *Very high excess risk* of diabetes
- *High excess risk* of coronary heart disease

ing debated by researchers, the answer in general is clear—being overweight or obese increases the risk of premature death.

When looking at this issue, we found that obese women in the Nurses' Health Study cohort had a greatly increased risk of premature death compared to the lean women (see Figure 16-12). Much of this increase seemed to be due to deaths from cancer and coronary heart disease. The obese women were twice as likely to die from cancer and four times more likely to die from coronary heart disease than their leaner counterparts.

Gaining weight in adulthood also increased risk of premature death. Women who had put on twenty-two pounds or more since age eighteen, re-

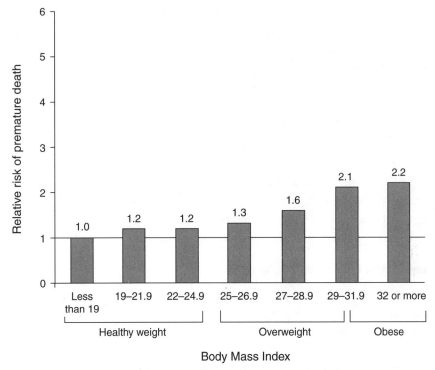

FIG. 16-12. The risk of premature death is low in the healthy range and increases as weight increases. (Source: Nurses' Health Study)

gardless of their starting weight, were at an increased risk of premature death compared to women whose weight had stayed steady over the same time period. Women who had gained more than forty-five pounds were at the highest risk—60 percent greater than women whose weight had remained steady.

While some large cohort studies have shown that higher rates of premature death occur not only in the overweight but also in the very lean, we have found in the Nurses' Health Study that all women in the healthy weight range who had maintained a stable weight had very similar low rates of premature death. Smoking and undiagnosed disease (such as cancer), which are linked to leanness as well as to an increased risk of premature death, can complicate the study of weight and premature death. Not adequately taking these two factors into account can give a false impression that being lean increases the risk of dying prematurely. In the Nurses' Health Study, when we took smoking and undiagnosed disease into account, we found that the risk of dying prematurely was low for all women in the healthy weight range and increased steadily in the overweight and obese.

Obviously, there is such a thing as being too thin. Women who are extremely underweight can experience a number of health problems, including osteoporosis, fatigue, and menstrual and reproductive disorders. In the Nurses' Health Study, however, so few women fall into this category that we are unable to assess the impact that being underweight has on long-term health.

## WHAT IT ALL MEANS

Although the details of the individual studies can seem confusing at times, the general conclusion about the link between weight and health is very basic: carrying excessive weight and gaining weight as an adult is generally bad for health. The evidence also shows, though, that the achievable goals of avoiding significant weight gain as you age and losing a modest amount of weight (if you are overweight) can have significant health benefits.

### Benefits of Maintaining a Steady Weight

Many women may find particularly encouraging our findings that simply maintaining a steady weight through adulthood, whether it is in the healthy range or not, can have many health benefits. The goal of maintaining a steady weight is much easier to achieve for many women than losing weight and keeping it off. And the benefits for doing so are substantial. The risk of premature death, coronary heart disease, diabetes, hypertension, and breast cancer are all lower in women whose weight has stayed steady throughout adulthood compared to women who have put on weight. Numerous other studies have confirmed these findings, which led the *U.S. Dietary Guidelines for Americans* to refocus its recommendations in 1995 and again in 2000 to put emphasis first on maintaining a stable weight and secondly on weight loss.

### Benefits of Weight Loss

Although harder to achieve for some than maintaining a stable weight, weight loss also has its many benefits. If you are overweight, losing weight—even a modest five to ten pounds—can improve your quality of life, blood glucose levels, blood cholesterol levels, and blood pressure as well as lower your risk of diabetes and coronary heart disease.

### Body Shape

We have shown that apple-shaped women, those with large waist measures, have a greater risk of developing coronary heart disease and adult-onset diabetes. Moreover, it seems that in some instances a woman's shape may be increasingly important as she ages past sixty-five, a time when most women begin to lose weight due to loss of muscle. If a woman loses weight but still retains or develops an apple shape, she is still likely at increased risk of developing coronary heart disease and adult-onset diabetes, even though her overall BMI has dropped. It is also possible for a woman to maintain the same weight but to carry her weight differently, changing from pear-shaped to apple-shaped or vice versa. Keeping track of body shape, therefore, becomes especially important for this group of women since the risk of coronary heart disease increases a great deal as women age. Regular physical activity has been shown in some studies to help women control the amount of weight they carry around their waists.

## A Healthy Weight: The Nurses' Health Study Perspective

The 1998 federal guidelines recommend these BMI ranges for healthy weight, overweight, and obesity:

*Healthy weight* is a BMI between 18.5 and 24.9

*Overweight* is a BMI between 25 and 29.9

*Obesity* is a BMI of 30 and over

But do these categories match the findings from the Nurses' Health Study? Is a BMI between 18.5 and 24.9 truly a healthy weight?

In general, yes. Our data do support these categories. We have found that a BMI between 18.5 and 24.9 is linked to lower rates of numerous disorders and premature death. In fact, data from the Nurses' Health Study were partially responsible for defining the healthy ranges used in both the 1995 and 1998 federal guidelines.

However, we have also found that women who are well within the healthy weight range described above can begin to exhibit health problems. Most notably, women with BMIs of 22 or more had an increased risk of developing adult-onset diabetes or dying from coronary heart disease, and those with BMIs of 20 or more had an increased risk of developing hypertension. Based on such data, it seems that a prudent BMI for some women, especially those at high risk of coronary heart disease, may be lower than those that are acceptable in the 1998 guidelines. When solely looking at the health consequences studied in the Nurses' Health Study, the optimal BMI for an adult woman may be between 18.5 and 23. Women in this range developed the fewest chronic disorders and had the lowest risk of premature death.

## The Good News

- Simply maintaining a steady weight through adulthood, whether in the healthy range or not, can have many health benefits.
- Some weight-related health risks, such as diabetes, are reduced almost immediately when excess weight is lost.
- The focus of weight loss should be on moderate changes that you can sustain over the long term. Don't aim for or expect overnight results.
- Slowly working up to thirty to forty minutes of moderate activity three to five days a week is a good way to begin a program of regular physical activity.
- Successful dietary changes do not need to be complicated. Weight gain occurs when too many calories are eaten for the amount of energy expended, so that real weight loss simply depends upon a decrease in the total amount of calories eaten.

## WHAT I TELL MY PATIENTS ABOUT WEIGHT CONTROL

DR. NANCY RIGOTTI

Remember the "freshman fifteen" we complained about in college—those fifteen extra pounds many women put on during their first year away from home? Well, the sad fact is that it's all too easy to put on extra weight. This is especially true at certain times in life, such as after pregnancy. And it can seem impossible to take the weight off or even to maintain a constant weight rather than continue to gain.

But you are not alone if you have gained weight since reaching adulthood. About half of the women in this country are overweight. Fortunately, there are steps you can take to reduce your weight.

The benefits beyond the obvious (looking and feeling better) are enormous. There are clear health advantages to maintaining a healthy weight: you reduce your risk of hypertension, adult-onset diabetes, high blood cholesterol, cardiovascular disease, and certain types of cancer.

So if you want to lose weight, how do you begin? This is what I tell my patients:

1. **Calculate your BMI, using the formula in Table 2 in Appendix C.** If your BMI is between 18.5 and 24.9, your weight is healthy and your goal should be to maintain it. If your BMI is 25 or over, you are overweight and should take steps to reduce your weight.

2. **Determine whether your body shape is apple (with weight accumulating around your waist) or pear (with fat accumulating in your hips and thighs).** Sometimes you can tell just by looking at yourself in a mirror. If not, take a tape measure and measure the circumference of your waist. If your waist is thirty-five inches around or more, or has grown by two to three inches in the past year, and you have a BMI of 25 or higher, losing weight will help reduce your risk of disease (particularly cardiovascular disease and adult-onset diabetes). And if you are sixty-five or older, pay particular attention to the size of your waist. We tend to lose muscle mass as we grow older, so even if your BMI is within the healthy range, but your waist size is large, you'll need to take steps to protect your health.

3. **Set reasonable goals for weight reduction.** Sometimes the first thing you should do is merely to maintain your weight. Only later, as you begin adopting the healthy diet and exercise plan that I'll outline next, should you aim for losing weight. A reasonable goal is to reduce your weight by 10 percent over six months. Then you may need to maintain that weight before attempting to lose more weight—because your metabolic rate (the rate at which you burn calories) decreases as you lose weight.

4. **Change what you eat and how much you eat.** The first step in losing weight is to begin reducing the number of calories you consume every day. The best way to do this strikes many women as boring. But it works! Eat less red meat and fewer high fat items and consume more fruits, vegetables, and fibers. Pay attention to the amount of food—even healthy food—that you eat. American life has accustomed us to ever larger portions. Many women who can't understand why they can't lose weight when they eat healthy food are eating portions that are just too big.

5. **Exercise more.** The number of calories burned through physical activity is as important as the number you consume every day by eating. The key to adopting a good exercise plan is to start slowly and then build gradually. Start with thirty to forty minutes of moderate activity three to five days a week; then build to thirty to forty-five minutes of moderate activity on most or all days of the week. You don't have to go to a gym to exercise.

6. **Find support and different ways of dealing with stress.** The most successful weight-loss plans take our minds and spirits into account, as well as our bodies. Food often provides comfort after a long stressful day, or when we're depressed or feeling lonely. Exercise is a much better way to handle stress. Find a support group or experiment with different tension relievers. You might find a complementary approach helpful, such as yoga or tai chi.

7. **Watch out for weight gain during the holidays.** They are a time of celebration and should be enjoyed, but it's also important not to overdo it and eat too much. Measure your weight going into Thanksgiving and again after New Year's Day, and resolve to lose any weight you have gained over the holidays by the beginning of spring. It's far easier to lose a small amount soon after the holidays than a large amount that's built up over a number of years.

8. **A few helpful rules to remember:**

- Low fat items still have calories: many cookies and pastries advertise themselves as low in fat—and they are. But they are so loaded with sugar that they still contain many calories. You can actually gain weight by eating such items, so watch the calories as well as the fat content.

- Don't focus on what you can't eat—this will only make you feel deprived and lead to overeating in the long run. Instead, think about the foods that you like that are also good for you. For example, if you like fruit, make sure you fit several servings into your day's diet. If you focus on getting five servings of the fruits and vegetables you like into your day, you may find yourself not craving the sweets and fats that lead to weight trouble.

- Do everything in moderation—even moderation! If you have a day or two where you go off your diet and don't exercise, don't agonize or feel guilty about it. We all need breaks sometimes. Pick yourself up and get back on track. All too often, women feel that if they've stopped dieting for a few days, all is lost—and so they stop dieting permanently. That's a bad idea. Remember, this is a process that goes on for a long time—the rest of your life. Being constant, hanging in there for the long haul, is much more important than being perfect.

# Smoking

## Key Lifestyle Message

- Not smoking (or quitting if you do) is one of the best things you can do for your overall health and quality of life.

## BACKGROUND

It is no longer news that smoking kills. From the time that the first *U.S. Surgeon General's Report on Smoking and Health* was released in 1964, there has been increasing public awareness that smoking is the main cause of many serious diseases—such as lung cancer, oral cancer, chronic obstructive pulmonary disease (COPD), coronary heart disease, and stroke. Consequently,

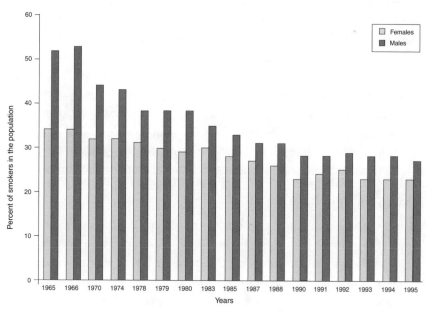

FIG. 17-1. The percentage of women and men in the United States who smoke has declined steadily since the mid-sixties. (Source: Centers for Disease Control and Prevention)

rates of smoking have steadily declined since the mid-sixties (see Figure 17-1) as more and more men and women weighed the health risks of tobacco use and either stopped smoking or never started. Where 34 percent of all women in the United States smoked in 1965 shortly after the release of the Surgeon General's report, only 23 percent did so in 1995. The decline in men has been even greater, dropping from 52 percent to 27 percent over the same period.

Despite these declines, smoking is still a huge health burden in the United States. A quarter of the population (approximately 46 million people) still smokes. Most smokers begin when they are young—almost all before twenty years old and many well before that—responding to a variety of social pressures and becoming unwittingly addicted to the nicotine contained in the tobacco. Once smokers are addicted, quitting is difficult.

If you are a female smoker, quitting may be particularly difficult for you. Some research shows that women are more likely than men to resume smoking in the long term after they have tried to stop, possibly due to unique barriers to quitting—for example, concerns about weight and stresses related to family care. Although hard, quitting smoking for good has undeniable benefits that begin shortly after stopping: your risk of developing many diseases drops, your life expectancy on average increases, and your overall quality of life improves. Quitting also benefits those close to you. Babies of nonsmokers are more likely to be born a normal weight and are less likely to develop breathing problems (such as lung infections) later in life than babies of smokers. In addition, you will no longer expose those around you to the smoke from your cigarettes—known as passive smoke—which can increase the risk of lung disease (such as asthma and bronchitis) in children as well as increase the chances of developing coronary heart disease and lung cancer in later life. Finally, and possibly most important, you will be a good role model for the young people around you. If you smoke, they are more likely to smoke. By stopping for good, you help them avoid an addiction that causes at least one out of every five deaths in the United States.

## Tobacco and Your Body

What is it about smoking that affects your body and contributes to the development of such a long list of health disorders? The woman who smokes a pack of cigarettes a day takes more than 50,000 puffs a year, repeatedly exposing herself to the more than 4,400 chemicals contained in tobacco smoke. As many as 42 of these chemicals are known carcinogens (cancer-causing agents).

Three particularly dangerous substances in tobacco smoke are tar, nicotine, and carbon monoxide. Each has major harmful effects throughout the body.

- Tar is the name given to a large group of cancer-causing chemicals that become a sticky substance in the lungs. In addition to contributing to the development of chronic bronchitis and emphysema, these irritants' impact on the airways is believed to be a key factor in initiating the disease process that eventually results in over 90 percent of lung cancers.
- Nicotine is an addictive chemical that, when absorbed through the lungs, affects the cardiovascular and nervous systems. A smoker smokes cigarettes to maintain a particular level of nicotine in the bloodstream.
- Carbon monoxide is a gas that robs the body of oxygen by decreasing the amount of oxygen red blood cells can carry throughout the body. It has detrimental effects on the cardiovascular system.

Smoke's adverse effects are not limited to the smoker, however. Even non-smokers who regularly breathe a smoker's passive smoke can experience many of the same reactions to the chemicals in the tobacco.

## LESSONS FROM THE NURSES' HEALTH STUDY AND OTHER STUDIES

When most people think of diseases that are related to cigarette smoking, lung cancer is the one that most likely comes to mind first. And while lung cancer deserves this top billing, it is only one of a large number of serious disorders—ranging from heart disease and numerous cancers to cataracts and osteoporosis—caused by smoking.

## Smoking: The Larger Picture

- Smoking is the main cause of many serious diseases, including lung cancer, oral cancer, chronic obstructive pulmonary disease (COPD), coronary heart disease, and stroke.
- Smoking kills more than 430,000 people each year in the United States, the equivalent of three nearly full jumbo jets crashing every day (with no survivors) for an entire year.
- Despite a significant decline in the percentage of smokers since 1965, a quarter of the population still smokes.
- There are more than 4,400 chemicals contained in tobacco smoke, including numerous carcinogens.
- While quitting smoking can be very difficult, over a thousand people quit for good every day!

## The Risks of Smoking

### INCREASED RISK OF LUNG CANCER

For over thirty years, research has shown that cigarette smoking dramatically increases the risk of lung cancer—the leading cancer killer in the United States. Although other risk factors have been linked to the disease, smoking is by far the most important—accounting for almost 90 percent of lung cancers that develop. Not surprisingly, when we looked at this issue in the Nurses' Health Study, we found that women who smoked had a very large risk of lung cancer, and that the more they smoked, the greater their risk was (see Figure 17-2). Compared to nonsmokers, women who smoked about two packs of cigarettes a day had about 22 times the risk of the disease.

The extent to which smoking increases the risk of lung cancer is unique and eclipses most other relationships between a risk factor and a disease that appear throughout this book. To compare: eating excessive amounts of red meat increases the risk of colon cancer approximately 1.5 times; high blood cholesterol increases the risk of coronary heart disease approximately 3 times, and hypertension increases the risk of stroke approximately 5 times. Even the

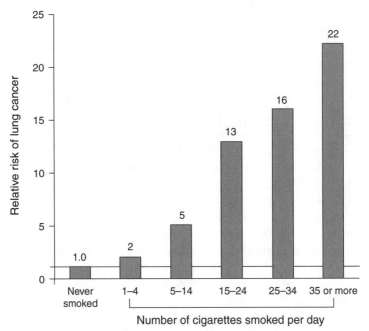

FIG. 17-2. The relative risk of lung cancer increases steadily with the number of cigarettes smoked per day. (Source: Nurses' Health Study)

15-fold increase in the risk of breast cancer associated with the often feared BRCA 1 gene mutations (the "breast cancer gene") does not equal the 22-fold increase in the risk of lung cancer associated with being a two-pack-a-day smoker.

Although extremely large, this risk can be reversed. We found that once a woman quits smoking, her risk of lung cancer will drop over time. Risk begins to decrease around two years after quitting, and by fifteen or more years of not smoking, a woman's risk almost equals that of a woman who has never smoked (see Figure 17-3). For virtually all women who smoke, it is never too late to benefit from quitting.

Cigarette companies run advertisements implying the contrary, but neither low tar nor low nicotine cigarettes seem to protect women from developing lung cancer. Women smoking such "lite" cigarettes often smoke more or inhale more deeply to compensate. Once we took into account the amount that women smoked, we found that tar content of cigarettes bore no relationship to the risk of lung cancer.

Smoking likely causes lung cancer by repeatedly exposing the cells in the lungs to the damaging effects of the tar and other carcinogens in tobacco smoke. Once damaged, the cells are more likely to become cancerous.

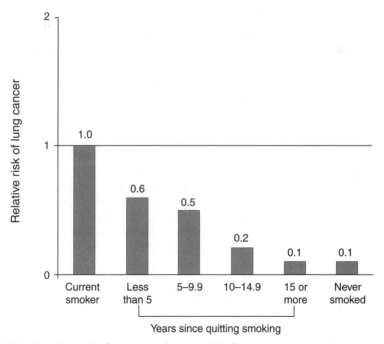

FIG. 17-3. The relative risk of lung cancer drops steadily after a woman quits smoking. Over time it nearly equals the risk of a woman who never smoked. (Source: Nurses' Health Study)

## Smoking: Understanding the Cancer Risks

- On average, smokers die seven years earlier than nonsmokers, but the risk of premature death drops to nearly that of a nonsmoker ten to fifteen years after quitting smoking.
- Fortunately, the risks of lung cancer, cardiovascular disease, and many other smoking-related diseases drops significantly over time once a woman quits smoking for good.
- Smoking "lite" cigarettes with lower tar and nicotine levels does not reduce a woman's risk of lung cancer or cardiovascular disease.
- The risk of cancer of the mouth and throat increases dramatically when smoking is combined with drinking alcohol.

## The Benefits of Quitting Smoking—A Time Line

The benefits of quitting begin almost immediately and continue on for the rest of a person's life. For someone who has smoked twenty cigarettes a day, here is what happens in the hours, weeks, and years after quitting:

- **After two hours:** Nicotine begins to leave the system.
- **After twelve hours:** Carbon monoxide has completely left the system, and blood now carries oxygen more efficiently.
- **Within a week:** The senses of taste and smell sharpen. Breath, hair, fingers, and teeth are cleaner. Circulation improves. All the nicotine is gone from the system, along with the worst of the withdrawal symptoms.
- **Within a month:** The cilia (the hairlike structures that line your airways) begin to recover and remove more mucus from your system, which cleans the lungs and reduces the chance of infection. Coughing, sinus congestion, fatigue, and shortness of breath decrease.
- **After a year:** The risk of having a heart attack or stroke is reduced and falls substantially over the first two to four years; the risk of lung and other cancers falls, but more slowly; lung function improves (but never quite returns to normal).

### INCREASED RISK OF ORAL AND PHARYNGEAL CANCER

Smoking is the primary cause of oral cancer and pharyngeal cancer. Oral cancer includes cancers of the lip, mouth, and tongue. Pharyngeal cancer is cancer of the pharynx, the part of the throat between the mouth and vocal chords. Although not yet assessed by the Nurses' Health Study, many other studies have found the overall risk of oral and pharyngeal cancer is 3 to 4 times greater in women who smoke than in women who do not. And the more a woman smokes and the longer she smokes, the greater is her risk of these diseases (see Figure 17-4). Women who both drink and smoke are at particular risk of oral and pharyngeal cancer. The risks linked with each individual activity increase dramatically when the two are combined. One study found that a woman who drank two to four alcoholic drinks a day and smoked a pack or two a day for twenty or more years had 12 times the risk of oral and pharyngeal cancer compared to that of a nonsmoker and nondrinker. Again, as in the case of lung cancer, the risk of oral and pharyngeal cancer is reversible with time. About ten years after quitting, a woman will find that her risk of these diseases drops to near that of a nonsmoker.

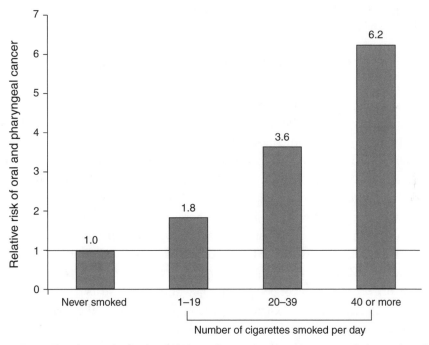

FIG. 17-4. The relative risk of oral and pharyngeal cancer in women increases with the number of cigarettes smoked per day. (Source: National Cancer Institute)

## INCREASED RISK OF PANCREATIC CANCER

Cancer of the pancreas—an organ next to the stomach that helps produce enzymes and hormones essential for digestion and maintenance of blood sugar levels—is the fifth leading cause of cancer death in the United States. Unfortunately, very few lifestyle factors have been linked to its development, limiting the steps people can take to try to prevent the disease.

Along with a number of other studies, we have found that smoking is one habit that is linked to the risk of pancreatic cancer. Compared to women who had never smoked, those women in the Nurses' Health Study who currently smoked had nearly 2.5 times the risk of this cancer. Strikingly, if a person stops smoking, this risk seems to drop dramatically after just two years. When we combined our data with that of a similar study of male health professionals, we discovered that just two years after stopping, the risk of pancreatic cancer drops to half that of a current smoker, and ten years after a person stops smoking, the risk equals that of someone who had never smoked.

The exact mechanisms by which smoking might cause pancreatic cancer are currently unknown. One possibility is that nitrosamines, a group of chemicals found in tobacco smoke, might play a part in a process that causes pancreatic cells to turn cancerous.

## INCREASED RISK OF COLON CANCER

Although not all studies are consistent, a growing body of evidence suggests that smoking can increase the risk of colon cancer, particularly if a woman starts smoking early in life and does so for more than twenty years.

In the Nurses' Health Study, we found that the risk of colon cancer did not increase until thirty-five years after a woman had started to smoke more than ten cigarettes a day. At that point, whether she had quit or not, she was twice as likely to develop the disease as a woman who had never smoked. We also found that smoking increases the risk of developing noncancerous growths in the colon—called adenomatous polyps—that can eventually turn into cancer. The increased risk of polyps linked to smoking, though, develops over a much shorter period than does the increased risk of colon cancer. Instead of a lag of thirty-five years, the risk of polyps goes up within twenty years after a woman starts smoking. The more cigarettes she smokes per day, and the longer she smokes, the higher her risk.

These results suggest that tobacco actually initiates the development of colon cancer. It may cause cells to grow abnormally, which may then lead to small adenomatous polyps. These polyps may become larger, and finally, after a period of several decades, cancerous. Thus, years may pass between the time a woman takes up smoking and the time that she actually develops colon cancer.

Unlike its relationship with other cancers, smoking seems to have an irreversible effect on the colon: women who quit smoking still have an increased risk of colon cancer decades after they started.

## INCREASED RISK OF CERVICAL CANCER

There is good evidence that smoking approximately doubles the risk of cervical cancer. The cervix, about one inch around, connects the vagina to the uterus (womb), and it is through the cervix that sperm travels to fertilize a woman's egg during conception. Cigarette smoke contains chemicals that can damage the DNA of cells in the cervix, which can cause them to become cancerous. The increase in risk, though, appears reversible. After a woman stops smoking, the risk of cervical cancer appears to drop, as new cells likely replace damaged ones.

## INCREASED RISK OF OTHER CANCERS

Smoking also increases the risk of a number of other cancers, including kidney, bladder, and liver cancer (see box below). As with most other cancers linked to cigarette smoking, the risk of almost all of these increases with the amount smoked and decreases after a person has quit smoking.

Perhaps surprisingly, there appears to be no link between smoking in adulthood and breast cancer. And although it may seem counterintuitive—

## Cancers Definitely or Probably Linked to Smoking

- Lung
- Oral (lip, mouth, and throat)
- Pancreas
- Colon
- Cervix
- Larynx (part of the throat containing the vocal cords)
- Pharynx (part of the throat between the mouth and vocal cords)
- Esophagus (the muscular tube leading from the pharynx to the stomach)
- Bladder
- Kidney
- Liver
- Stomach
- Leukemia

given that smoking increases the risk of many cancers—a number of studies have actually shown that smoking may lower the risk of endometrial cancer, which occurs in the lining of the uterus. Being overweight and having high estrogen levels increase the risk of the disease, and because smokers tend to be leaner and to have lower estrogen levels, they also tend to have a lower risk of endometrial cancer. However, given smoking's devastating effect on the rest of the body, no one should consider smoking as a means to lowering the risk of the disease. Maintaining a healthy weight and eating a healthy diet are much more effective approaches that also lower the risk of many other diseases.

## INCREASED RISK OF CHRONIC BRONCHITIS AND EMPHYSEMA

Smoking is a major cause of chronic bronchitis and emphysema, two conditions often grouped under the name chronic obstructive pulmonary disease (COPD)—a leading cause of death in the United States. In emphysema, the air sacs (alveoli) in the lungs lose their elasticity and cannot shrink or expand effectively. In chronic bronchitis, the airways in the lung become inflamed and clogged with mucus. Only rarely does a smoker experience just one or the other disorder. If one is present, the other likely is as well to some degree. In advanced stages of these disorders, breathing becomes severely obstructed, drastically limiting the supply of oxygen to many organs. The effect on the heart is particularly pronounced and eventually leads to significant heart failure.

Numerous studies show that the risk of chronic obstructive lung disease is more than 10 times greater in smokers than in nonsmokers. And while the risk linked to chronic bronchitis appears to be reversible after a person quits smoking, much of the serious damage to the lungs from emphysema is not. In the Nurses' Health Study, when we assessed the link between smoking and chronic bronchitis, we found that women who currently smoked had a large risk compared to women who had never smoked, and the more the women smoked, the greater their risk (see Figure 17-5). Only five years after quitting, however, a woman's risk of chronic bronchitis dropped to that of a woman who had never smoked.

In contrast, the risk of emphysema linked to smoking is larger than that of chronic bronchitis and does not decrease after a woman has quit.

## INCREASED RISK OF CARDIOVASCULAR DISEASE

Cardiovascular disease—which includes coronary heart disease, stroke, and peripheral arterial disease—is the number one killer of women. More than 500,000 women die from the disease each year. Characterized by the buildup

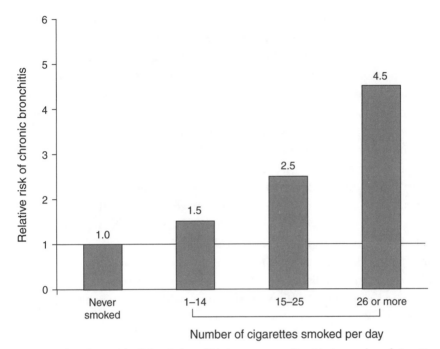

FIG. 17-5. The relative risk of chronic bronchitis increases steadily with the number of cigarettes smoked per day. (Source: Nurses' Health Study)

## Smoking Can Affect Nonsmokers, Too

- Regular exposure to passive smoke—the smoke from someone else's cigarette—increases the risk of serious disease in nonsmokers. Lung cancer, coronary heart disease, sudden infant death syndrome, and respiratory illnesses in children are all more common in those regularly exposed to passive smoke.
- A mother who does not smoke or who quits smoking helps to protect her children from asthma and other childhood lung diseases.
- Children of nonsmokers are less likely to become smokers.

of cholesterol and fat in the arteries, cardiovascular disease occurs when the arteries become too narrow, blocking the flow of blood. Numerous studies have found that smoking greatly increases the risk of the cardiovascular diseases. Tobacco smoke not only promotes the dangerous buildup of fat and cholesterol on artery walls, it can also promote the formation of blood clots that can be the ultimate cause of a stroke or heart attack.

As in the case of lung cancer, "lite" cigarettes and menthol cigarettes do not lessen the risk of cardiovascular disease linked to smoking.

*Coronary Heart Disease.* Coronary heart disease occurs when the arteries that supply oxygen and nutrients to the heart (the coronary arteries) become blocked. As with many other large cohort studies, we found in the Nurses' Health Study that women who currently smoke have a large risk of coronary heart disease compared to women who have never smoked, and the more a woman smokes, the greater her risk (see Figure 17-6). Women who smoked more than two packs of cigarettes a day had nearly 11 times the risk of coronary heart disease than those who had never smoked. Again, after quitting, a woman's risk of coronary heart disease dropped. Two years after quitting, the risk in former smokers was cut in half. Ten or more years later it nearly equaled that of women who had never smoked (see Figure 17-7).

There is also a great deal of evidence that smoking exacerbates the effect of other coronary heart disease risk factors—such as hypertension, diabetes, and high blood cholesterol. We found that smokers with hypertension had 22 times the risk of coronary heart disease than nonsmokers with normal blood pres-

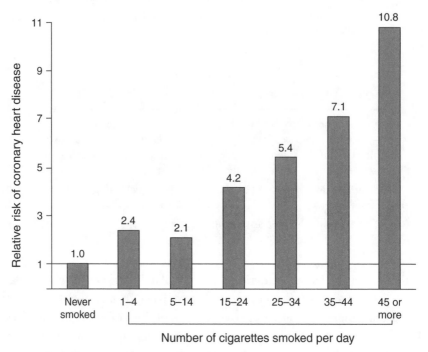

FIG. 17-6. The relative risk of coronary heart disease increases steadily with the number of cigarettes smoked per day. (Source: Nurses' Health Study)

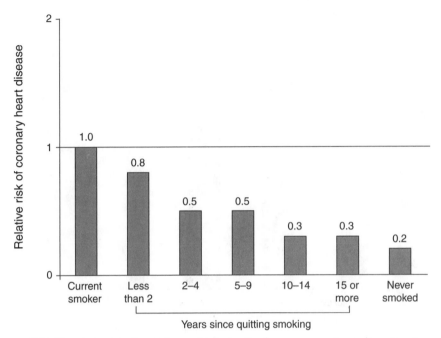

FIG. 17-7. The relative risk of heart disease drops steadily after a woman quits smoking. Over time it nearly equals the risk of a woman who never smoked. (Source: Nurses' Health Study)

sure. Similarly large increases in risk were also seen in smokers with diabetes or high blood cholesterol.

*Stroke.* There are two main types of stroke—ischemic and hemorrhagic. An ischemic stroke occurs when the arteries that supply blood to the brain become blocked. A hemorrhagic stroke occurs when there is bleeding (hemorrhaging) in a blood vessel in the brain. We were one of the first to study the link between smoking and stroke in women, finding that smoking increases the risk of both types of stroke—a result many other studies have since corroborated. Compared to women in the Nurses' Health Study who have never smoked, those who currently smoked were almost three times more likely to experience a stroke of any type. As the number of cigarettes smoked per day increased, so did the risk of stroke (see Figure 17-8).

When assessing the different kinds of stroke, we found that the risk of ischemic stroke was very similar to that for all strokes: about 3 times the risk for current smokers compared to those who never smoked. However, when assessing one particular subgroup of hemorrhagic stroke, called subarachnoid hemorrhage, we found that the risk for a current smoker compared to someone who never smoked was nearly fivefold higher. A subarachnoid hemor-

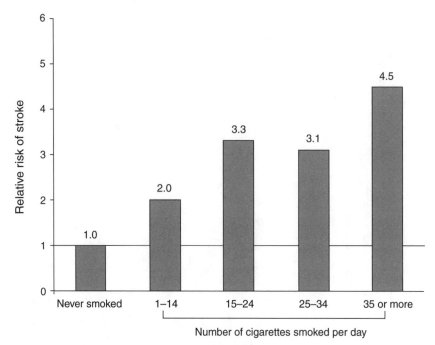

FIG. 17-8. The relative risk of stroke (both ischemic and hemorrhagic) increases with the number of cigarettes smoked per day. (Source: Nurses' Health Study)

rhage occurs when a blood vessel on the outer part of the brain bleeds into the space between the brain and inner skull (the subarachnoid space).

The effects of smoking on both ischemic and hemorrhagic stroke appear reversible. For all types of stroke combined, we found that the risk of the disease dropped by a quarter only one to two years after a woman had quit smoking. Five or more years after she had quit, the risk of a former smoker nearly equaled that of a woman who had never smoked.

*Peripheral Arterial Disease.* Peripheral arterial disease occurs when the ar-

## Smoking and Birth Control Pills

Smoking and using birth control pills is a potentially deadly combination. It has been well established that smokers who currently use birth control pills have a large increase in the risk of blood clots, heart attacks, and strokes compared with that of nonsmokers, especially after the age of thirty-five. For nonsmokers, there appears to be little or no such risk linked to using the pill, further highlighting the benefits of quitting smoking.

teries that supply oxygen and nutrients to the legs become blocked. Though not usually fatal, it can be a serious, disabling condition that results in leg pain, gangrene, and possibly amputation. People who suffer from peripheral arterial disease often have trouble walking even short distances before they experience severe leg pain caused by inadequate blood flow to the muscles. We have not yet assessed peripheral arterial disease in the Nurses' Health Study, but numerous other studies have. The Framingham Heart Study has found that both men and women who smoke have about double the risk of the disease as do nonsmokers, and the more they smoke, the greater their risk.

## Tobacco's Effect on the Cardiovascular System

Tobacco has both short- and long-term negative effects on the cardiovascular system. Over the long term, it can promote the buildup of fat and cholesterol on artery walls by lowering the blood level of "good" cholesterol (HDL) and causing injury to the inner lining of arteries. Over the short term (during and shortly after smoking a cigarette), it can promote changes in the blood and arteries that increase the likelihood that blood clots will form, often the ultimate cause of a heart attack or stroke.

## PROBABLE INCREASED RISK OF ADULT-ONSET (TYPE 2) DIABETES

Diabetes can contribute to a number of health problems, including coronary heart disease, stroke, blindness, skin ulcers, nerve disorders, and kidney dysfunction.

Most large cohort studies done to date have found a link between smoking and an increased risk of diabetes. In the Nurses' Health Study, we found that those women who smoked twenty-five or more cigarettes a day had a risk of the disease 50 percent greater than that of women who had never smoked. We also found that smoking exacerbates the risk of cardiovascular disease associated with diabetes. Smokers with diabetes had about 3 times the risk of coronary heart disease and stroke compared to nonsmokers with diabetes.

## PROBABLE INCREASED RISK OF EYE DISEASE

Smoking has been proposed as a possible cause of two types of eye disease— cataracts and macular degeneration. Cataracts occur when the lens in the eye becomes cloudy, which blurs and can eventually completely block vision. Macular degeneration occurs when the middle part of the retina (macula) begins to break down, which mars a person's central area of sight while peripheral vision remains unchanged. Most studies have found a link between smoking and each of these diseases.

*Cataracts.* In the Nurses' Health Study, when we assessed the link between cataracts and smoking we found that the heaviest smokers—those who had smoked the most cigarettes throughout their lives—had a 60 percent greater risk of the disease than nonsmokers. Although it is unclear exactly how smoking might cause cataracts, it may be that substances in tobacco smoke cause oxidation in the lens.

*Macular Degeneration.* When we assessed macular degeneration, we found that smoking was related to a moderate to large increase in risk for both current and past smokers. The more a woman smokes, the greater the increase in risk.

## PROBABLE INCREASED RISK OF HIP FRACTURES AND OSTEOPOROSIS

Breaking a hip can be a life-threatening event in the elderly and is usually associated with the bone-weakening effects of osteoporosis. Although all women lose bone mass after menopause, smokers appear to lose more than nonsmokers. In a large analysis combining the results of nearly thirty studies, researchers found that by age eighty, smokers had lost 6 percent more of their bone mass than nonsmokers. Although the reason for this is uncertain, it may be that smoking lowers estrogen levels in the body, which leads to more rapid bone loss.

When we studied the link between smoking and the risk of hip fracture in the Nurses' Health Study, we found that women who smoked were 20 percent more likely to break a hip than those who did not smoke. The more cigarettes women smoked, the greater their risk. We also found that smoking has long-lasting effects on bone. After women stopped smoking, it took at least ten years for their risk of fracture to drop to that of women who had never smoked.

A large analysis that combined the results of twenty studies reported similar results to ours. In that analysis, researchers also found that smoking had more of an impact on the risk of hip fracture among older women than among middle-aged women. This is of particular concern, since older women are already at increased risk because of their age.

## INCREASED RISK OF HEALTH PROBLEMS
## DURING PREGNANCY AND EARLY LIFE

Although not yet assessed in the Nurses' Health Study, a large amount of evidence links smoking during pregnancy with a number of health problems in infants and newborns, including premature delivery, low birth weight, and sudden infant death syndrome. Smoking may contribute to these problems by reducing the amount of oxygen the fetus gets during pregnancy. Although it is best for the mother to be a nonsmoker from conception to birth, evidence shows that mothers who start their pregnancy as smokers but stop during the pregnancy have higher birth weight babies than women who continue to smoke.

## The Dangerous Effects of Smoking Go Well Beyond Lung Cancer

Most people know that smoking causes lung cancer, but many may not be aware that smoking is also directly linked to a wide variety of other serious diseases. For example, compared to women who don't smoke, women who do have a:

- *Very high* risk of coronary heart disease and chronic obstructive pulmonary disease, which includes asthma, chronic bronchitis, and emphysema
- *High* risk of oral cancer, pharyngeal cancer, colon cancer, pancreatic cancer, stroke, and peripheral arterial disease
- *Moderate* risk of cataracts, macular degeneration, and diabetes
- *Small* risk of osteoporosis

Evidence also suggests that smoking in pregnancy is linked to health problems in infants, including premature delivery, low birth weight, and sudden infant death syndrome.

### POSSIBLE INCREASED RISK OF SUICIDE

In the Nurses' Health Study, we have discovered a link between cigarette smoking and suicide. Compared to women who do not smoke, those who smoke one to twenty-four cigarettes a day have a moderate risk of committing suicide, and those who smoke twenty-five or more a day have a large risk of suicide. It is unclear exactly how the two are related. However, it is very unlikely that smoking actually causes women to commit suicide. A more probable explanation is that people who experience depression are more likely to be regular smokers than people who do not. Because the nicotine in tobacco can alleviate some of the symptoms of the condition, smoking is a way for depressed people to try to self-medicate their condition. It may be that the more depressed a woman is, the more she is likely to both smoke and to commit suicide.

## PASSIVE SMOKING

For more than a decade, passive smoking has been identified as an important health risk. Breathing the smoke from other people's tobacco products has been linked to lung cancer and coronary heart disease in adults and sudden infant death syndrome and breathing problems in children. While great strides have been made to make public areas—such as restaurants, airplanes, and office buildings—free from smoke, large numbers of people are still exposed to passive smoke on a regular basis. One large study conducted by the federal government found that almost 90 percent of individuals who do not use tobacco have a chemical in their system that indicates they have been exposed to tobacco smoke during the previous two to three days. Children, particularly those living in a household with a smoker, experienced particularly high rates of exposure.

*Lung Cancer.*  Overall, regular exposure to passive smoke increases a non-smoker's risk of lung cancer by 25 to 50 percent. As with many diseases linked to active smoking, the longer and more intense the nonsmoker's exposure to passive smoke, the greater his or her risk. One analysis, which combined the result of thirty-seven studies, found that the risk of lung cancer in a nonsmoker who had a smoking spouse was small if the spouse smoked less than ten cigarettes a day but grew to be large if he or she smoked a pack or more a day. In the Nurses' Health Study, we found that women who were regularly exposed to passive smoke had a 50 percent greater risk of lung cancer than those not regularly exposed.

*Coronary Heart Disease.*  Based on the results of numerous studies, passive smoking appears to increase the risk of coronary heart disease in nonsmokers by about 20 to 30 percent. In the Nurses' Health Study, we found the risk associated with passive smoking to be slightly larger and to increase with the amount of exposure (see Figure 17-9).

*Sudden Infant Death Syndrome.*  Both active smoking by a mother during pregnancy and passive exposure to cigarette smoke by the child in infancy have been linked to increased risk of sudden infant death syndrome. Compared to infants not exposed to passive smoke, those who are exposed have about twice the risk of sudden infant death.

*Breathing Problems and Infections in Children.*  Children regularly exposed to passive smoke are more likely to experience middle ear infections, repeated respiratory illnesses, wheezing, and slightly decreased lung function.

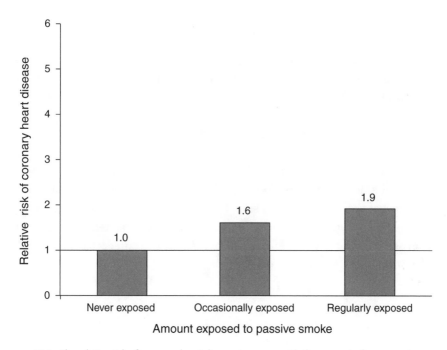

FIG. 17-9. The relative risk of coronary heart disease increases with the amount of exposure to passive smoke. (Source: Nurses' Health Study)

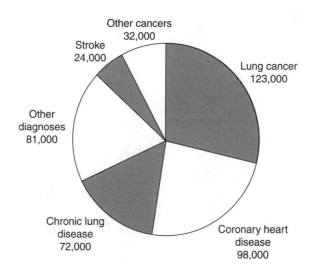

FIG. 17-10. 430,000 U.S. deaths are attributable to cigarette smoking each year. (Source: Centers for Disease Control and Prevention)

## How Does Smoking Affect Length of Life?

More than 430,000 individuals die each year in the United States from smoking-related causes (see Figure 17-10). Smoking causes one out of every five deaths in the United States, and on average, smokers die seven years earlier than nonsmokers. In the Nurses' Health Study, we found that women who smoke have nearly double the chances of dying prematurely than women who have never smoked (see Figure 17-11).

Such statistics are staggering given that the disability and premature death caused by smoking is entirely preventable. But current smokers can still reduce their risk of premature death by stopping smoking as soon as possible. A number of large cohort studies, including ours, have found that ten to fifteen years after she quits, a former smoker's risk of premature death drops to nearly that of a woman who has never smoked.

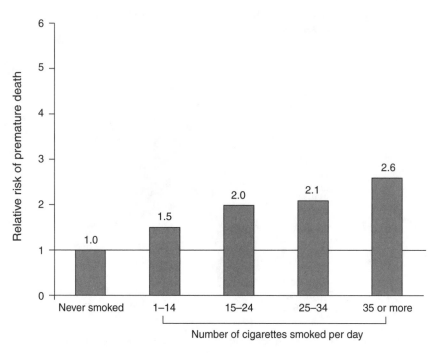

FIG. 17-11. The relative risk of premature death increases steadily with the number of cigarettes smoked per day. (Source: Nurses' Health Study)

## Cigars, Pipes, and Smokeless Tobacco

Even though cigarette smoking dominates most of the health messages related to tobacco use, all forms of tobacco have large health risks associated with them. Cigars, pipes, and smokeless tobacco (snuff) are often perceived as safer either because they do not involve smoke (smokeless tobacco) or because the smoke is not inhaled as deeply into the lungs (cigars and pipes). Despite this, cigars, pipes, and smokeless tobacco are associated with many serious health risks and should be avoided as carefully as cigarettes.

| TYPE OF TOBACCO | HEALTH RISKS |
| --- | --- |
| Cigars and pipes | Coronary heart disease |
| | Lung cancer |
| | Oral cancer |
| | Esophageal and laryngeal cancer |
| | Chronic obstructive pulmonary disease |
| Smokeless tobacco (snuff) | Oral cancer |

## WHAT IT ALL MEANS

Smoking is the single most important cause of premature death among women and men, which makes the overall health messages related to smoking very clear and concise.

- It is best never to start using tobacco.
- People who currently use tobacco should stop for good as soon as possible.

The benefits of quitting smoking are enormous and cannot be overstated. The increased risk of nearly all serious diseases linked to tobacco use drop over time after the smoker quits, most to levels that equal that of someone who has never smoked.

## WHAT I TELL MY PATIENTS ABOUT SUCCESSFULLY QUITTING SMOKING

DR. NANCY RIGOTTI

All my patients know that smoking is bad for them, even though they may not know about all of the risks involved. Still, most of those who smoke wish that they didn't, and many have tried to quit. But as every smoker knows, quitting can be difficult. Only rarely is a patient successful on the first try. Most often, it takes several tries before she quits for good.

In my experience, most smokers think that what it takes to quit is a hefty dose of willpower, and they worry that they will not have the toughness. I disagree. I think of quitting smoking as a learning process. Just as most smokers once had to learn to enjoy inhaling cigarette smoke, they have to learn how to live without cigarettes as daily companions. Learning any new skill involves trying something new and making some mistakes. So it's no surprise that many smokers who make the effort to quit end up back on cigarettes. The secret to success is to learn from past mistakes. If you do and you keep trying to stop smoking, you can succeed.

Understanding what motivates you to smoke and the obstacles that you'll encounter along the way can help you discover the approach that will work best for you. Usually you need to combine multiple approaches. There is no single magic approach. If your first (or second or third) attempt fails, you can learn from the experience and use that knowledge to stop for good on your next try. Even though it's tough to quit smoking, it is far from impossible. Over a thousand people quit for good every day.

## Preparing to Quit

Take some time to prepare your plan to quit. Start by thinking about why you want to quit and why you keep smoking. For most smokers, addiction to nicotine is the main reason to keep smoking. Though a smoker may enjoy the first cigarette of the day, after that, most of her smoking is done to prevent the discomfort of the symptoms of nicotine withdrawal: irritability, restlessness, anxiety, or difficulty concentrating. Smokers also use cigarettes to cope with stress and such unpleasant feelings as anger, frustration, and boredom. To quit, a smoker needs to break the nicotine addiction and learn how to cope with these feelings without using cigarettes.

Make a list of the reasons to quit and post it in a visible place. Besides the medical benefits listed above, smokers who quit save money, set a good example for their children, free themselves from addiction, smell better, and so on. In the end, only you can make the decision to stop. Once you do, you can get help from medicines, family and friends, special programs, and health professionals. Quitters who use these techniques and build these skills are 60 percent more likely to be successful than those who do not. Some of the most important skills to develop relate to breaking the habit of smoking and developing a smoke-free lifestyle. These tips can help.

## Monitor Your Smoking Habits

Start by learning about when and why you smoke. Keep a diary for one week that tracks when, where, and how much you smoke. Attach a small index card or piece of paper to each pack of cigarettes. Every time you smoke a cigarette, write down the time you smoked, where you smoked, and what events or feelings immediately preceded your smoking, and how badly you wanted that particular cigarette on a scale of 1 to 5. Reviewing your week-long diary can help you identify and address circumstances linked to your smoking.

## Setting a Date to Quit

However you plan to quit smoking, set a quit date and prepare for it in a way that minimizes the symptoms of nicotine withdrawal. Make sure everyone close to you knows your plan: they can be invaluable in helping you succeed.

## Prepare a Tobacco-Free Environment

Try to make your home smoke-free, even if your spouse is a smoker. Not only will it eliminate passive smoke—and the health risks associated with it—from the place in which you spend most of your time, it may also entice the smoker(s) you live with to quit.

Here's how to do it:

- Eliminate all ashtrays, matches, and lighters from the house.
- Tell all smokers they need to go outside to smoke. No exceptions— not even for spouses, close relatives, or best friends.
- Stand firm with your policy. It will help those in your family, and it will be a good example for your friends and neighbors.

Of course you want to make your own home a tobacco-free environment. You also want to avoid any place or situation where people are likely to be smoking. If close friends and coworkers are smokers, try to avoid them in situations when they are most likely to be smoking. Also avoid situations where many people will be smoking, such as bars, clubs, or rock concerts.

## Monitor Your Mood

Smokers tend to be more depressed than nonsmokers. Suffering from depression, even mild depression, can make it harder to quit. Feeling overwhelmed at the thought of quitting or approaching it negatively may be signs of depression. People who are successfully treated for depression are more likely to succeed at quitting. Getting counseling, as I discuss below, can greatly help you with depression and make it easier to quit smoking.

## Avoid Alcohol and Caffeine

Alcohol can promote the desire for nicotine. Because smoking is often associated with drinking, it helps to limit alcohol consumption or to stop using alcohol altogether for a while during the time when you are quitting smoking.

The same is true of coffee and other caffeine-containing drinks. If you regularly drink caffeinated coffee (or other caffeine-containing drinks), slowly reduce your consumption so that you can avoid caffeine withdrawal symptoms—headache and fatigue. You want that behind you before you start to quit smoking.

## Exercise

Practically all of my patients who want to quit smoking have a fear of gaining weight. And they're right: most people do tend to gain some weight when they quit smoking. But even though becoming overweight causes health problems, in general the benefits of quitting far outweigh any risks this amount of weight gain may have.

Quitting can cause you to gain weight in two ways. First, when nicotine is withdrawn, there is a decrease in the rate at which the body metabolizes (processes) nutrients. So many former smokers may actually be eating the same amount of food as before, but because they use those calories at a slower rate, they put on weight. Second, many people substitute food for cigarettes, consuming more food than they did previously.

Regular exercise can minimize the amount of weight you put on while in the process of quitting smoking. In the Nurses' Health Study, women who added two or more hours a week of vigorous exercise gained only an average of five pounds over two years. Incidentally, the women in the study who continued to smoke also put on weight over the same period—approximately one and a half pounds.

With weight gain an important obstacle to quitting, all smokers should consider adopting an exercise program before beginning the process. Regular exercise before, during, and after actually makes it more likely that you will be successful at quitting.

## Healthy Diet

Some of my patients tell me that changing their diet to a more healthy one—particularly snacking on raw fruits and vegetables and drinking eight glasses of water a day—actually makes it easier for them to quit smoking. They find that being disciplined in one way helps them to be more disciplined in another. But don't overdo it. Going on a weight-loss diet at the same time that you try to quit smoking is not a good strategy. You are likely to fail at both. To control your weight, focus on maintaining a healthy diet and getting regular exercise.

## Plan How to Deal with Nicotine Withdrawal

Tobacco creates an addiction, a physical dependence. You are hooked. Your body needs nicotine and develops symptoms when levels of nicotine in your blood get low. When a smoker quits, she can develop the following symptoms of nicotine withdrawal: cravings for a cigarette, irritability, anxiety, depression, inability to concentrate, impatience, anger, excessive hunger, and difficulty sleeping. These withdrawal symptoms reach a peak two or three days after quitting and then wane gradually over several weeks. Many smokers have simply endured these discomforts and quit. But that is not necessary. Today there are effective ways to minimize the discomfort of quitting smoking.

Nicotine withdrawal can be treated both with nicotine replacement therapy and with a medicine, called bupropion, that reduces the cravings of any addiction. My patients often ask me why doctors would prescribe a toxic substance like nicotine. I explain that it is other components of tobacco smoke, not nicotine, that damages the heart, lungs, and other organs. Nicotine causes addiction, and addiction can be treated by gradually lowering the amount of the addicting substance that is in the body. Nicotine replacement therapy does this in a way that smoking a cigarette does not.

### NICOTINE REPLACEMENT THERAPY

Some people are able to quit cold turkey. That is hard. I'm not sure I could have done it if I had become addicted to tobacco. Many of my patients have found nicotine replacement therapy to be helpful in overcoming the initial withdrawal from nicotine. The four different types of nicotine replacement therapy currently available—nicotine patch, nicotine gum, nicotine nasal spray, and a nicotine inhaler—all release nicotine into your bloodstream in amounts large enough to block the discomfort of withdrawal. In contrast to smoking, they produce relatively constant blood levels of nicotine. Therefore, they do not produce the pleasure or hit that smokers notice, but they do blunt the pain of withdrawal and they do not contain any of the other toxic chemicals in tobacco.

Using any nicotine replacement product will approximately double your chances of quitting successfully compared to using none of them. Both the patch and the gum are available without a prescription and are safe for most people when used correctly. The nasal spray and inhaler require a doctor's prescription.

You should never smoke or use snuff or chewing tobacco while using the patch or gum; this increases your risk of nicotine overdose. If you have heart disease or are pregnant or breast-feeding, talk to your health care provider before starting nicotine replacement.

### Nicotine Patch

The patch contains a fixed amount of nicotine that is released in doses and absorbed by your bloodstream throughout the day. On the day you plan to quit, you apply a nicotine patch to a hairless spot on your upper arm or torso. A typical patch is worn for sixteen or twenty-four hours and replaced the next morning.

The patch is most often available in three strengths, though some come in two. This allows you to start with the highest dose of nicotine, when your withdrawal symptoms are heaviest, and over time switch to lower doses as your symptoms start to wane. Most smokers start with the highest dose unless they weigh less than a hundred pounds or smoke less than half a pack a day. Most people should use the patch for eight weeks. The major side effect is skin irritation at the site where the patch is worn. To avoid this, apply the patch to a different area of skin each day. Do not use any tobacco products while wearing the patch.

In most cases, the patch is the preferred method of nicotine replacement therapy because it is easy to use, generally requiring only one application a day.

### Nicotine Gum

When nicotine gum is chewed, it releases nicotine, which is absorbed through the lining of the mouth and then passes into the bloodstream. The gum is available in two strengths—2 milligrams per piece and 4 milligrams per piece. The lower strength version is recommended for lighter smokers (who smoke less than one pack a day), while the higher strength is reserved for those who smoke more than a pack a day.

When using the gum, chew it only long enough to release the nicotine, which will produce a peppery taste. Then place it between your gums and cheek to allow the nicotine to be absorbed. When the taste disappears, chew the gum again just enough to produce the distinctive taste. Then push it back into the corner of your mouth. If you chew it too fast, nicotine will be released faster than it can be absorbed and it will do you no good. Each piece should be kept in the mouth for thirty minutes and then discarded. Keep in mind that it takes twenty minutes for the nicotine in the gum to fully reach the bloodstream. In contrast, when you smoke a cigarette, it takes only seconds for nicotine blood levels to rise.

People who use nicotine gum often chew too few pieces per day, and for too few weeks, to receive the gum's maximum benefits. In general, I recommend to my patients a fixed schedule of at least one piece every one to two hours for one to three months. Some people develop side effects such as hiccups, upset stomach, a sore jaw, or a burning sensation in the mouth. Often these are the results of improper chewing technique.

Most of my patients find the patch easier to use than gum, but some prefer gum. One reason is that nicotine gum provides the smoker with an oral activity to replace the act of smoking, which can help break the urge to smoke in response to certain cues. People with dentures have trouble chewing the gum and often do better with another type of nicotine replacement.

Occasionally, nicotine gum users become dependent on the gum. To avoid this, do not use the gum for longer than six months, and reduce your use gradually when you decide to quit. Never use any tobacco products while chewing nicotine gum.

### Nicotine Nasal Spray and Inhaler

Nicotine nasal sprays and inhalers require a prescription from your doctor. The nicotine nasal spray is absorbed through the mucous membrane of your nose and into the bloodstream within five to ten minutes. The nicotine in the inhaler is absorbed through your mouth, throat, and lungs and has its peak effect in twenty minutes.

Nicotine levels are maintained one to two hours, but there is a more dramatic rise in blood nicotine levels with the nasal spray than with the patch, gum, or inhaler. This produces more rapid relief of withdrawal symptoms and better stimulates the nicotine rush a smoker gets from a cigarette, but it also poses greater potential for becoming dependent on the spray.

Side effects of the nasal spray include nose and throat irritation, watery eyes, sneezing, and coughing. Side effects of the inhaler include coughing and mouth and throat irritation.

The studies done thus far of the inhaler and spray show them to be about as effective as the patch and gum. However, there are fewer studies of these techniques than of the patch or gum.

## Non-Nicotine Drug Treatment

In contrast to quitting aids that release nicotine into the bloodstream, there are some drug therapies currently being studied that do not do so. One of these is the antidepressant drug bupropion. Like nicotine replacement therapy, bupropion approximately doubles your chances of quitting successfully. Symptoms of depression or negative moods have been linked to nicotine dependence, and antidepressants can help relieve such symptoms, possibly making it more likely that an attempt at quitting will be successful.

Bupropion is started one week before a smoker's planned quit day and is continued for eight to twelve weeks. Because the drug does not contain nicotine, it can be used in combination with nicotine replacement therapy. A side effect of bupropion is having a seizure, although this is rare at the low doses generally used to help you quit smoking. Other more frequent side effects of bupropion are insomnia, agitation, anxiety, dry mouth, headache, and skin rash.

## Getting Support from Family and Friends

Most hard things are easier when you have the support of the people closest to you. Getting support from them will help you be successful with your quit attempt. Compared to people who do not get such support, those who do have a 30 to 50 percent greater chance of quitting successfully. Let those around you know you are attempting to quit. By providing encouragement, helping you work through particular obstacles, and not enticing you to smoke, they will help you through the process. One of the key supporters is your partner, especially if he or she does not smoke. It is really hard to succeed at quitting if your partner continues to smoke throughout the process. Try to quit together. If he or she resists, prepare a plan to cope with his or her smoking. Ask your partner to refrain from smoking in your home, at least for the first month or two after you quit, and ask him or her to keep ashtrays, cigarettes, and other temptations out of sight.

## Getting Counseling from Health Care Professionals

Counselors can be an important source of support and can provide insight different from that given by friends and family. You would likely benefit from attending some sort of cessation counseling, either one-on-one with a counselor or in a group situation. Overall, cessation counseling doubles the chances of quitting successfully. It provides you with an opportunity to develop the skills necessary to overcome obstacles to quitting, and group counseling also gives you a source of social support.

The longer and more frequent the counseling sessions, the more effective they are in aiding quitting. At a minimum, you should look for these elements in a counseling program:

- Session length: at least twenty to thirty minutes
- Number of sessions: at least four to seven
- Number of weeks: at least two

Smoking cessation groups are usually organized by local hospitals and by local chapters of the American Lung Association (website: www.lungusa. org; phone: 212-315-8700), the American Heart Association (website: www. americanheart.org; phone: 800-AHA-USA1), and the American Cancer Society (website: www.cancer.org; phone: 800-ACS-2345).

## Alternative Medicine Methods for Quitting

Many of my patients who want to quit smoking are interested in alternative medicine approaches. Many therapies, including acupuncture, hypnosis, and herbal remedies, are offered to help smokers quit. None of these has been proven through scientific study to be effective, and acupuncture has been shown not to work for stopping smoking. However, the health risks of continuing to smoke are so great that if an alternative therapy helps you quit, it may be worthwhile. Discuss any alternative anti-smoking program you are considering with your physician before you undergo treatment. If an alternative method does not work, try one of the conventional treatments. Do not give up.

## Helping Your Kids Avoid Tobacco

Some of the patients who ask my help in quitting smoking are not smokers themselves, but are worried about someone else in the family, often their kids. Children explore and experiment. That's a part of being a kid. Unfortunately, for many youth, experimentation with tobacco can lead to lifelong nicotine addiction and serious health problems.

Most smokers begin using tobacco before the age of twenty, and many do so much younger. Helping young people reason through their actions and the consequences (both in the long and short term) can give them the skills they need to successfully avoid tobacco use. As early as elementary school, parents should start talking to their children about tobacco.

Some recommendations from a federal report on smoking cessation include: Make sure your kids know that they will come into contact with peers who will want them to experiment with tobacco. Discuss ways they can resist and counter such peer pressure by giving them information about tobacco and its effects. For example:

- Most kids do not smoke or use smokeless tobacco.
- All forms of tobacco are addictive, even more so than many drugs.
- Smoking makes a person smell bad, stains the teeth and skin, hinders athletic performance, and ruins clothes.
- Smoking can cause a long-term cough and sore throat.
- Tobacco is expensive and requires money that could be spent on items much more fun (concert tickets, books, posters, or CDs).
- There are many other ways to assert one's independence than smoking, which has many negative consequences.

Helping our children avoid tobacco use is one of the best means we have to ensure their good health and improve the overall health of the nation. And the trends are encouraging. For over thirty years the rate of smoking in the United States has been decreasing. Even though nicotine is extremely addictive, over 1,000 people are able to quit smoking for good every day—something I frequently remind my smoking patients about. But the real hope lies in the future, with our children, who with adequate knowledge and skills and the help of a caring society may be able to avoid tobacco use altogether and eliminate it from the public health landscape.

# CHAPTER EIGHTEEN

# The Major Nutrients—
# Fat, Carbohydrates, Fiber,
# and Protein

## Key Lifestyle Message

- Eating a diet rich in fruits, vegetables, whole grains, and fiber and low in saturated and trans fats is one of the best ways to improve your overall health.

## BACKGROUND

Food plays several roles at once in our daily lives. At its most basic, it provides the nutrients we need to survive and to thrive. But as you well know, food is also much more than just sustenance. It is the backdrop for many social occasions and is a source of enjoyment in its own right. We gather at meals with our friends, family, and colleagues to socialize and to celebrate, and we often eat simply for the wonderful taste of a well-prepared meal. However, it is the health aspects of food that often come to the fore when we think about what we eat, how we prepare our food, and how our diets make us feel. One nationwide survey found that close to 70 percent of people in the United States are significantly concerned about the link between the food they eat and their future health.

Over the next four chapters, we will try to answer that often vexing question: What should I eat to be healthy? This chapter discusses how the major nutrients—fats, carbohydrates, fiber, and protein—relate to health. Chapters 19 and 20 review what is known about the relationship between specific foods and beverages and health. And finally, Chapter 21 discusses the potential health benefits and risks of selected vitamins and minerals—both those found in food and in dietary supplements.

## THE MAJOR NUTRIENTS

Every day you are likely inundated with health messages about the major nutrients. As in no time previously, these messages seem to appear almost everywhere, from grocery store aisles and school cafeterias to bookstore shelves and Internet websites. And the messages run the spectrum: *Eat low carbohydrate. Eat high carbohydrate. Eat high protein. Eat low protein.* Figuring out how you should try to eat—what it is about the major nutrients you should focus on—can be a challenging, even maddening task.

In this chapter, we will review what the research says about the link between the major nutrients and health, and try to dispel some outdated, or simply incorrect, messages about them.

The major nutrients (also called macronutrients) are so called because the body needs them in relatively large quantities to function properly. The big three—fat, carbohydrates, and protein—are the primary sources of calories in the body, but they also have many other roles. For example, fat aids in the absorption of certain vitamins and is necessary to maintain the structure of cells, and protein is a main constituent of muscle and other tissue and is needed for a healthy nervous system. Fiber, which does not provide any calories, can affect blood clotting and modify how the body uses other nutrients.

## LESSONS FROM THE NURSES' HEALTH STUDY AND OTHER STUDIES

A large amount of research has assessed the link between the major nutrients and health, and over the past decade, the thinking behind this relationship has become more refined. Blanket statements such as *fat is bad* and *carbohydrates are good* rarely apply anymore. Data now show us that issues such as the relationship between fat intake and heart disease or that between carbohydrates and diabetes are much more complex than originally thought.

Over the course of the Nurses' Health Study, we have spent a great deal of time teasing out the influence the major nutrients have on the risk of disease. Overall, the most powerful findings show that some types of fat and carbohydrates can increase the risk of coronary heart disease and diabetes and that other types of fat and carbohydrates—as well as fiber—can lower risk. Possibly surprisingly, we (as well as many other researchers) have found only a few links between the major nutrients and cancer.

## Dietary Fat

Next to smoking, no health-related activity has been vilified more than eating a high fat diet. It is said by many to cause heart disease, cancer, and weight gain. But what do the data really show about the link between fat in the diet and health? More and more, the data show that it is the *type* of fat—rather than the amount of total fat—that is linked to illness.

When properly assessed in studies, a high total fat intake seems to have no real bearing on the risk of cancer or cardiovascular disease. As for a high fat intake causing weight gain, there is also very little evidence of this. It is true that fat carries with it a lot of calories—9 calories per gram compared to 4 calories per gram for carbohydrates and protein—but studies show that people tend to adjust the amount of food they eat to meet their normal calorie intake. Calories seem to act no differently whether they come from fat, protein, or carbohydrate. The primary cause of weight gain is simply eating more calories (no matter what the source) than are burned through activity. A good example: even though the average total fat intake has dropped over the last ten years in the United States, the prevalence of overweight and obesity has increased dramatically.

### Types of Fat, Plus Cholesterol

Fat is a rich source of energy for the body, and it has other important functions as well. It provides structure to cells, is a precursor to many hormones, and is a component of the sheath that surrounds nerves. Fat adds a lot of flavor to food and provides a sense of satiety after a meal, staving off the sense of hunger for a longer period than is the case with a meal with little or no fat.

As discussed earlier (see Chapter 4), there are four main types of fat: saturated fat, trans-unsaturated fat (also simply called trans fat), polyunsaturated fat, and monounsaturated fat. Each type has a distinct chemical structure, which is one reason they can have a varied effect on the risk of disease. Most foods that have fat generally contain more than one type. Red meat, for example, is high in saturated fat but also contains a good deal of monounsaturated fat. Canola oil is high in polyunsaturated and monounsaturated fat but also contains a little bit of saturated fat (see table).

• **Saturated fats** come primarily from animal sources and are solid at room temperature in their pure form, such as butter and lard. Other sources of saturated fat are red meat, cheese, nonskim milk, and tropical vegetable oils, such as palm kernel oil and coconut oil.

## Percentage of Specific Types of Fat in Common Oils and Fats*

| | Saturated | Mono-unsaturated | Poly-unsaturated | Trans | Alpha-linolenic acid |
|---|---|---|---|---|---|
| *Oils* | | | | | |
| Canola | 7 | 58 | 29 | 0 | 12 |
| Safflower | 9 | 12 | 74 | 0 | 0 |
| Sunflower | 10 | 20 | 66 | 0 | 2 |
| Corn | 13 | 24 | 60 | 0 | 1 |
| Olive | 13 | 72 | 8 | 1 | 1 |
| Soybean | 16 | 44 | 37 | 0 | 7 |
| Peanut | 17 | 49 | 32 | 0 | 1 |
| Palm | 50 | 37 | 10 | 0 | 0 |
| Coconut | 87 | 6 | 2 | 0 | 0 |
| *Cooking Fat* | | | | | |
| Crisco | 22 | 29 | 29 | 18 | 2 |
| Lard | 39 | 44 | 11 | 1 | 0 |
| Butter | 60 | 26 | 5 | 5 | 1 |
| *Margarines/Spreads* | | | | | |
| Imperial, Soybean Stick | 18 | 2 | 29 | 23 | 4 |
| Fleishman Spread Corn & Soybean Tub | 16 | 27 | 44 | 11 | 1 |
| Shedd's Country Crock Spread, Soybean Tub | 17 | 24 | 49 | 8 | 6 |
| Promise Tub; Sunflower, Soybean, and Canola | 18 | 22 | 54 | 5 | 1 |

*Values expressed as percent of total fat; data are from analyses at Harvard School of Public Health Lipid Laboratory and U.S.D.A. publications.

- **Trans fats** are vegetable fats that have been altered during a heating process and, like saturated fats, are solid at room temperature. Stick margarine and vegetable shortening are examples of trans fats, and they are widely used in commercial baking products—cookies, cupcakes, pies—often appearing on food labels as *partially hydrogenated vegetable oil*. Commercially fried foods, such as the French fries and onion rings from fast food restaurants, are also major sources.

- **Polyunsaturated fats** come primarily from plant and fish sources—though there are some animal sources as well—and are liquid at room temperature. Common sources are liquid vegetable oils, oil-based salad dressings, and fatty fish (like salmon and tuna). There are two specific polyunsaturated fats, called essential fats, that the body must get in the diet. These are linoleic acid and alpha-linolenic acid.

- **Monounsaturated fats,** like polyunsaturated fats, are liquid at room temperature. Major sources include olive oil, peanut oil, canola oil, and in the American diet, meats and dairy products.

- **Cholesterol,** which is often lumped together with fats, is more of a fat-like substance than a true fat. It does not provide any calories, but it does serve some important functions, including being a precursor to certain hormones and bile salts that aid in digestion. Only foods of animal origin contain cholesterol. Egg yolks, shellfish, whole milk dairy products, and certain organ meats (such as liver, kidney, and brain) are particularly high in cholesterol. However, cholesterol is not a required part of the diet. The body can make all it needs in the liver and intestines.

## Potential Risks and Benefits of Fat Intake

### Coronary Heart Disease

Coronary heart disease is a leading cause of death among American women, claiming more than 230,000 lives each year. A low fat diet has long been recommended as a way to lower the risk of coronary heart disease. However, this now seems to be an oversimplification. In the Nurses' Health Study, we have found that it is not the total intake of fat that affects the risk of heart disease, but rather the level of intake of the different kinds of fats. Both saturated fat and trans-unsaturated fat increase the risk of coronary heart disease, while polyunsaturated fat and monounsaturated fat lower risk.

Fats are thought to influence the risk of coronary heart disease primarily by affecting low density lipoprotein (LDL) ("bad") and high density lipoprotein

(HDL) ("good") cholesterol levels. LDL cholesterol can promote heart disease by contributing to the buildup of fat and cholesterol in the coronary arteries (called atherosclerosis). HDL cholesterol has the opposite effect, removing cholesterol from the walls of arteries and from the blood, and helping to eliminate it from the body. A low LDL level and a high HDL is the best combination when it comes to lowering the risk of heart disease. Aside from their influence on blood cholesterol, fats may also affect other factors linked to coronary heart disease, such as blood clotting, sensitivity to insulin, and the chances of having a fatally irregular heartbeat following a heart attack.

*Saturated Fat.* Saturated fat is well known as a "bad" fat, but when it comes to its effect on the risk of coronary heart disease, it does not increase risk as much as many people might think. While saturated fat does increase total cholesterol, it does this by raising both the LDL cholesterol *and* HDL cholesterol. In the Nurses' Health Study, we found that increases in saturated fat intake only slightly increased the risk of coronary heart disease.

*Trans Fats.* Like saturated fats, they are solid at room temperature. Gram for gram, trans fats are the worst fats for the heart. Studies have found that they not only raise LDL levels but also lower HDL levels, a worst-case scenario when it comes to blood cholesterol and heart disease. In the Nurses' Health Study, we found that replacing only about 30 calories a day of carbohydrates with about 30 grams of trans fats could nearly double the risk of coronary heart disease.

*Polyunsaturated Fat.* Studies have consistently found that polyunsaturated fats lower LDL cholesterol while they either slightly lower or have no effect on HDL cholesterol. In the Nurses' Health Study, we found that replacing about 80 calories a day of carbohydrates with about 80 calories of polyunsaturated fat lowered the risk of coronary heart disease by about 40 percent. We also found that one specific type of polyunsaturated fat, alpha-linolenic acid, was particularly effective at preventing death from coronary heart disease. Women whose diets contained the greatest proportion of alpha-linolenic acid—found in many vegetable oil–based salad dressings—had almost half the risk of dying from heart disease than women whose diets contained the lowest proportion of alpha-linolenic acid. In addition to improving cholesterol levels, alpha-linolenic acid may also help protect against the deadly irregular heartbeats that can follow a heart attack. However, before drastically changing family eating habits to include more alpha-linolenic acid, women may want to know that some studies have found that alpha-linolenic acid may increase the risk of serious prostate cancer. In our study of 51,000 male health professionals, we found that men eating the most alpha-linolenic acid had over three times the risk of advanced prostate cancer as men eating the least.

Some studies have also shown that the polyunsaturated fat found primarily in fatty fish (omega-3) may help lower the risk of coronary heart disease, particularly sudden death caused by irregular heartbeats. Although studies to date have not consistently found a benefit, in the Nurses' Health Study we found a 20 percent reduction in the risk of heart disease among women who ate fish at least once a month. Those who ate fish more frequently received even greater protection.

*Monounsaturated Fats.* Just as trans fats are particularly bad for cholesterol levels, monounsaturated fats seem particularly good, both lowering LDL levels and increasing HDL levels. In the Nurses' Health Study, we found that replacing about 80 calories a day of carbohydrates with about 80 calories of monounsaturated fats lowered the risk of coronary heart disease by about 30 percent. Even though red meat is a major source of monounsaturated fat in the United States, increasing meat intake is not a recommended way to increase the amount of monounsaturated fat in the diet. In addition to containing a good deal of saturated fat, a high red meat intake may also increase the risk of colon cancer. Olive oil, peanut oil, and canola oil are much healthier choices, as they contain very little saturated fat.

*Cholesterol.* Cholesterol in the diet is often confused with cholesterol in the blood. While it would seem to make sense that eating a lot of cholesterol would have a particularly bad effect on blood cholesterol levels, this is not the case for most people. Overall, the amount of cholesterol in the diet has only a small influence on blood cholesterol levels. It is actually the intake of saturated and trans fat that has a more profound effect on blood cholesterol. But cholesterol in the diet does seem to slightly affect the risk of coronary heart disease. Studies show that adding an extra 200 milligrams of cholesterol a day to the diet (about the amount found in an 8-ounce steak) increases the risk of developing heart disease by about 10 percent.

A major source of cholesterol, eggs seem to have been unduly maligned over the past thirty years. While it is true that the 200 milligrams of cholesterol in the average egg yolk may slightly increase the risk of heart disease if eaten very frequently, eggs contain many other nutrients that may actually be good for the heart, including protein, folic acid, some polyunsaturated fats, vitamin E, and some B vitamins. In the Nurses' Health Study, we found that the risk of coronary heart disease and stroke was the same for healthy women who ate one egg a day as it was for those who ate fewer than one egg a week.

## ADULT-ONSET (TYPE 2) DIABETES

Adult-onset diabetes is a very serious disorder that affects approximately 16 million people in the United States. The high blood glucose levels and hormonal abnormalities that result from diabetes contribute to a number of health problems, including coronary heart disease, stroke, blindness, skin ulcers, nerve disorders, and kidney dysfunction. Although studies comparing different countries throughout the world have found a link between high total fat intake and diabetes, most large cohort studies—including the Nurses' Health Study—have not. Some different types of fat, however, may be linked to risk. We found that a high intake of trans fat increased the risk of adult-onset diabetes and that a high intake of vegetable fat could lower the risk by as much as 40 percent, comparing women with the highest intake of these fats to those with the lowest intake and keeping calorie intake constant. And there is even some evidence that a high intake of monounsaturated fat may improve the body's ability to efficiently use insulin, the hormone that helps the body properly regulate blood glucose levels.

## BREAST CANCER

Although women frequently hear the message that a high fat diet increases the risk of breast cancer, most of the evidence suggests that a high fat diet in adulthood has little, if any, effect on the risk of developing breast cancer. When we assessed this issue in the Nurses' Health Study, we found that neither a high fat nor a low fat diet had any influence on breast cancer risk.

As with heart disease, however, type of fat may be important when it comes to breast cancer. One large Swedish study found that women eating the greatest amount of monounsaturated fat had a 20 percent lower risk of the disease than women eating the least. In the Nurses' Health Study, our most recent results showed no benefit from a high intake of monounsaturated fat, but one reason for this may have to do with the source of the monounsaturated fat. Most of the studies that have shown monounsaturated fats to protect against breast cancer have been performed in Europe and have specifically evaluated olive oil intake. In our study, animal products (such as red meat and cheese) have been the primary source of monounsaturated fats. That the fat comes from such different food sources could account for the difference in findings.

Some unanswered questions still remain about fat intake and breast cancer, however. It is unclear how fat intake in youth may affect risk later in life. It is also unclear how a very low fat diet throughout adulthood affects risk. Studies such as the Women's Health Initiative and our Nurses' Health Study II should help answer such questions in the future.

## Non-Hodgkin's Lymphoma

About 55,000 people a year in the United States develop non-Hodgkin's lymphoma, a cancer that starts in the lymph nodes and can spread to other lymphatic tissues. Although the other main type of lymphoma—Hodgkin's lymphoma—primarily affects children and young adults, 95 percent of non-Hodgkin's lymphoma cases occur in adults. Some studies have found a link between fat intake and the risk of non-Hodgkin's lymphoma, possibly because of a connection between dietary fat and the health of the immune system. When we studied this issue in the Nurses' Health Study, we found that women who ate the most trans fat had more than double the risk of the disease than women eating the least. This study, though, only suggests that there may be a link between trans fat and non-Hodgkin's lymphoma. Other studies are needed before we can come to any firm conclusions.

## Endometrial Cancer

Endometrial cancer develops in the endometrium, the inner lining of the uterus. A high fat diet appears to have little, if any, effect on the risk of developing endometrial cancer. Although some smaller studies have shown that eating high amounts of fat might increase risk, most larger studies—including ours—have not. Saturated fat intake, however, may be linked to risk. We found in the Nurses' Health Study that the more saturated fat postmenopausal women ate, the more likely they were to develop endometrial cancer. Saturated fats are thought to alter the body's natural production of certain hormones that can increase the risk of endometrial cancer.

## Carbohydrates

Carbohydrates are the main source of calories in the U.S. diet—contributing about half of all calories—and run the range from table sugar to whole oats. Although all types of carbohydrates provide energy, the way in which they provide energy and the reaction they cause in the body can vary drastically.

One popular way to categorize carbohydrates is into *simple* and *complex*. Simple carbohydrates are sugars. The most basic simple carbohydrates are glucose (sometimes called dextrose), fructose (also called fruit sugar), and galactose (also called milk sugar). And the other sugars found in food can be made from these three. Table sugar contains sucrose, made by joining a molecule of glucose with one of fructose, and milk contains lactose, made by joining a molecule of glucose with one of galactose. Complex carbohydrates are made up of long chains of these simple sugars. Although there are many types of complex carbohydrates in food, the main one is starch, which is a long chain of glucose. In the digestive system, complex carbohydrates such as starch are broken down into their component sugars. Some complex carbohydrates, though, are indigestible and pass largely unchanged through the stomach and the intestines. These indigestible carbohydrates are called fiber and are a key part of the diet.

The most important carbohydrate to the body is glucose. It is the preferred energy source for most tissues, and maintaining normal levels of glucose in the blood is essential to the body's functioning optimally. During digestion, the body breaks down the carbohydrates in food to release glucose so that it can be absorbed into the bloodstream. This causes blood glucose levels to rise. In response to this, the pancreas, an organ in the abdomen, releases the hormone insulin. Insulin allows the glucose in the blood to enter the body's cells, where it is either used immediately for energy or stored for use at a later time. As the glucose is taken up by the tissues, its level in the blood drops. When the blood glucose level drops back down to normal, insulin is released at a much lower rate.

Not all foods, however, affect this process in the same way. While insulin levels rise and fall following a meal with any kind of carbohydrate, how drastically they react differs according to the type of carbohydrate. A food that causes a quick influx of glucose into the bloodstream will cause insulin levels to rise very rapidly and to very high levels. This can occasionally cause cells to take up too much glucose, dropping blood glucose levels to below normal. This in turn can trigger the body to feel hungry (even if a meal has just been consumed) because it is being told by the brain that it needs more glucose. Foods that are converted more slowly to glucose have a mellower influence on insulin levels. They are less likely to cause such big ups and downs in glucose and insulin levels that can cause false sensations of hunger and other more chronic problems.

## GLYCEMIC INDEX

How quickly and strongly a food raises blood glucose levels is estimated by its glycemic index. A high glycemic index means that a food has a strong effect on blood glucose levels; a low glycemic index means the food has only a small effect. Pure glucose is often used as the reference point for the glycemic index and is given a score of 100. All other foods have glycemic index scores under 100 that are based on how quickly they raise blood glucose levels compared to pure glucose.

While on the surface it would seem that foods made up of simple carbohydrates would always have a higher glycemic index than those made up of complex carbohydrates, this is not the case. There are some foods that contain a good deal of simple carbohydrates (such as many fruits) that have only moderate effects on blood glucose, and there are some foods that contain a good deal of complex carbohydrates (such as white rice) that have a large effect on blood glucose levels. See Table 1 in Appendix C for a glycemic index of a selection of foods.

Several things determine how rapidly the carbohydrates in a particular food are broken down and the resulting glucose absorbed into the bloodstream. One important factor is the level of processing a food has been through. Refined grains—those that have been processed a great deal—have a higher glycemic index than grains that have been left largely intact. Brown rice, for example, has a lower glycemic index than more refined white rice—the glycemic index of which is fairly close to pure glucose. The fiber content of the food also has a large influence on its glycemic index. Fiber, which cannot be digested, can help slow down the release of glucose by surrounding carbohydrates and shielding them from immediate digestion. Other factors that affect glycemic index include the acid and fat content of the food. The higher in fat and more acidic a food is, the slower it is converted to glucose.

Why be concerned with the glycemic index of foods? Aside from the effect that high glycemic index foods may have on stimulating false hunger and thereby contributing to weight gain, there is very strong evidence that a diet containing a lot of high glycemic index foods increases the risk of diabetes and coronary heart disease, two of the leading causes of death in American women. Most of the carbohydrates Americans eat come from refined sources—bread, soft drinks, sweets, white potatoes, ready-to-eat cereals, and milk. Thus Americans could lower the risk of these serious illnesses by switching to less processed grains.

It is important to point out, though, that an entire diet should never be based just on the glycemic index. If this were the case, ice cream, which has a glycemic index of 30, would frequently be chosen over carrots, which have a glycemic index of 92. Rather, the focus should be on choosing low to medium glycemic index foods overall, but not at the expense of other important nutrients. The good news: fruits, vegetables, beans, and unrefined grains are usually rich in nutrients while also having a moderating effect on blood glucose levels.

## Potential Benefits of Low Glycemic Index and Whole Grain Foods

### LOWER RISK OF ADULT-ONSET (TYPE 2) DIABETES

Adult-onset diabetes, which is characterized by sustained high blood glucose levels, begins to develop when the cells in the body stop using insulin efficiently. This inefficiency forces the body to produce an ever-increasing amount of insulin to compensate, which eventually causes the cells in the pancreas that produce insulin to fail from overwork. With insufficient insulin produced to help cells take up glucose, blood glucose levels rise to high levels.

A diet filled with high glycemic index foods may increase the risk of diabetes by further burdening the pancreas to produce large amounts of insulin in response to the resulting high levels of glucose in the blood. In the Nurses' Health Study, we found that those women who ate the most foods with a high glycemic index—which results in what is called a high glycemic load—had a 50 percent greater risk of diabetes compared to those women who ate the least (see Figure 18-1). The risk was even greater in women who also ate very little cereal fiber, the kind found in whole grain foods (see Figure 18-2).

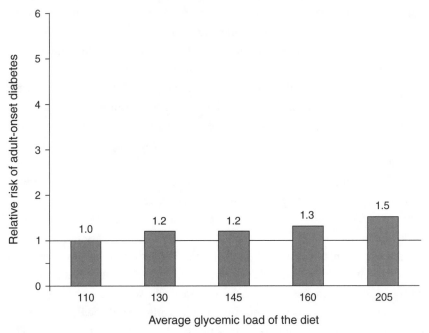

FIG. 18-1. The relative risk of adult-onset diabetes increases as the glycemic load of the diet increases. A high glycemic load generally indicates a diet with a lot of carbohydrates that have a high glycemic index. (Source: Nurses' Health Study)

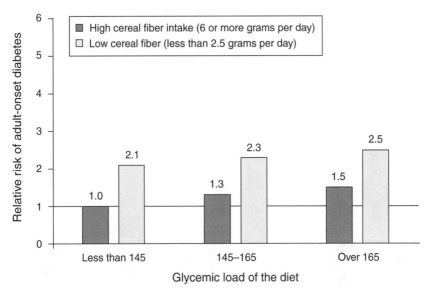

FIG. 18-2. The increased risk of adult-onset diabetes linked to a high glycemic load diet is made even greater when combined with a low cereal fiber diet. (Source: Nurses' Health Study)

## LOWER RISK OF CORONARY HEART DISEASE

Several large studies have shown that whole grain foods can reduce the risk of coronary heart disease. In addition to having a lower glycemic index than more refined grains, these foods tend to be packed with heart-healthy vitamins and nutrients, including fiber, folate, and vitamin E. In the Nurses' Health Study, we found that the more frequently women ate whole grains, the less likely they were to develop heart disease. Brown rice, whole grain breakfast cereal, and bran seemed to offered the most protection.

When we specifically assessed how the glycemic index of foods related to the risk of coronary heart disease, we found that overweight women whose diets had the highest glycemic load were twice as likely to develop heart disease as overweight women whose diets had the lowest glycemic load (see Figure 18-3). The high insulin levels caused by a high glycemic load may not only increase the risk of diabetes (a major heart disease risk factor) but also adversely affect blood cholesterol levels, triglyceride levels, and blood pressure, each of which can increase the risk of coronary heart disease. For normal weight women, glycemic load seemed to have no appreciable effect on risk. This may be because the effect of high glycemic index foods on insulin levels may be more pronounced if a woman is already experiencing insulin resistance, something strongly linked to being overweight.

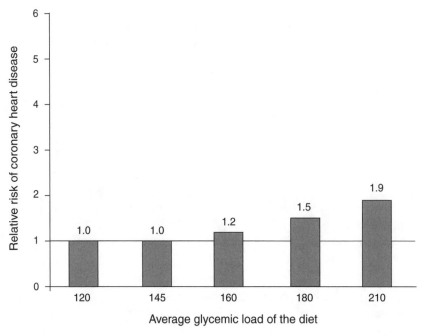

FIG. 18-3. The relative risk of coronary heart disease increases as the glycemic load of the diet increases. A high glycemic load generally indicates a diet with a lot of carbohydrates that have a high glycemic index. (Source: Nurses' Health Study)

Because complex carbohydrates are often touted as being a healthier choice for the heart, we also assessed how simple and complex carbohydrates each separately affected the risk of coronary heart disease. What we found was that neither simple nor complex carbohydrates had any influence on risk, suggesting—in our study, at least—that measures of a food's glycemic index are much better at predicting the risk of coronary heart disease than distinguishing between the specific kinds of carbohydrates in the food. We are, however, one of the first large studies to assess the link between glycemic index and heart disease. As more researchers study this issue, we will get a better sense of where our findings fit into the total body of evidence.

## Fiber

Fiber is a favorite of food marketers. Since it was found to help improve blood cholesterol levels in the 1980s, fiber content has been listed on food packages throughout grocery store aisles. And there *are* many benefits to a high fiber diet. In addition to helping improve blood cholesterol levels, it can reduce the risk of coronary heart disease and diabetes and help prevent constipation.

However, fiber is not the panacea some would make it seem. Despite many statements to the contrary, fiber intake seems to have little, if any, influence on the risk of cancer, including cancers of the colon or breast. One possible exception to this is endometrial cancer.

What is fiber? It is the general name given to carbohydrates that cannot be digested. All fiber comes from plant sources and can divided in a number of different ways. One way is by the source of the fiber—the type of plant from which it comes. Cereal fiber is fiber from grains. Fruit and vegetable fiber is, obviously, fiber from fruits and vegetables. Fiber can also be categorized as soluble and insoluble, depending on how it reacts with fluid. Soluble fiber partially dissolves in the fluid in the intestines, forming a gel, and may help lower blood cholesterol levels in some people by capturing cholesterol and carrying it out of the body. Insoluble fiber does not dissolve in fluid and helps form bulk in the intestines, which aids in regularity and preventing constipation. Most foods that contain fiber have both soluble and insoluble fiber, though the amount of each can vary a great deal. Good sources of soluble fiber include oat bran, whole oats, beans, peas, oranges, grapefruit, and strawberries. Good sources of insoluble fiber include whole wheat bread, wheat bran, cabbage, carrots, brussels sprouts, and cauliflower.

The processing of food, especially grains, has a big impact on fiber content. Whole or minimally processed grains, such as whole oats, tend to have many times the fiber of highly processed grains, such as oatmeal. During processing, the outer bran layer of a grain—the layer that contains most of the fiber as well as a lot of vitamins and minerals—is removed. The more a grain is processed, the less fiber (and the fewer vitamins and minerals) it will have.

Recommendations for fiber intake generally set a goal of around 20 to 35 grams of fiber every day for adults, about twice the amount in the average American diet. In addition to whole grain products, beans, nuts, and many fruits and vegetables are also good sources of fiber. See Table 3 in Appendix C for the fiber content of selected foods.

## Potential Benefits of High Fiber Foods

### LOWER RISK OF CORONARY HEART DISEASE

A good deal of research has shown that a high fiber diet may lower the risk of coronary heart disease, something we have found in the Nurses' Health Study as well. Overall, we discovered that a 10-gram-a-day increase in total fiber intake could lower the risk of coronary heart disease in women by nearly 20 per-

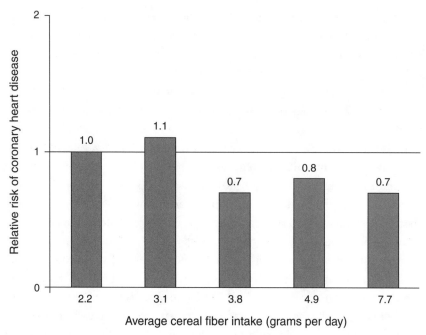

FIG. 18-4. As cereal fiber intake increases, the risk of heart disease decreases. (Source: Nurses' Health Study)

cent. One type of fiber, though, was particularly effective—cereal fiber. Women who ate the greatest amount of cereal fiber were approximately 35 percent less likely to develop heart disease than women who ate the least (see Figure 18-4).

Probably the most well known way in which fiber may lower the risk of heart disease is by improving blood cholesterol levels—lowering total cholesterol and LDL cholesterol. But there seems to be more to fiber's influence on the risk of heart disease than its effect on cholesterol levels. A large study that combined the results of twenty studies on cholesterol and oat bran (which is rich in cereal and soluble fiber) found that while a high fiber diet was definitely linked to better blood cholesterol levels, it had only a small impact on them. Therefore, a high fiber diet likely provides other heart health benefits as well. These possibly include lowering the risk of high blood triglycerides, blood clots, and diabetes.

## LOWER RISK OF ADULT-ONSET (TYPE 2) DIABETES

A number of studies have shown that a high fiber diet can help lower the demand for insulin in patients who already have diabetes, and it may also lower the risk of initially developing the disease. Fiber helps delay the digestion of carbohydrates, essentially making a high glycemic index food act more like a medium or low glycemic index food. Avoiding the spikes in blood glucose and insulin caused by high glycemic index foods can lower the risk of diabetes. In the Nurses' Health Study, we found that women who ate the most fiber had a 20 percent lower risk of developing adult-onset diabetes compared to women eating the least amount of fiber. As with coronary heart disease, most of this benefit was from one particular type of fiber: cereal fiber. Compared to women eating the least amount of cereal fiber, those eating the most were nearly 30 percent less likely to develop diabetes.

## Possible Lower Risk of Endometrial Cancer

In some small studies, high fiber intake has been linked to a reduced risk of endometrial cancer. However, large cohort studies, including the Nurses' Health Study, have yet to find a link between the two. High levels of estrogen in the body increase the risk of endometrial cancer by promoting the growth of cells in the endometrium. Fiber may help protect against the disease by affecting the way in which estrogen is absorbed in the intestines.

### Protein

There is an increasing interest in the link between protein and long-term health. Once thought to be of concern only to weight lifters and other athletes wanting to put on muscle, protein intake is coming to the fore as research shows links to certain chronic diseases and some popular weight-loss books push the benefits of high protein diets. Despite great interest in the topic, research into the link between protein and long-term health is still in its early stages. The best data show that a high protein intake may increase the risk of osteoporosis while possibly lowering the risk of coronary heart disease and stroke. But many more studies are needed before researchers can reach any solid conclusions.

Protein is the main component of tissue throughout the body, including muscle, skin, and hair. It is also an essential part of enzymes and antibodies, playing key roles in both the immune system and in chemical reactions going on throughout the body. Although the body can be very efficient at using protein, it needs some new protein in the diet every day to replace that lost in chemical reactions and in sloughed-off hair and skin. If it does not get what it needs from food, the body draws protein from muscle, and over time, this can cause significant muscle loss.

For most adult women, the recommended daily intake of protein is 0.8

grams day for every kilogram of body weight. This translates to about 50 grams a day for a 143-pound woman. Pregnant and lactating women (as well as youth) have greater protein needs. Pregnant women need approximately 10 extra grams of protein every day on top of their normal needs. Lactating women need about 15 extra grams a day during the first six months of breastfeeding and 12 extra grams a day thereafter.

In addition to the total amount of protein you consume, the quality of the protein in your diet is also important. Protein is made up of building blocks called amino acids—twenty in all. After a meal, the protein in food is broken down into its component amino acids. The body then uses these amino acids (as well as those made by other means) to create the specific proteins it needs. While the body can make most of the amino acids it needs for protein production, there are nine that it cannot and must get from food. These are called essential amino acids, and they occur in varying amounts depending on the food source of the protein. The protein from animal sources (meat, fish, and milk, for example) is complete protein, meaning that it supplies all of the essential amino acids. The protein from most vegetable sources, on the other hand, is incomplete, meaning it does not contain all the essential amino acids. (The grain quinoa is one exception.) Vegetarians must therefore consume different sources of vegetable protein to make sure they get all the essential amino acids they need. Popular vegetarian food combinations, such as beans and rice, and beans and corn tortillas, often serve this function well, providing all of the essential amino acids.

## Potential Risks and Benefits of a High Protein Diet

### PROBABLE INCREASED RISK OF OSTEOPOROSIS

One downside to eating a high protein diet may be an increased risk of osteoporosis. Diets high in protein cause an increase in acids in the bloodstream, a result of protein digestion. To neutralize these acids, the body leaches calcium from the bones. Over an extended period, this can lead to an increased risk of osteoporosis and the bone fractures that can result from it. In the Nurses' Health Study, we found that the more protein a woman consumed, the more likely she was to suffer a wrist fracture. Women who ate at least five servings of red meat a week were 20 percent more likely to have a wrist fracture than those who ate less than one serving a week. There is also some evidence that animal protein may cause greater calcium loss from bone than vegetable protein. Although it is unclear exactly why this might be, it may be that the specific types of amino acids in animal protein increase the acid level in blood to a greater extent than those found in vegetable protein. This relationship needs to be further studied, however.

This potential link between high protein diets and an increased risk of fracture may have a potentially disturbing implication for popular weight-loss plans that tout low carbohydrate, high protein diets. What many people find appealing about these diets is that foods typically viewed as taboo for weight loss—such as steak, bacon, and sausage—are a centerpiece of the program. This focus on a high intake of protein (specifically animal protein) may over the long term result in enough calcium loss from bone to cause osteoporosis. While the true risks and benefits of high protein weight loss programs are not currently known, it is always best to choose a high quality diet, especially when cutting back on calories to lose weight. The red meat and high fat dairy products people often choose to eat on high protein weight loss plans are high in saturated fat and not particularly rich in vitamins and minerals, suggesting they may increase the risk of coronary heart disease as well as colon cancer.

## POSSIBLE LOWER RISK OF CORONARY HEART DISEASE

Some research suggests that a high protein diet may help lower risk of coronary heart disease, though only a few studies have assessed this issue. In the Nurses' Health Study, we found that when fat intake (which is often linked to protein intake) was taken into account, women who ate the greatest amount of protein had a 25 percent lower risk of coronary heart disease than women eating the least. And the type of protein in the diet—whether animal or vegetable—did not seem to make a difference. Although it is unclear exactly how protein might lower the risk of coronary heart disease, there is some evidence that increases in protein intake can improve cholesterol levels, lowering LDL as well as raising HDL.

## POSSIBLE INCREASED SURVIVAL AFTER BREAST CANCER

Although the findings are very preliminary and need to be confirmed by others, we observed in the Nurses' Health Study that women diagnosed with breast cancer who ate the greatest amount of protein survived longer than women eating the least amount of protein. Those women eating over 81 grams of protein per day were 35 percent less likely to die of breast cancer during the eighteen-year study period than women eating less than 61 grams per day. It seems that most of the benefit from protein likely came from dairy foods and poultry, as we found no link between red meat and increased survival.

## What About Total Calories?

There has been a good deal of research assessing the relationship between the total amount of calories in the diet and long-term health, with some intriguing results. Studies of rodents have found that cutting calories by 30 to 60 percent can greatly reduce the risk of cancer and lengthen the average life span by nearly 50 percent. Among other possible mechanisms, the restriction in calories is thought to reduce cell damage from oxygen free radicals that can contribute to aging, cancer, and coronary heart disease. With such promising results in animals, does this mean that humans would benefit as well from such a drastic regimen? This is unclear, and given how lengthy and complicated (not to mention unrealistic) it would be to perform similar studies in humans, we will likely never have a complete answer. However, results from calorie restriction studies being done in monkeys are expected in a number of years and may help shine light on how limiting calories in the diet may affect human health.

In the real world, properly studying the link between total calories in the diet and long-term health is fairly complicated. Calories are closely associated with many different risk factors—such as weight, physical activity, and intake of the major nutrients—which often makes it difficult to tease out what is caused by the calories themselves and what is caused by those factors directly related to calories. For example, one of the most consistent findings from cohort studies assessing coronary heart disease is that the more calories a woman eats, the less likely she is to develop heart disease. While this may seem strange—giving women carte blanche to eat whatever they want—when physical activity is taken into account, the reason becomes clear. It is not that people who eat more and gain weight have a lower risk of coronary heart disease—because they would actually be at increased risk from the weight gain. Rather, people who are physically active and therefore need to eat more calories to replace those they burn are at a lower risk of the disease. A higher intake of calories is simply a marker for a higher level of physical activity in these studies.

Disentangling the interplay of all these factors is essential to studying the link between total calories and disease. And while early international studies found some associations between total calories and certain diseases, more recent, well-designed studies have found few, if any, links between total calories themselves and illness. The risk of diabetes, colon cancer, breast cancer, and gallstones may somehow be directly related to total calories consumed, but each of these must to be more thoroughly studied before researchers can draw any firm conclusions.

## A Calorie Is a Calorie Is a Calorie

Trying to lose weight, or even maintain a certain weight, is very difficult for many people, leaving them open to trying a wide range of weight-loss diets— high protein, low protein, high carbohydrate, low carbohydrate. What often gets lost in the publisher's or producer's fight to catch consumers' eyes, though, is one simple fact: when it comes to weight control, a calorie is a calorie is a calorie. No matter what the source, whether carbohydrates, proteins, or fats, a calorie always provides the same amount of energy. The key is balance, eating only as much as is burned during the day. Eating more than is burned causes weight gain. Eating less causes weight loss. And the source of the calories makes no difference to the body, whether it is gourmet ice cream or nonfat frozen yogurt.

## WHAT IT ALL MEANS

You should take one clear message from this chapter and the three that follow: *the quality of your diet matters*. Eating a diet containing high quality fats and carbohydrates as well as a good amount of fiber can significantly lower the risk of coronary heart disease, diabetes, and possibly a number of other diseases. When it comes to fat, minimize the amount of trans fat in the diet, cut down on saturated fat, and replace these with polyunsaturated or monounsaturated fats. Olive, canola, and peanut oils are always good choices. Fruits, vegetables, and whole grains should make up a large part of what you eat. Not only do they contain a good deal of fiber and tend to have less drastic effects on blood glucose and insulin levels, they are also rich in vitamins and minerals. Finally, eating only as much food as you need is also an important part of a high quality diet. Weight gain caused by regularly consuming too many calories is one of the most important contributors to chronic disease in the United States. Making physical activity an integral part of daily life can help you balance the amount you eat and the amount you burn each day.

## WHAT I TELL MY PATIENTS ABOUT THE MAJOR NUTRIENTS

DR. CELESTE ROBB-NICHOLSON

Too often we view a particular food group as all bad or all good: fat is bad; protein is good, for instance. New information about nutrients is released piecemeal, and it's hard to get the full story, which is more complex. The most reasonable approach is to eat a variety of foods from all groups to obtain essential vitamins and minerals, while avoiding the particular types of food that may increase your risk of disease later on. To do so, I generally advise the following:

## Watch Overall Calorie Count

However they divide up their nutrients, women need to take in the number of calories they will burn. Sometimes patients lose the forest for the trees. They are so concerned with avoiding fat that they load up on "low fat" desserts that are high in carbohydrate calories, only to find that they still gain weight. To maintain a healthy weight, eat a varied diet that includes more fruits, vegetables, and whole grains, only moderate amounts of meats and dairy products, and minimizes sugar and fats. And count your calories.

## Know Your Fats

It's a good idea to limit your overall fat calories to 30 percent of your daily total. But try to get as many of those fat calories as possible from monounsaturated or polyunsaturated fats. Watch your level of saturated fats, and avoid trans fats as much as possible. Packaged food labels are reliable guides to the types of fats in a food except for trans fats. However, if you scan the "Nutrition Facts" box on the labels, the term "hydrogenated" is a giveaway that trans fats are present in some quantity.

If you have difficulty reading labels, there are a few rules of thumb that might help. Trans fats tend to lurk in snack foods and packaged baked goods. When choosing fats, the softer, the better, because liquids are less likely to contain saturated or trans fats. Another method is to eat certain types of foods rarely, while eating others on a more regular basis.

## Think Glycemic Index

Research has found that a food's glycemic index—the measure of how quickly and to what degree it raises your blood glucose levels—can affect your risk of diabetes and heart disease, especially if you are overweight. Most of us do not readily know the glycemic index of the foods we eat, and it's not a number I recommend you memorize for each item. Rather, familiarize yourself with the foods listed the Glycemic Index of Selected Foods (Table 1 in Appendix C) and generally try to eat more of those in the low glycemic column than in the high glycemic column. Eating foods high in fiber will also help regulate your blood glucose levels.

## Fiber Is Essential but Not a Cure-all

Fiber, although not the panacea we once thought, still has many benefits. It helps to prevent constipation, improves blood cholesterol levels, and reduces the risk of diabetes and heart disease. But recent research has shown it does not affect the risk of either breast or colon cancer. In addition, getting most of your fiber from high fiber supplements, rather than food, can lead to loss of minerals. So the best strategy is to obtain about 20 to 35 grams of fiber each day, by eating fruits, vegetables, beans, and whole grain products. Whole oats, black beans, and whole wheat spaghetti are especially high in fiber. Make simple substitutions: choose whole grain breads over white, and brown rice over white. See Table 3 in Appendix C for more examples, or read the dietary labels on packaged food carefully.

## Put Protein in Perspective

As essential as protein is to our health, we are still learning a lot about it. Research has shown that too much of it (especially from red meat) can increase your risk of osteoporosis. On the other hand, protein is essential for your health and high levels may reduce your risk of heart disease and increase your chances of survival after breast cancer, according to other research. We know enough to offer a few guidelines. High protein diets are all the rage now, but over the long run, it is healthier to eat protein in moderation (50 grams a day for the average woman). Vary your sources of protein so that you get more from vegetable sources and less from meats and dairy products. If you are a vegetarian, make sure your diet is varied so that you get all the essential amino acids that enable your body to use the protein you digest.

## Exercise As Well As Eat

Exercise is never very far from any discussion about food and nutrition. We need to expend as many calories as we eat or we will gain weight. It would be far too great a burden to add up the energy we burn in calories each day and try to match the total in our diets. There would be no time for the rest of daily living. However, if you go through the process of estimating your calorie expenditure on an average day and an active day, you can keep those totals in mind as you choose the foods you eat throughout the week.

# CHAPTER NINETEEN

# Foods

## Key Lifestyle Message

- Eating a diet rich in fruits, vegetables, and whole grains is one of the best ways to improve your overall health.

## BACKGROUND

Reports on health and diet are constantly appearing in the media, touting the benefits of a new "miracle food" or declaring the risks of a food once thought healthy. It's no wonder that trips to the supermarket have become increasingly time-consuming, as women ponder each item on the shelf, wondering if it will cause heart disease or prevent cancer. Fortunately, there are some familiar and consistent messages in the ever-turning tide of diet information, with *eat your fruits and vegetables* being at the top of the list. There are also some new messages that are both exciting and scientifically sound. In this chapter, we will try to clarify exactly what those messages are by reviewing the links between food and women's health.

### Why Foods?

Why think about whole foods when we are scientifically savvy enough to study the specific components of foods? There are a few reasons. First is the obvious one: we eat foods, not nutrients, and this has implications for the way we approach changes in our diet. Eating one food instead of another is often easier than counting daily calories or calculating percentages of fat. The second reason is more complicated. Although scientists can now isolate many of the specific components of different foods, they can't necessarily tell which component is responsible for which risk or benefit. And even when they can, it is not always clear whether the component is working alone (and so could be taken as a supplement) or whether it functions only in concert with other ingredients in the food. For example, beta-carotene was thought to be the ingredient in vegetables that offered protection against lung cancer. But when researchers gave beta-carotene supplements to smokers, they found no reduction in the risk of lung cancer. In fact, they found a somewhat elevated risk. This may be because researchers identified the wrong component of vegetables—or because beta-carotene does not have the same effect on lung cells when it is taken alone as when it is taken with the other vitamins and minerals in vegetables. It may also be that the combination of carotenoids is more important than beta-carotene alone. Studies now suggest that a wide range of carotenoids offers the greatest protection. Thus, it is important to understand not only how specific nutrients affect health but also how whole foods influence risk.

## LESSONS FROM THE NURSES' HEALTH STUDY AND OTHER STUDIES

Although it is relatively new as a formal area of research, the study of diet and health has been going on for hundreds of years. In the first century A.D., poor nutrition was thought to be a cause of what we now call esophageal cancer, and by the mid-1600s, at least one physician had reported a connection between red meat and the overall risk of cancer. By the early 1900s, there was a diet recommended to reduce the risk of cancer, a diet not unlike one we would recommend today: rich in plant-based foods and moderate in meat and alcohol. The difference is that today we have solid evidence to back this recommendation.

*In the Nurses' Own Words . . .*

I had always enjoyed participating in the Nurses' Health Study, but being relatively healthy, I felt I would not especially benefit from it. My beliefs were radically altered, however, when the study questions began asking about dietary habits. As I read the questions referring to the different types of food I ate and the frequency with which I ate them, I thought, "I can never answer these questions." The only solution was to keep a temporary food diary. I was amazed. I thought I had maintained good eating habits. I was wrong. Since then, I have paid more attention to my diet. Not only has this helped me maintain an ideal body weight, but I feel great.

—From JH

## Foods from Plants

Plant-based foods are a rich source of vitamins, minerals, and a variety of other essential nutrients. In addition, they tend to be low in saturated fat and calories. For these reasons, they are thought to be extremely beneficial, offering protection against both cancer and cardiovascular disease.

Researchers are not yet sure which particular component of plant-based foods offers protection. It may be the very combination of vitamins and nutrients, or it may be one particular ingredient. Of the specific components that have been investigated to date, folate, fiber, potassium, and antioxidant vitamins appear to be most important.

- **Folate** is a vitamin found naturally in green leafy vegetables, citrus fruits, nuts, seeds, and beans. It is also now added to the grain supply in the United States in the form of folic acid and can be found in bread, cereal, rice, and pasta. This vitamin is essential not only for basic cell growth and function but also for the moderation of homocysteine levels. Homocysteine is a protein that at high levels can damage the artery walls and raise the risk of cardiovascular disease. It can also be harmful for unborn babies; pregnant women who have elevated levels of this protein are at increased risk of having a baby with birth defects. Eating folate-rich foods or taking supplements with folic acid can help ensure that homocysteine remains at a normal level.

- **Fiber,** found only in plant foods, fiber provides the bulk necessary to help move waste through the large intestine and out of the body. One particular type of fiber, called soluble fiber, may also lower the level of blood cholesterol in some people. It does this by forming a gel that binds cholesterol in the intestines and carries it out of the body.

- **Potassium** is a mineral that helps maintain the proper amount of fluid inside and around the cells. It also plays a role in metabolism, muscle contractions, and the transmission of signals in the nervous system.

- **Antioxidants** are a special group of vitamins and minerals that counter damage done to the cells by free radicals, molecules formed naturally by cells but defective because they are missing an electron. When a free radical tries to replace its missing electron by grabbing one from a cell, it damages the cell in a process called oxidation. Oxidation is thought to be partially responsible for the effects of aging and for diseases such as cataracts, cardiovascular disease, and cancer. Antioxidants can help prevent this process by giving their electrons to free radicals before the radicals attack the cells. Vitamin C, vitamin E, and carotenoids (like beta-carotene) are all examples of antioxidants.

## FRUITS AND VEGETABLES

"Eat at least five servings of fruits and vegetables every day." This is the one of the best-recognized dietary recommendations for women's health. More than 250 studies have assessed the impact of fruits and vegetables on cancer risk, and hundreds more have been done on cardiovascular risk. These studies generally support a protective effect against cardiovascular disease and possibly several types of cancer.

### The Benefits and Risks of Fruits and Vegetables

LOWER RISK OF HIGH BLOOD PRESSURE. More than 30 million Americans, including half of all women over the age of forty-five, suffer from high blood pressure. Also called hypertension, high blood pressure is a major risk factor for coronary heart disease. Diets rich in fruits and vegetables may help lower blood pressure, especially if combined with a low fat diet. In a large randomized controlled trial completed by the National Institutes of Health, women were placed randomly on one of three diets: an average American diet, a fruit-and-vegetable diet, and a fruit-and-vegetable diet that was also low in saturated fat. Over the course of the eleven-week study, women on the fruit-and-vegetable diets had decreases in blood pressure, while women on the average American diet did not. The diet that combined fruits and vegetables with low saturated fat offered the greatest benefit.

LOWER RISK OF CORONARY HEART DISEASE. Although not all studies are consistent, eating fruits and vegetables seems to offer at least modest protection against coronary heart disease. In the Nurses' Health Study, women who ate an average of three servings of fruits and vegetables a day were about 20 percent less likely to develop heart disease than women who rarely ate fruits and vegetables. A serving is a medium-sized piece of fruit, a cup of raw vegetables, or six ounces of juice. Green leafy vegetables (such as spinach and kale), cruciferous vegetables (such as broccoli and cauliflower), and vitamin C–rich foods (like oranges and green peppers) seemed particularly beneficial.

LOWER RISK OF ISCHEMIC STROKE. Ischemic stroke is a common form of cardiovascular disease that occurs when a blood vessel in the brain is blocked by a blood clot or some other particle. If the vessel is blocked for more than two hours, the part of the brain that was nourished by that vessel will die, causing permanent disability and possibly death.

Eating a diet rich in fruits and vegetables may lower the risk of ischemic stroke in the same way that it lowers the risk of heart disease. In the Nurses'

## Salad Dressing

Eating a spinach salad is an excellent way to lower your risk of coronary heart disease—but you can get double the benefit by also choosing a heart-healthy salad dressing. Data from the Nurses' Health Study suggest that topping your salad with oil and vinegar (or Italian dressing) might be more beneficial than a creamy dressing. We found that using oil and vinegar dressing at least five times a week cut women's risk of heart disease in half. This is probably because oil and vinegar salad dressings are usually made with unhydrogenated soybean oil, which contains an unsaturated fat called alpha-linolenic acid. This fatty acid reduces the risk of irregular heartbeats, which in turn lowers the risk of fatal heart disease. Oil and vinegar dressings may also be made with olive oil, a key component of the heart-healthy Mediterranean diet.

Health Study, we found that eating five or more servings of fruits and vegetables a day could lower the risk of ischemic stroke by as much as 30 percent (see Figure 19-1). Citrus fruits, cruciferous vegetables, and green leafy vegetables again seemed to be most beneficial.

*POSSIBLE LOWER RISK OF BREAST CANCER.* Although many different foods have been thought to influence the risk of breast cancer, few have been supported by epidemiologic data, including fruits and vegetables. In the Nurses' Health Study, we found that eating at least two servings of these foods a day slightly lowered the risk of breast cancer in premenopausal women but not among postmenopausal women. When researchers combined our study results with those

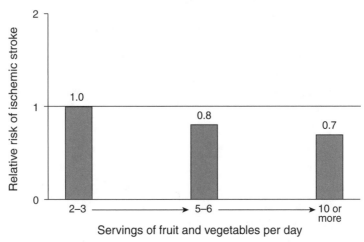

FIG. 19-1. The risk of ischemic stroke is modestly reduced among women who eat at least five servings of fruits and vegetables a day. (Source: Nurses' Health Study)

of seven other large studies, they found similar results: total intake of fruits and vegetables had very little effect on the risk of breast cancer. However, specific types of fruits and vegetables, such as those rich in carotenoids, do appear to reduce risk modestly, primarily in premenopausal women.

POSSIBLE LOWER RISK OF LUNG CANCER. Lung cancer is the leading cancer killer in the world. There is absolutely no doubt that this disease is caused predominantly by smoking: women who smoke are about 25 times more likely to develop lung cancer than women who never smoke. Clearly, the most effective way to prevent this disease is to never start smoking, and if you do start, to quit as soon as possible.

To a much lesser extent, the risk of lung cancer may also be modestly reduced by eating fruits and vegetables. This has been confirmed in several large cohort studies, including the Nurses' Health Study and the Iowa Women's Health Study. In our study, women who ate at least four servings of fruits and vegetables a day had about a 20 percent lower risk of lung cancer than those who rarely ate fruits and vegetables.

Although fruits and vegetables contain a number of vitamins and nutrients that could benefit the lungs, researchers have focused primarily on vitamin A. This vitamin has been shown to be important for cell growth and also serves as an antioxidant. However, clinical trials to test the effectiveness of a precursor of vitamin A (beta-carotene) have been largely unsuccessful. This may be because the beta-carotene was taken as a supplement, rather than in combination with the many other healthful ingredients contained in fruits and vegetables.

POSSIBLE LOWER RISK OF COLON CANCER. Although smaller studies have long suggested that eating vegetables and fiber might lower the risk of colon cancer, larger studies have not confirmed this. In two short-term randomized controlled trials, researchers found that the risk of polyps (precursors to colon cancer) was the same among those who ate a fiber-rich diet and those who did not. A number of large cohort studies, including the Nurses' Health Study, have shown similar results.

POSSIBLE LOWER RISK OF ENDOMETRIAL CANCER. Several small studies have shown that fruits and vegetables protect against endometrial cancer. However, this relationship is not yet well established. Only one large cohort study has examined it, and that study found no link.

POSSIBLE LOWER RISK OF OVARIAN CANCER. Eating vegetables may reduce the risk of ovarian cancer, although few studies have addressed the issue and results have not been consistent. In the Iowa Women's Health Study, vegetables in general were not related to ovarian cancer, but green leafy vegetables were.

Women who ate at least six servings a week of these vegetables were half as likely to develop ovarian cancer as women who ate less than two servings a week. One smaller study reported similar findings, though others, including the Nurses' Health Study, observed no relationship.

LOWER RISK OF OTHER CANCERS. In addition to the more common cancers discussed above, fruits and vegetables may reduce the risk of several other kinds of cancer. Of these, the evidence is strongest for cancers of the esophagus, mouth, pharynx, and stomach. Women may be able to cut their risk of these cancers in half by adding 2 or more servings of fruits and vegetables to their daily diet.

## NUTS

Nuts have traditionally been perceived as an unhealthy food because of their high fat content. In the United States, nut consumption has been declining steadily since the mid-eighties, perhaps because of an increased concern about the effect of dietary fat on health. But as Nurses' Health Study data have helped to show, nuts such as almonds, walnuts, and peanuts might be more nutritious than we once thought. Though they are high in fat, they contain mostly unsaturated fats, which can help lower the level of low density lipoproteins ("bad" cholesterol) in the blood. In addition, the nutrients in nuts (vitamin E, potassium, magnesium, folate, and fiber) may help prevent atherosclerosis and hypertension.

### The Benefits and Risks of Nuts

PROBABLE LOWER RISK OF CORONARY HEART DISEASE. Five large cohort studies have examined the link between nuts and coronary heart disease, and they have shown strikingly consistent results: the risk of coronary heart disease is substantially reduced among women who eat nuts regularly. In the Nurses' Health Study, we found that the more nuts a woman ate, the less likely she was to develop heart disease (see Figure 19-2). Similar findings were reported in the Iowa Women's Health Study.

## WHOLE GRAIN FOODS

Grains such as wheat, rice, corn, barley, and rye form the basis of most diets worldwide. They are usually milled into flour and consumed in the form of bread, cereal, and pasta. Some grain products, like wheat bread and popcorn, remain in the whole grain form, while others, like white bread and muffins, are more refined. Since most of the vitamins and minerals are removed from

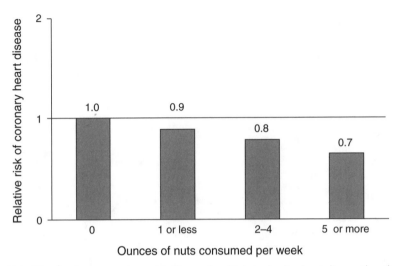

FIG. 19-2. Women who eat nuts in moderation are less likely to develop heart disease than those who never eat nuts. (Source: Nurses' Health Study)

grains during the refining process, whole grain foods tend to be more nutrient-rich than refined foods. They include dark bread, whole grain breakfast cereal, cooked oatmeal, wheat germ, brown rice, bran, and other grains such as kasha and couscous.

### The Benefits and Risks of Whole Grain Foods

LOWER RISK OF CORONARY HEART DISEASE. Several large studies have shown that whole grain foods can reduce the risk of coronary heart disease. These foods tend to be packed with heart-healthy vitamins and nutrients, including fiber, folate, and vitamin E. Fiber, in particular, has been studied extensively and has been shown to influence three of the most important factors linked to heart disease: cholesterol, diabetes, and blood clots.

In the Nurses' Health Study, we found that the more often women ate whole grains, the less likely they were to develop heart disease (see Figure 19-3). When we looked at specific whole grain foods, we found that whole grain breakfast cereal, bran, brown rice, and popcorn offered the most protection.

LOWER RISK OF ISCHEMIC STROKE. Whole grain foods may have a similar effect on ischemic stroke. In the Nurses' Health Study, we found a 30 to 40 percent reduction in the risk of ischemic stroke among women who ate at least one serving of grains a day. A serving of grains is equivalent to a slice of wheat bread or

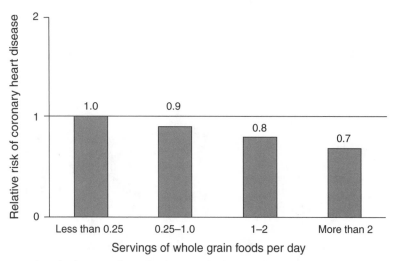

FIG. 19-3. The risk of coronary heart disease is modestly reduced among women who eat at least one serving of whole grains a day. (Source: Nurses' Health Study)

a cup of brown rice. We also found that refined grains (like white bread and muffins) offered little to no benefit. These results suggest that women can

## Margarine

For a number of years, experts recommended that people choose margarine over butter. This was because the saturated fat in butter was known to raise the risk of coronary heart disease. However, research has now shown that some forms of margarine may be worse than butter when it comes to heart health. Margarine that is hard at room temperature (that is to say, stick margarine) contains high amounts of trans-unsaturated fat, which can substantially increase the risk of heart disease. Soft margarine also contains this type of fat, but in smaller amounts. In the Nurses' Health Study, women who ate at least four teaspoons of stick margarine a day were 50 percent more likely to have a heart attack than those who rarely ate margarine. Based on this evidence and that from other studies, it is now recommended that people use liquid vegetable oil whenever possible or trans-free margarine. If margarine is used, it should be one that is also low in saturated fat.

How can you tell what type of fat is in your margarine? Check the label for the amount of saturated fat. In addition, most manufacturers that make a margarine free of trans fats advertise this on the package. In the near future, the trans fat content of foods will be added to product labels, making it easier to identify and thus avoid this harmful fat.

## Soy

As a natural source of estrogen, soy has been touted as an all-purpose answer to women's health. It has been suggested to lower the risk of breast cancer and heart disease, as well as other conditions. However, as we describe below, there is yet not enough evidence to support either of these health claims or to make dietary recommendations about soy.

The proposed link between soy and breast cancer has been based largely on results from international studies, which have shown lower rates of breast cancer among Japanese women than American women. Since the Japanese diet is much richer in soy than the American diet, researchers assumed that the soy was responsible for the lower breast cancer rates. Unfortunately, it is not that simple: Japanese women and American women tend to have different childbearing patterns, levels of physical activity, and rates of obesity, and all of these may contribute to the differences in breast cancer rates. So far, the epidemiologic studies that have looked carefully at the link between soy and breast cancer have yielded mixed results, with some showing a benefit and others no relationship. While laboratory studies do show that soy-based estrogens might protect breast cells from becoming cancerous, there will need to be many more epidemiologic studies conducted before we can reach any firm conclusions about soy and breast cancer.

Another health benefit that has been attributed to soy is a lower risk of heart disease. This is based on data from numerous studies showing that a high intake of soy protein (about 50 grams a day) in place of animal protein lowers both total blood cholesterol and LDL cholesterol (the "bad" cholesterol). Based on these studies, the Food and Drug Administration has authorized that soy products can be labeled as potentially heart-healthy. However, additional research is needed to confirm whether the cholesterol-lowering effects of soy actually translate into a lower risk of heart disease.

With soy products growing in popularity in the United States, we will soon be able to study their health effects more thoroughly. Until that evidence is available, however, women should probably consume soy foods and soy beverages only in moderation.

lower their risk of ischemic stroke by simply substituting whole grain cereal for refined each morning.

## Foods from Animals

Though animal products can be grouped together by their source, they tend to be very different from each other in nutrient and fat composition. Thus, they have very different effects on women's health. Some, like red meat, can be harmful when consumed in excess, while others, like fish, may be eaten more freely.

## Red Meat

Once considered a sign of social status, diets high in red meat have recently fallen out of favor in the United States. Consumption of beef, pork, and lamb has declined dramatically in the past forty years, probably because of increasing concern about the effects of meat on health. While red meat is an excellent source of protein and iron, it also contains large amounts of saturated fat, which can raise the level of cholesterol in the blood. In addition, when cooked at high temperatures, red meat may generate cancer-causing chemicals.

### The Benefits and Risks of Red Meat

INCREASED RISK OF COLON CANCER. Colon cancer is one of the most preventable forms of cancer, yet it is also one of the most common. In the past two decades, scientists have identified many factors linked to this disease and have found red meat to be among the most important. This may be because of the saturated fat in red meat or the carcinogens potentially present in cooked meat.

Most studies that have examined the link between red meat and colon cancer have seen a strong relationship: eating red meat frequently can double the risk of colon cancer. However, each study has its own definition of *frequently*, which makes it difficult to tell how much is too much. What we found in the Nurses' Health Study is that women who eat red meat once a week are at slightly increased risk, while those who eat it once a day are at much greater risk (see Figure 19-4).

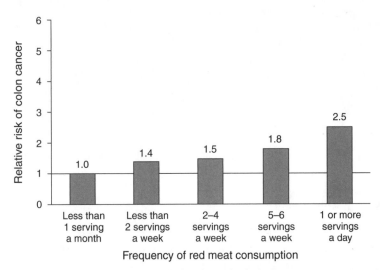

FIG. 19-4. The more meat women eat, the higher their risk of colon cancer. (Source: Nurses' Health Study)

## Fish

Like red meat, fish is an excellent source of protein. Moreover, it contains very little saturated fat and is instead rich in unsaturated fats called omega-3 fatty acids. These fatty acids have been shown to lower blood pressure, inhibit blood clotting, and reduce irregular heartbeats and triglyceride levels.

### The Benefits and Risks of Fish

LOWER RISK OF CORONARY HEART DISEASE. Because the unsaturated fat (omega-3) in fish is thought to help declog the arteries, researchers have speculated that eating fish might reduce the risk of heart disease. To date, most of the studies on this topic have been done on men and have been fairly inconsistent. In the Nurses' Health Study, however, we found a 20 percent reduction in the risk of heart disease among women who ate fish at least once a month. Those who ate fish more frequently received even greater protection (see Figure 19-5).

There is also some evidence that eating fish might reduce the immediate risk of sudden cardiac arrest. Cardiac arrest occurs when a woman's pulse suddenly stops. In one study, researchers found a 50 percent reduction in the risk of sudden cardiac arrest among women who ate at least one serving of fish a week.

POSSIBLE LOWER RISK OF MACULAR DEGENERATION. Macular degeneration occurs when the middle part of the retina (macula) begins to break down, marring a

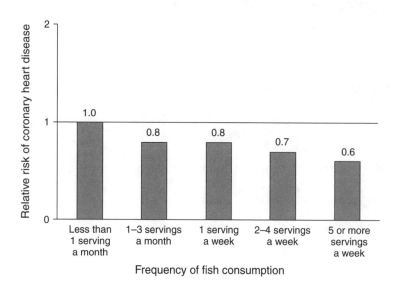

FIG. 19-5. The more fish women eat, the lower their risk of heart disease. (Source: Nurses' Health Study)

person's central area of sight while peripheral vision remains unchanged. In the Nurses' Health Study, we found that eating less animal fat and more fish might lower the risk of macular degeneration. This is the first report of a possible link, however, and needs to be confirmed in other studies.

## EGGS

Eggs were once considered the perfect food, being rich in protein, iron, B vitamins, folate, vitamin E, and unsaturated fats. But when reports began to emerge in the 1960s about the harmful effects of cholesterol, people began to think twice about their egg consumption. A single egg yolk contains more than 200 milligrams of cholesterol, and at that time, it was thought that this was enough to raise the level of cholesterol in the blood.

While we have certainly not come full circle to thinking that eggs are the perfect food, scientific evidence now suggests that concerns about eggs and cardiovascular disease may have been overstated. In the Nurses' Health Study, we found that the risk of cardiovascular disease was the same among women who ate one egg a day as it was among those who ate fewer than one egg a week. The only group for whom eggs appeared to increase risk was women with diabetes. Among these women, eating one egg a day was associated with a 50 percent increase in the risk of cardiovascular disease. Although this finding needs to be confirmed, it would be prudent for diabetic women to limit their egg consumption, since they are already at increased risk of cardiovascular disease.

## Foods and Cancer

- Although researchers have studied many aspects of diet in relation to cancer, only two types of foods have been shown to be related to risk: fruits and vegetables, and red meat.
- Eating a diet rich in fruits and vegetables lowers the risk of several types of cancer.
- Eating red meat more than once a week can increase the risk of colon cancer.

## Foods and Cardiovascular Disease

- Women can lower their risk of cardiovascular disease by eating a diet rich in fish and plant-based foods.
- Eating fish regularly lowers the risk of both heart disease and cardiac arrest.
- Eating fruits and vegetables daily lowers the risk of high blood pressure, coronary heart disease, and ischemic stroke. Topping a salad with oil and vinegar dressing may offer additional protection against heart disease.
- Eating nuts in moderation—and whole grain foods in abundance—also lowers the risk of heart disease.
- Although eggs were once thought to raise the risk of heart disease, current evidence suggests that there is no link between the two.

## Coffee

Known for its caffeine kick, coffee is one of the most commonly consumed drinks in the world. However, caffeine is an addictive drug that in excess can cause nervousness, irritability, sleeplessness, and the jitters. At high levels of intake, it may also affect women's health in a more significant way by raising the risk of hip fracture.

Caffeine can indirectly promote the loss of bone by increasing the amount of calcium that is excreted in the urine. Several studies have suggested that women who consume large amounts of caffeine, such as four or more cups of coffee a day, have lower bone mass than those who consume little.

In the Nurses' Health Study, we found a similar relationship: the more caffeine a woman consumed, the more likely she was to fracture a hip. Coffee appears to be the main culprit, probably because it contains more caffeine than tea or cola drinks and is consumed much more frequently.

Though coffee has long been thought to also increase the risk of heart disease and certain types of cancer, there is little evidence to support this. In the Nurses' Health Study, we found no difference in the risk of heart disease among women who drank six cups of coffee a day and women who never drank coffee. Overall, drinking coffee in moderation appears to have few if any adverse consequences.

## WHAT IT ALL MEANS

Overall, diets that are rich in plant-based foods appear to be most beneficial. Fruits, vegetables, whole grain foods, and nuts contain nutrients that not only sustain basic cell growth but also offer protection against cardiovascular disease and cancer. Moreover, with the exception of nuts, they are low in calories, which means that they will probably not contribute significantly to weight gain. Animal-based foods, on the other hand, cannot be given the same blanket seal of approval. These foods differ from each other in their fat composition and thus differ in their effects on women's health. Beef, pork, and lamb tend to be high in saturated fat and can raise the risk of colon cancer, while fish is generally high in unsaturated fat and may protect against heart disease. While beef, pork, and lamb do not need to be abolished from the diet, they should be eaten only in moderation.

### How Overall Dietary Habits Affect Health

While it is helpful to know which particular foods are good for you, it is also important to examine your overall dietary habits. In the Nurses' Health Study, we looked at how the diet as a whole affects women's risk of cancer and cardiovascular disease. We did this by giving each woman in the study a "healthy eating score." This was based on how often women ate grains, fruits, vegetables, milk, and meat and on how much their diets consisted of total fat, saturated fat, cholesterol, and sodium. The higher the score, the healthier the diet—and the lower the risk of cardiovascular disease. The women who scored the highest had a 20 percent lower risk of cardiovascular disease than the women who scored the lowest. Although several of the individual components are linked to cancer, we did not see an association between this composite score and the risk of cancer.

Using a similar scoring system, researchers have also found that overall diet affects length of life. During a five-year study period, researchers found a 30 percent reduction in mortality among those who scored highest versus those who scored lowest. Taken collectively, these results suggest that it is wise to incorporate as many of the elements of a healthy diet as possible into your daily regimen.

## WHAT I TELL MY PATIENTS ABOUT FOODS

DR. CELESTE ROBB-NICHOLSON

You'd think that something we do every day, such as eating, would be simple. But of course it's not. I find that many of my patients are concerned about the latest study on some type of food, and what they should do about it. For instance, should they drink more wine to protect against heart disease? And if so, should it be red wine or white? One moment, oat bran is in and the next it's out. With so many changing messages out there, selecting a healthy diet is not so simple at all.

Many of the details about how best to eat and drink have been discussed in this chapter. But I find it's helpful to provide a framework so patients can sort through the details and decide for themselves which foods to eat. There are three things to keep in mind when trying to eat a more healthy diet.

## The Big Picture

All too often, we focus on one particular food rather than on the range of foods and beverages we consume every day. When it comes to diet, the big picture is what matters. There is no single perfect food that will supply your body's needs. And it's not what you eat in a single meal or even a single day that counts over time. Think of your diet over a longer period—say, a week—and try to get nutrients from all of the major food groups: fruits and vegetables, grains, dairy, and protein. Try to get your grains from whole grain foods and your dairy from low fat sources, such as low fat yogurt, cheese, or skim milk. Substitute fish, poultry, or beans for red meat to get enough protein. And aim for at least five servings of fruits and vegetables each day. Consume alcohol and caffeine in moderation, and use fats, oils, and sweets sparingly.

## Balance

The other mistake we often make is to approach the whole issue of diet as an all-or-nothing black-and-white proposition. We decide to eat only the "good" foods and eliminate the "bad" ones. But there are very few foods that are all good or bad. Some food, such as red meat, appears to be good for you when consumed in moderation but bad if consumed in excess. Others, such as fruits, vegetables, and grains, seem to be good for you no matter how much you eat. However, unless you are cautious, you can get into trouble with a purely vegetarian diet. Red meat, fish, and poultry are all excellent sources of protein, iron, and vitamin $B_{12}$, and fish is loaded with omega-3 fatty acids.

And eliminating the "bad" foods, as in many fad diets, can give rise to cravings for them. A week of eating garden salad without dressing and drinking nothing but water will turn most of us into fast food addicts, yearning for those fat-laden fries. Eat a variety of foods.

Another key to balance is portion control. Research has shown that we

Americans have been increasing the sizes of our portions both when we eat out and at home. A serving of rice or pasta is half a cup, which looks pretty scanty on a plate that usually holds four to six servings. Keep an eye on the size of your servings.

## Begin Now

Another common misperception, especially among my patients who are in their forties or older, is that it's too late to begin eating a healthy diet. In fact, it's never too late. And the more often you eat a healthy diet, the better off you'll be.

## Tips for a Healthy Diet

First and foremost, make fruits and vegetables part of every meal. Whether they're fresh, frozen, or canned, these foods should be the basis of your diet. Often called the "original fast food," fruits and vegetables can be prepared quickly and easily. Here are some ideas for boosting your fruit and vegetable intake at breakfast, lunch, and dinner—and of course, in between.

At breakfast:

- Top your cereal with berries, bananas, or peaches.
- Drink 100 percent fruit or vegetable juice.
- Add fruit to your yogurt, pancakes, or waffles.
- Add diced vegetables such as peppers, tomatoes, and onions to your omelette.

## The Vegetarian Diet

Given the overwhelming health benefits of a plant-based diet, should women just stop eating meat and become vegetarian? Most diet researchers answer with a qualified no. It is not so much a matter of forsaking meat altogether, they say, but of adding a vegetarian twist to your current diet.

Eating moderate amounts of meat can also be beneficial. A middle-of-the-road strategy may be to balance the meat you eat with vegetarian meals. Some studies have tested this approach with good results. In one such study, researchers compared the blood cholesterol levels of people who ate red meat daily and of those who limited their meat intake to fewer than four servings a week. Those who limited their meat consumption had substantially lower levels of "bad" cholesterol in their blood.

At lunch and dinner:

- Add lettuce and tomato to your sandwich.
- Choose juice with your meal instead of soda.
- Eat a salad as the main course instead of as a side dish.
- Try tossing fruit—like oranges, grapefruit, and nectarine slices—onto your green salad.
- Have fresh fruit for or with dessert.

For your snacks:

- Blend yourself a smoothie, using low fat yogurt, fruit juice, and fresh, canned, or frozen fruit.
- Snack on grapes, carrots, celery sticks, or pepper slices.
- Dried fruit makes a great snack, too: dates, figs, prunes, raisins, apricots, etc.

In addition to fruits and vegetables, eat plenty of whole grain foods. Try to add at least one serving of these foods to your weekly diet by:

- Choosing dark bread instead of white bread for your toast or sandwich.
- Eating cooked oatmeal or cereal for breakfast.
- Snacking on popcorn instead of chips.
- Having a side of couscous or wild rice with your meal.

Cut back on red meat, substituting with fish, poultry, and other sources of protein whenever possible. If you choose to make red meat a part of some meals, make it a side dish rather than the entrée. The less you eat of this food, the better. Finally, keep an eye on the size of your servings so your portions are in the right proportion.

# CHAPTER TWENTY

# Alcohol

## BACKGROUND

Alcohol has been used by humans for at least 4,000 years and occupies a unique place in most societies. It is often a sacred part of religious ceremony and is a focal point of many social celebrations and everyday interactions. Yet it is an addictive drug that, when abused, has potentially severe short-term and long-term health consequences. These consequences depend largely on how much a person drinks—and on how much he/she can tolerate physiologically.

Alcohol tends to be less well tolerated by women's bodies than men's, and thus the effects can be more dramatic among women. A central nervous system depressant, alcohol acts like a sedative or tranquilizer, slowing down motor coordination and reaction time. It also impairs judgment, memory, reasoning, and self-control. Drink for drink, women accumulate more alcohol in their bloodstream than men and so experience these effects much more rapidly. This is due to several physiologic differences between men and women. First, in order for alcohol to be moved out of the bloodstream, it must be neutralized by a certain enzyme in the stomach. Women inherently have lower levels of this enzyme than men. Second, women tend to have a higher proportion of body fat than men, and body fat does not absorb alcohol; it allows alcohol to accumulate in the bloodstream. Finally, despite having more body fat, women tend to have smaller bodies than men. As a result, they have less blood circulating in their bodies, so that the ratio of alcohol to blood rises much more rapidly than it does in men.

The other factor obviously influencing the health consequences of alcohol is how much is consumed. A committee of the Institute of Medicine has defined three levels of alcohol intake based on their health consequences: low, moderate, and heavy. For women, low alcohol intake means drinking less than half a drink a day, with a drink defined as a 12-ounce bottle of beer, a 5-ounce glass of wine, or a 1.5-ounce shot of 80-proof liquor. This is about what the average American woman drinks (that is, two to three drinks a week) and is still considered a relatively safe amount. Moderate drinking is the next step up and involves having up to two drinks a day. Though considered safe in the short term, moderate drinking comes with both risks and benefits in the long term. Heavy drinking, on the other hand, has no benefits. It can lead to cirrhosis, alcoholism, accidents, violence, and a number of different cancers. In this chapter, we examine the risks and benefits of moderate drinking, where, unlike low and heavy intake, the line is not always clear in terms of safe versus unsafe.

## The Benefits of Moderate Alcohol Consumption

### Lower Risk of Coronary Heart Disease

Thanks to extensive media coverage, most women now recognize that moderate alcohol consumption can lower the risk of coronary heart disease. Although red wine was initially thought to be the most beneficial type of alcohol, it is now apparent that beer, white wine, and liquor also offer protection. In the Nurses' Health Study, we found that drinking one drink a day—be it a glass of wine, bottle of beer, or shot of liquor—cut women's risk of coronary heart disease by about half (see Figure 20-1). Similar results have been reported in numerous other studies.

One of the questions that remains about this relationship is whether women can receive the same benefit by drinking two drinks on three days of the week as by drinking one drink on each day of the week. Few studies have looked at this, but those that have have suggested that the answer is no. In one

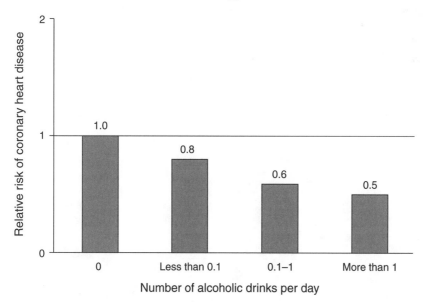

FIG. 20-1. The risk of heart disease is substantially lower among women who drink small amounts of alcohol each day compared to those who do not drink at all. (Source: Nurses' Health Study)

large study, researchers looked at the number of drinks women consumed per day and the number of days they drank per week. The lowest risk was seen among women who drank one to two drinks per day on five to six days per week. Those who averaged the same number of drinks per week but consumed them on fewer days had either less benefit or none at all.

The reason for this is that the effects of alcohol on the cardiovascular system are thought to be only temporary. For example, alcohol may increase the level of "good cholesterol" in the blood and lower the level of a blood-clotting substance, but only for about twenty-four hours. By drinking a small amount of alcohol each day, a woman may keep these substances in the blood at the optimal level for protection against heart disease.

## Lower Risk of Ischemic Stroke

Given that ischemic stroke is similar in nature to coronary heart disease (both being caused by clogged blood vessels), it is not surprising that alcohol has the same effect on ischemic stroke that it does on heart disease. When consumed in moderate amounts, alcohol can substantially reduce the risk of both conditions. In the Nurses' Health Study, we found that the risk of ischemic stroke was about 50 percent lower among women who drank one drink a day compared to those who did not drink at all (see Figure 20-2). These results have been replicated in many other large studies.

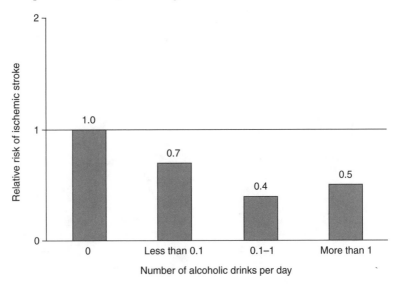

FIG. 20-2. Women who drink small amounts of alcohol each day are much less likely to have an ischemic stroke than women who do not drink at all. (Source: Nurses' Health Study)

## The Risks of Moderate Alcohol Consumption

### INCREASED RISK OF BREAST CANCER

Alcohol is one of the most consistent dietary factors related to the risk of breast cancer. More than twenty-five studies have shown that it increases risk, most likely by raising the level of estrogen in the bloodstream or making the breast more vulnerable to carcinogens.

In the Nurses' Health Study, we found that the type of alcohol consumed was not as important as the amount consumed. Women who drank half a drink a day—be it beer, wine, or liquor—had a slightly elevated risk of breast cancer, while those who drank a whole drink a day had an even higher risk (see Figure 20-3). When researchers combined our data with those from other large studies, they found similar results: a woman's risk of breast cancer rose by about 10 percent for every additional drink she consumed per day. In other words, a woman who averaged two drinks a day had a 10 percent greater chance of developing breast cancer than a woman who averaged one drink a day. This was true regardless of the type of alcohol consumed.

Because breast tissue may be particularly vulnerable during adolescence and early adulthood, researchers have speculated that drinking alcohol during these time periods might be more harmful than drinking alcohol later in life. To date, studies on this topic have been inconsistent.

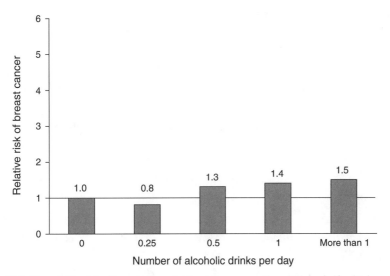

FIG. 20-3. The relative risk of breast cancer begins to increase with as little as half a drink per day. (Source: Nurses' Health Study)

## INCREASED RISK OF HIP FRACTURE

Hip fractures become increasingly common as women age. Prior to menopause, the body produces enough estrogen to keep bones healthy and strong. However, after menopause, estrogen levels drop, and bones can become brittle and vulnerable to fracture. About 90 percent of all hip fractures occur in those over the age of sixty-five, and most are the result of a bad fall.

Although alcohol increases estrogen levels in postmenopausal women, and moderate alcohol consumption has been linked to higher bone mass, it is more likely that alcohol actually leads to fractures. Drinking alcohol, even in moderate amounts, can make a person less steady and increase the likelihood that they will fall and injure themselves. In the Nurses' Health Study, we found that women who consumed about a drink a day were twice as likely to fracture their hips as women who did not drink at all. Similar results have been reported in several other studies, including the Framingham Study.

## PROBABLE INCREASED RISK OF COLON CANCER

Only a handful of long-term studies have examined the relationship between moderate alcohol consumption and the risk of colon cancer. To date, results have been inconsistent. Several studies have shown that alcohol does not alter colon cancer risk, while others have demonstrated a modest increase in risk. Overall, the epidemiologic evidence suggests that alcohol probably does increase the risk of colon cancer. This may be because alcohol lowers the level of folate in the body, which may in turn influence the risk of colon cancer.

## PROBABLE INCREASED RISK OF HEMORRHAGIC STROKE

Hemorrhagic stroke is much less common than ischemic stroke but tends to be more severe. It occurs when a small blood vessel in the brain ruptures, causing bleeding (hemorrhaging) into or around the brain. Although every stroke is serious, brain hemorrhages are often devastating because they can affect younger people and are more likely to cause death.

It has been suggested but not confirmed that moderate alcohol consumption might increase the risk of hemorrhagic stroke. In the Nurses' Health Study, we found a doubling of risk among women who drank even small amounts of alcohol each day (see Figure 20-4). However, few studies have confirmed these results.

If alcohol does in fact have an effect on the risk of hemorrhagic stroke, it is

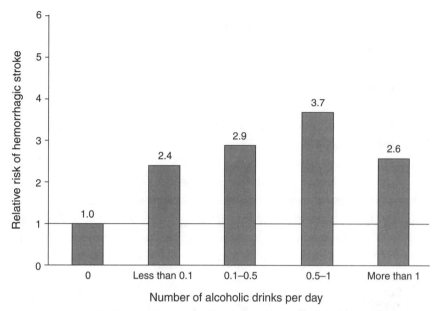

FIG. 20-4. Women who drink small amounts of alcohol each day are about three times more likely to have a hemorrhagic stroke than women who do not drink at all. (Source: Nurses' Health Study)

most likely indirect. Alcohol can raise a woman's blood pressure, enhance blood flow to her brain, and increase the chance of having irregular heartbeats, all of which make it more likely that a blood vessel in the brain will burst and bleed. In addition, high levels of alcohol intake have been shown to increase the tendency for bleeding.

## Alcohol and Pregnancy

There is no safe level of drinking during pregnancy. Women who are trying to get pregnant or who are already pregnant should not drink. During the first trimester, regular drinking—or even one period of heavy drinking—can damage the fetus. Women who drink as few as one or two drinks a day while pregnant may give birth prematurely, and their children may have a low birth weight or neurological problems. Even occasional social drinking can increase the risk of miscarriage, particularly in the first trimester. Heavy drinking is not safe for any woman, but is especially harmful to pregnant women. Women who drink alcohol heavily during pregnancy may give birth to babies with fetal alcohol syndrome, a group of birth defects that includes irreversible mental retardation.

### How Alcohol Use Affects Length of Life

Drinking in moderation can *decrease* a woman's risk of dying from some diseases, but *increase* her risk of dying from others. The best evidence of this to date comes from the American Cancer Society Cancer Prevention Study II. In that study, women who drank in moderation were about 20 percent less likely to die during the nine-year study period than women who did not drink at all. When researchers looked at specific causes of death, they found that moderate drinkers were much less likely than nondrinkers to die of coronary heart disease and stroke. However, moderate drinkers were also more likely to die of breast cancer. Results in the Nurses' Health Study were similar. Overall, these findings suggest that while moderate drinking does confer an overall mortality benefit—and a great benefit in terms of heart disease—women must still consider the increased risk of breast cancer and possibly other cancers.

## Moderate Alcohol Consumption: Weighing the Risks and Benefits

- Drinking alcohol in moderation consists of drinking less than two alcoholic beverages a day.
- This amount of alcohol can substantially lower the risk of heart disease and ischemic stroke.
- However, it also raises the risk of breast cancer, hip fracture, and probably colon cancer and hemorrhagic stroke.
- Beer, wine, and liquor all appear to have the same effects on women's health.

## WHAT IT ALL MEANS

Alcohol can have a wide range of effects on your health, depending on how much you consume. If you drink heavily (two or more drinks a day), you are at increased risk of cancer, heart disease, alcoholism, cirrhosis, and fatal accidents. This type of drinking has no benefits and is not recommended for women at any age. Moderate drinking, on the other hand, does have some benefits, although it too has risks. If you drink one drink a day, you receive some protection against heart disease and ischemic stroke. However, you are also at increased risk of breast cancer, hip fracture, and probably colon cancer and hemorrhagic stroke. These risks and benefits are the same whether you drink beer, wine, or liquor.

In the face of such competing risks and benefits, how can you decide whether moderate alcohol consumption is right for you? For women under the age of forty, there are few benefits to drinking, and these are strongly outweighed by the risks. Since most young women are at extremely low risk of heart disease, the protection afforded by moderate drinking will most likely have little impact at this age. In addition, the effects of alcohol on the cardiovascular system are thought to be acute (or short-term); thus, it is unlikely that drinking in early adulthood will offer any protection against heart disease later in life, when the risk becomes substantial. In addition to there being few benefits to drinking at this age, there are risks. Accidents are the leading cause of death among women under the age of forty, and alcohol, even when consumed in moderation, can increase the likelihood of a fatal accident.

For women over the age of forty, there is a great deal of debate about how to balance the risks and benefits of moderate alcohol consumption. Some health care providers argue that the benefits in terms of heart disease outweigh the risks in terms of breast cancer. This argument is based on two things. First, heart disease kills more American women each year than all cancers combined, and women should take action against the disease that poses the greatest threat to their lives. Second, alcohol raises the risk of breast cancer only slightly (about 30 percent) when consumed in moderation. Since most women are at relatively low risk of breast cancer anyway (compared to the risk of heart disease), this modest increase in risk will most likely not have much impact.

Other health care providers argue that the increased risk of breast cancer associated with alcohol is substantial, and that this risk outweighs the benefits in terms of heart disease. This argument is based on the fact that while there are a number of ways that women can reduce their risk of heart disease, there are very few ways that they can lower their risk of breast cancer. One way to lower that risk modestly is to avoid alcohol.

## WHAT I TELL MY PATIENTS ABOUT DRINKING ALCOHOL

DR. CELESTE ROBB-NICHOLSON

Most women do not drink alcohol for medicinal reasons or to prevent chronic illnesses. They drink alcohol because they like the taste and it is one of their social rituals. However, they do ask about how much alcohol is safe and what kinds are more healthful than others. And my patients have a wide variety of attitudes about alcohol. Some women avoid alcohol altogether, because they have a family history of alcohol or drug addiction. I support this strongly, because the risk of alcohol addiction is increased in women whose first-degree relatives have been addicted to alcohol.

Others are cautious because alcohol adds to their end-of-the-day fatigue, reduces their productivity, and dulls their relationships with family members. Some women who enjoy alcohol are cautious about how much they drink because of the fear that it will significantly increase their risk of breast cancer. Others drink a significant amount on a regular basis, convinced that it is the best way to reduce their risk of coronary heart disease. I am always quick to remind these women that they can reduce the risk of coronary disease through diet and exercise, which do not add to any risk of cancer.

Your own decision about alcohol should be based upon personal preference, your age, and your medical history. Less than half a drink a day, or two to three drinks a week is safe, if you are not prone to addiction and are not pregnant. Heavy drinking (two or more drinks a day) is not safe for any woman: it can increase your risk of cirrhosis, alcoholism, accidents, violence, and cancer. For my patients who are moderate drinkers, who drink at least one glass of alcohol a day and sometimes as much as two, I discuss these factors.

## Age Matters

If you are under forty, don't drink on a regular basis: the benefits of moderate drinking are far outweighed by the risks, mainly because women in this age group are not likely to suffer from coronary heart disease. At the same time, drinking can increase your risk of being in an automobile accident, and accidents are the leading cause of death in women younger than forty. For women forty and older, though, the risk/benefit equation becomes more complicated.

## Consider Your Medical History

If certain diseases and conditions run in your family, you may be at increased risk yourself. Here are the major conditions to be aware of:

- **Alcoholism.** If alcoholism has affected your family, especially your siblings, parents, or grandparents, then you may want to think twice about drinking at all. Alcohol is addictive, and if you are predisposed to become dependent, it may be best to avoid it altogether. If you decide to drink anyway, be aware of the early warning signs of addiction: an increased tolerance (having to drink more alcohol to feel the effects), a craving for alcohol, and a dependence on it. If you notice these signs, it is time to cut back or quit altogether.

- **Cancer.** Alcohol can modestly increase your risk of breast cancer, probably increases your risk of colon cancer, and has been loosely linked to increases in other types of cancer as well (notably that of the liver, mouth, and upper digestive tracts). If you have a family history of these cancers, you may already face an increased risk of them yourself. Drinking will only increase that risk, so you may want to avoid alcohol or drink only occasionally. On the other hand, if these diseases do not run in your family, moderate drinking should be safe. Even the risk of breast cancer, which seems to concern my patients most, increases only modestly (about 30 percent) in moderate drinkers.

- **Heart Disease.** If you are forty or older and concerned about your risk of heart disease, either because of your own medical history or your family's, then moderate drinking (one drink a day) may lengthen your life. The studies have shown consistently that moderate drinking can reduce the risk of coronary heart disease by half. However, alcohol should *not* be considered the major or only strategy for reducing risk of coronary heart disease. If you enjoy alcohol, are not at increased risk for addiction, and are already following a low fat diet and exercising, one drink each day may be a positive addition to your regimen.

## Watch Serving Sizes

Many of my patients are consuming more alcohol than they think. It's easy to do: some restaurants serve glasses of wine, for instance, that are so large they actually contain the equivalent of about a drink and a half. And a glass of beer is 12 ounces—not the 16-ounce serving you can get at some pubs. Try measuring a 6-ounce or a 12-ounce serving of water into a glass to help train your eye to recognize a single serving of wine or beer. Next time you eat out, you'll know when to stop pouring.

# CHAPTER TWENTY-ONE

# Vitamins and Minerals

## Key Lifestyle Message

- Eating a diet rich in fruits, vegetables, and whole grains is one of the best ways to improve your overall health.
- Taking a multivitamin every day can offer even more protection against disease.

## BACKGROUND

Just as your mother urged you to eat your fruits and vegetables, she probably also told you to eat a balanced diet so that you would get all your vitamins and minerals. Always looking out for your health, she was right once again. Vitamins and minerals *are* essential for good health. They perform vital roles throughout the body—from keeping the heart beating to helping heal injuries—and may even protect you from serious chronic diseases, such as diabetes and certain cancers.

As with many areas of health, however, it can be hard to separate fact from fiction when it comes to the health benefits of vitamins and minerals. Reading magazine articles, watching television, or walking down the dietary supplement aisle of a grocery store, you can come across a huge number of claims about the health benefits of vitamins and minerals, many of which, unfortunately, lack scientific credibility. Because vitamins and minerals (as well as other dietary supplements) represent "natural products," the U.S. Food and Drug Administration does not require them to follow the same strict regulations on labeling and health claims as drugs.

In this chapter, we will try to clarify exactly what the scientific evidence currently shows about the link between vitamins and minerals and many serious long-term disorders. Contrary to what you might think, when you weigh the current evidence, only a small number of chronic conditions can be confidently linked to the intake of specific vitamins and minerals.

## Vitamins and Minerals

Often referred to in scientific circles as micronutrients, vitamins and minerals are essential substances that the body needs only in small amounts to function properly. In addition to playing vital roles in the thousands of chemical reactions occurring throughout the body, vitamins and minerals are also key to strong bones, a healthy immune system, and fully functional red blood cells—to name only a few of their important functions. All told, there are over thirty currently known vitamins and minerals that the body needs regularly to work optimally and stave off disease.

Vitamins and minerals are called essential nutrients because the body needs them to function, yet aside from a few exceptions, cannot make them itself. This means that virtually all the vitamins and minerals the body requires must come from food, dietary supplements, or a combination of the two. Become deficient in a vitamin or mineral for a long enough time and a "deficiency disease" will develop. How severe the disease is depends on how long the deficiency has gone on and to what extent. A classic example is scurvy, a potentially fatal tissue disorder caused by vitamin C deficiency; scurvy was common in early maritime explorers who went for extended periods without access to vegetables and fruit, particularly citrus fruit. Similar disorders develop when almost any vitamin or mineral is lacking in the diet. For example, lack of iron causes anemia, lack of vitamin D causes rickets in children, and lack of vitamin A causes night blindness.

To help people avoid such deficiencies and the "deficiency diseases" associated with them, Recommended Dietary Allowances (RDAs) have been developed by the National Academy of Sciences that provide recommended levels of daily intake for vitamins and minerals. The first set of RDAs was published in 1943, and they are occasionally updated as more data are available on the nutrient needs of humans. The recommended daily levels specified by the RDAs protect you against the classic diseases, such as scurvy, that are caused by severe deficiency of these micronutrients.

In recent years, however, studies have shown that regular daily intake of vitamins and minerals above the RDA level may help protect against various chronic diseases such as atherosclerosis and cancer. This has led the National Academy of Sciences to propose a new set of standards called Dietary Reference Intakes (DRIs). While the DRIs include the RDAs, they also have a slightly broader mission. In addition to setting standards that focus on avoiding problems related to nutrient deficiencies, the DRIs will take into account broader issues of health as well, such as a nutrient's potential to lower the risk of various chronic diseases. See Table 4 in Appendix C for a list of recommended intakes for selected vitamins and minerals.

### Food Versus Supplements

A varied and well-balanced diet is all most people need to meet the DRIs. Vitamins and minerals are plentiful in fruits, vegetables, whole grains, and many dairy products. And every single food group provides some essential nutrients. Always eating a high quality diet, though, can be hard to do, with work, busy family schedules, and the lure of fast food around every corner. To combat this and to provide extra assurance against deficiencies, some foods in the United States have vitamins and minerals added to them, a process sometimes called fortification. For example, salt is fortified with iodine, flour is fortified with iron, and most breakfast cereals are fortified with folic acid.

Taking things a step further, vitamin and mineral supplements can provide added assurance that women are getting the nutrients they need to be healthy. However beneficial, supplements should be just that: supplements. Women should still eat a varied diet rich in fruits, vegetables, and whole grains. Because in addition to providing vitamins and minerals, a healthy diet also provides many other substances, some as yet unidentified, that help keep the body healthy and protect against disease.

## Too Good to Be True? Health Claims of Dietary Supplements

Vitamins and minerals are certainly essential for the body to function properly. But when it comes to dietary supplements, many in the industry regularly make health claims that are backed by little science. The manufacture and sale of supplements (including vitamins and minerals) is big business, and the industry has a great stake in making their products seem much more beneficial than they actually are. An important thing to remember: if a health claim sounds too good to be true, it probably is. One way to tell if the claim has overstepped what the scientific evidence currently shows? Check the label. Claims based on less-than-solid findings are required by the U.S. Food and Drug Administration to say: *This statement has not been evaluated by the Food and Drug Administration. This product is not intended to diagnose, treat, cure, or prevent any disease.*

## LESSONS FROM THE NURSES' HEALTH STUDY AND OTHER STUDIES

In the early part of the twentieth century in the United States, much of the science devoted to vitamins and minerals was focused on ways to identify and prevent severe deficiency-related disease. As economic prosperity and effective nutrition programs have brought such deficiency diseases under control in many countries throughout the world, the focus of research has now partially shifted to the link between vitamins and minerals and chronic diseases.

In the Nurses' Health Study, we began gathering in the early 1980s detailed information from participants about what they ate and the types of dietary supplements they took. This has allowed us to study the link between vitamins and minerals and a wide range of disease in women, from heart disease to cataracts. What we have found is generally in line with the results of other large studies: that low intake of a number of vitamins and minerals may be associated with certain chronic diseases, but the evidence for many others is still inconclusive.

### Vitamins and Chronic Disease

Vitamins can be divided into two categories: fat-soluble and water-soluble. Fat-soluble vitamins—such as vitamins A, D, E, and K—require some fat in the diet to be absorbed by the digestive system and to be stored in fat tissue. This has the advantage of providing a safety net against occasional deficiency—allowing the vitamins to be released as the body needs them—but the disadvantage of increasing the risk of toxicity. Regular intake of excessive amounts of vitamins A and D (especially in children) can cause dangerous levels to build up in fat tissue, causing toxic effects. In contrast, water-soluble vitamins—such as vitamins C, $B_6$, and folate—cannot be stored in fat tissue, and most of what is not immediately used by the body is lost in the urine. This makes the chances of toxicity from water-soluble vitamins much lower compared to fat-soluble vitamins, but it can still occur, especially with very high intakes.

One group of compounds that many people have heard discussed in the news or seen mentioned on food labels is the antioxidants. These substances, which include beta-carotene (which can be converted to vitamin A), vitamin C, and vitamin E, help protect cells and tissue from damage by oxygen free radicals, which can injure tissues. Oxidation caused by free radicals is thought to be partially responsible for the effects of aging and for certain diseases, such as cardiovascular disease, cancer, and cataracts. Antioxidant vitamins, in theory,

## Vitamins and Minerals: The Larger Picture

- Vitamins and minerals are essential for good health in general, and may offer some protection from chronic diseases.
- Nutrient deficiency, and in severe cases deficiency disease, can result when women don't get adequate levels of vitamins and minerals in their diets.
- A varied and well-balanced diet is an important source of vitamins, minerals, and other nutrients.
- Supplements, while often beneficial, cannot take the place of nutrient-rich fruits, vegetables, and whole grains.
- There is strong but not yet conclusive evidence that everyone should take a single multivitamin supplement daily.

may help prevent this damage and lower the risk of such diseases. While people who eat diets rich in these antioxidant vitamins have lower rates of cancer, coronary heart disease, and cataracts, research is still trying to determine whether it is actually the antioxidants that cause the lower rates or rather other substances in the same foods. It could also be other unrelated factors about such individuals that cause them to choose diets rich in these antioxidants.

### Fat-Soluble Vitamins

#### Vitamin A and Carotenoids

Vitamin A is a fat-soluble vitamin that performs vital roles in vision, cell growth, and the functioning of the immune system. It is found in two basic forms in food—retinol (which comes primarily from animal products) and carotenoids, such as beta-carotene (which come primarily from fruits and vegetables). Not all carotenoids, though, are related to vitamin A. Only a portion can be converted by the body into the vitamin. In addition to other functions, many carotenoids are also potent antioxidants, including beta-carotene, alpha-carotene, lycopene, lutein, and zeaxanthin.

Deficiency in vitamin A can lead to a range of vision problems, from difficulty seeing at night to permanent blindness. Despite being extensively studied as a means to lowering the risk of many chronic diseases—including cardiovascular disease and many cancers—to date, vitamin A and carotenoids appear to be linked to only two diseases pertinent to women: breast cancer and cataracts. And the evidence even for these is not completely solid.

*Breast Cancer*

CAROTENOIDS. There is some evidence that a moderate intake of certain carotenoids can lower the risk of breast cancer, particularly in premenopausal women. In the Nurses' Health Study, we found that compared to premenopausal women with the lowest intake of certain carotenoids (beta-carotene, lutein, and zeaxanthin), those with greater intake had a slightly lower risk of breast cancer. Although it is not known exactly how the carotenoids might lower risk, it may be that their antioxidant actions protect breast cells from damage that can promote cancer.

The Nurses' Health Study is one of the first large cohort studies to assess this issue, and more work needs to be done in this area before any solid conclusions can made about the link between carotenoids and the risk of breast cancer.

VITAMIN A. As with the carotenoids, there is some evidence that a moderate total intake of vitamin A can lower the risk of breast cancer among premenopausal women. In addition to its antioxidant properties (beta-carotene is included in total vitamin A intake), vitamin A's important role in cell growth may help protect breast cells from turning cancerous. We found in the Nurses' Health Study that premenopausal women who had a total vitamin A intake from food of about 7,590 IUs or more had a 10 to 30 percent lower risk of the disease compared to women with the lowest intake (under 7,590 IUs). Surprisingly, vitamin A supplements alone had no effect on the disease. This suggests that it may not be vitamin A itself that actually provides protection against cancer but some other substance found in vitamin A–rich foods. And not all studies have shown vitamin A to lower the risk of breast cancer. The Iowa Women's Health Study has found no link between the two.

*Cataracts*

CAROTENOIDS. Cataracts are an eye disease that occurs when the lens in the eye becomes cloudy, which blurs and can eventually completely block vision. One way cataracts are thought to develop is through oxidation of proteins in the lens, a process that the antioxidant properties of carotenoids may help protect against. In the Nurses' Health Study, women with the highest intake of the carotenoids lutein and zeaxanthin had a 20 percent lower risk of having cataract surgery than women with the lowest intake. Though not all studies are consistent, most have had similar results to ours, suggesting a protective link between carotenoids and cataracts. More studies are needed, however, before any solid recommendations can be made.

## Beta-Carotene and Lung Cancer

In the 1990s, two studies of beta-carotene supplements and chronic disease gained nationwide attention in the United States. The studies were randomized controlled trials assessing the potential benefits of taking beta-carotene supplements on the risk of lung cancer and cardiovascular disease in a population primarily made up of smokers. What made the studies remarkable was that not only did the beta-carotene not prevent disease, it actually slightly increased the risk of lung cancer. These findings were particularly striking because previous observational studies had shown that foods rich in beta-carotene (such as fruits and vegetables) were associated with a lower risk of lung cancer and cardiovascular disease in smokers. A large, twelve-year-long randomized trial published not long after these two, however, had more neutral results. In both smokers and nonsmokers, taking beta-carotene supplements still showed no benefit in lowering the risk of cancer or cardiovascular disease, but neither did it increase risk.

Why the apparent contradiction? There are a number of possibilities. It may be that the whole complex net of antioxidants—rather than a single antioxidant—delivered by fruits and vegetables is needed to decrease the risk of disease. Or it may be that both the antioxidants and other important nutrients found in fruits and vegetables is required to lower risk. It is also possible that we have not yet tested the right carotenoid or combination of carotenoids for long enough periods.

Although the exact link between carotenoids and chronic disease is still being worked out, the evidence as a whole suggests that both women and men should make it a priority to eat a diet rich in fruits and vegetables, which contain a good amount and range of antioxidants and other important nutrients.

VITAMIN A. Although some studies have found a link between total vitamin A intake and the risk of cataracts, much of the evidence suggests that it is carotenoids, rather than vitamin A per se, that offers protection. For example, while we found in early calculations that a high total vitamin A intake from food could lower the risk of cataracts, when we added information about specific carotenoids to more recent data, the benefit of vitamin A intake nearly disappeared. This issue, however, is still being studied.

## WHAT IT ALL MEANS—VITAMIN A AND CAROTENOIDS

Vitamin A and certain carotenoids may help lower the risk of breast cancer and cataracts. There is also some evidence that carotenoids are linked to other chronic diseases as well, such as cardiovascular disease. Currently, though, there

## Good Food Sources of Vitamin A and Carotenoids

| *Beta-carotene and other carotenoids* | *Retinol* |
|---|---|
| Carrots | Liver |
| Sweet potatoes | Fortified milk and eggs |
| Pumpkin | |
| Spinach | |
| Collards | |
| Turnip greens | |
| Broccoli | |
| Tomatoes | |
| Mangoes | |
| Cantaloupe | |
| Apricots | |

## Vitamin A and Carotenoids at a Glance

- Some vitamins, including vitamin A, are called fat-soluble vitamins and are stored in fat tissue. These can actually have toxic effects when present in excessive amounts. Other vitamins are water-soluble and leave the body if not used immediately.

- Antioxidants are nutrients that help to protect cells and tissues from damage that may be responsible for the effects of aging, cataracts, cardiovascular disease, and cancer.

- Vitamin A and carotenoids, found in foods such as carrots and green leafy vegetables, may help to lower the risk of breast cancer and cataracts.

seems to be no benefit to exceeding the DRI for vitamin A of 700 mcg a day for an adult woman. (This is equivalent to approximately 2,300 IU a day from a vitamin A supplement). In fact, intake above about 3,000 mcg a day (approximately 10,000 IU) can be toxic, especially for pregnant women. Toxic effects can include headache, hair loss, liver damage, miscarriage, and birth defects.

There are currently no recommendations set for carotenoid intake, but fruits and vegetables are rich in carotenoids and should always be a main part of any diet.

## VITAMIN D

Vitamin D plays an essential role in the health of the body's skeleton. It aids in the absorption of calcium (the main component of bone) and helps maintain bone density. Without adequate amounts of vitamin D, children can develop bone malformations (rickets) and adults can develop weakened bones, which can lead to osteoporosis. Some evidence also suggests that a high vitamin D intake may lower the risk of colon cancer.

Fortified milk is the major food source of vitamin D in the United States. Unlike other vitamins and minerals, though, the body can also make all the vitamin D it needs, given enough sunlight. Ultraviolet light from the sun reacts with a form of cholesterol in the skin that then forms vitamin D. Sun exposure, however, can be an unreliable source of the vitamin. With busy work schedules and seasonal changes—UV light in winter is not strong enough in northern climates to make vitamin D in the skin—many people do not get enough ultraviolet rays and need to obtain vitamin D from other sources. The elderly especially have an increased need for vitamin D. Production in the skin declines with age, as may the ability to absorb the vitamin.

*Osteoporosis.* Bone loss is a natural part of aging. In general, the process is gradual but can be accelerated by a number of dietary, hormonal, and lifestyle factors. Osteoporosis develops when the losses in bone mass become so extensive that bones become weak and prone to fractures. Given the role of vitamin D in calcium absorption and the maintenance of bone density, it seems logical that increasing its intake would lower the risk of osteoporosis in the elderly. But does the evidence bear this out? To date, studies have had mixed results, but there have been some promising findings. In one randomized controlled trial, women took either a placebo every day or a supplement containing vitamin D and calcium. After three years, the women on the supplement had not only lost less bone mass than those on the placebo, they also had a lower risk of fracture. Fractures occurred in only 6 percent of the women on supplements and in 20 percent of those on placebo.

Taken collectively, the current evidence does suggest that women can benefit from increasing their intake of vitamin D. However, there are many factors involved in bone loss, making it difficult to highlight any single nutrient as a means to lowering the risk of osteoporosis. In addition to vitamin D and calcium, physical activity, estrogen, vitamin K, and fluoride all interplay in the process of bone buildup and loss.

*Colon Cancer.* Although results to date are mixed on the topic, there is some evidence that a high vitamin D intake can lower the risk of colon cancer. In the Nurses' Health Study, we found that women who had the highest intake of vitamin D (over 550 IU) from food and supplements had a 60 percent lower risk of the disease compared to women with the lowest intake. It is not exactly clear how vitamin D might lower colorectal cancer risk, but some studies show that it can inhibit the rapid growth of cells in the colon, a condition that can lead to cancer.

## What It All Means—Vitamin D

There is promising evidence that getting adequate vitamin D can lower the risk of osteoporosis, while evidence is still emerging on the link between vitamin D and colon cancer. All women should try to get the Dietary Reference Intake for vitamin D—200 IU (5 mcg) a day for ages nineteen to fifty; 400 IU (10 mcg) for ages fifty-one to seventy; and 600 IU (15 mcg) for ages seventy-one and older. Most multivitamins contain 400 IU (10 mcg) of vitamin D. It is not clear, however, that getting more than the DRI, either through food or supplements, provides any additional benefits. As with excessive intake of other fat-soluble vitamins, a very high intake of vitamin D can actually have toxic effects on the kidneys and heart. And children, in whom problems can start with as little as 1,800 IU a day, are particularly prone.

## Good Sources of Vitamin D

Ultraviolet sunlight (except in winter months in northern areas)
Fortified dairy products
Eggs
Vitamin-fortified breakfast cereal

## Vitamin E

Vitamin E's primary function in the body is as an antioxidant. It helps prevent damage to cells by oxygen free radicals, which, among other things, keeps red blood cells and the nervous system healthy. Deficiency in vitamin E almost never occurs, especially in healthy adults

As with vitamin A, a great deal of research has been done on the link between vitamin E and certain chronic diseases. Because of vitamin E's powerful antioxidant qualities, there has been great interest in the potential of this vitamin to lower the risk of lung cancer, breast cancer, and cardiovascular disease. To date, however, there is no solid evidence that increasing one's intake of vitamin E can lower the risk of any type of cancer. There are more solid data that a high vitamin E intake may lower the risk of coronary heart disease, but even this seems unclear with the results of recent studies.

*Coronary Heart Disease.* One factor that can contribute to the narrowing of the arteries that feed the heart is the oxidation of LDL ("bad") cholesterol. The chemical change that occurs to LDL cholesterol when it is oxidized makes it more likely to promote atherosclerosis, or the buildup of cholesterol and fat in the arteries. Because vitamin E is carried in LDL, it may help prevent its oxidation and lower the risk of coronary heart disease.

Although some recent randomized trials—performed primarily in high risk men—have found no link between vitamin E and coronary heart disease, several observational studies have had encouraging results. We found in the Nurses' Health Study that women with the highest intake of vitamin E (an average of about 200 IU per day) had a nearly 35 percent lower risk of heart disease than women with the lowest intake. Vitamin E from food alone, however, was not enough. Women needed to supplement food with vitamin E capsules to see any benefit. Even women consuming the most vitamin E through food averaged only 7.7 IU per day and did not show any decrease in their risk of heart disease. It is not clear why the different studies have had such conflicting results. Additional studies—including randomized clinical trials in women—should help clarify the relationship in the future.

## WHAT IT ALL MEANS—VITAMIN E

Taking vitamin E supplements may help lower the risk of heart disease in women, although more studies are needed before this is known for certain. But because it is very unlikely to have toxic effects even at fairly high doses and may

## Good Food Sources of Vitamin E

Vegetable oil, margarine, shortening

Wheat germ

Nuts

Green leafy vegetables

prove beneficial, we do not think it is unreasonable that all women consider taking a single 400 IU vitamin E tablet each day or a multivitamin containing vitamin E. However, it is important to remember that no supplement can replace a good diet and other healthy lifestyle choices.

The DRI for vitamin E is 15 mg a day for an adult woman. For most vitamin E supplements, 1 mg of vitamin E equals 1 IU of vitamin E.

## Water-Soluble Vitamins
### Vitamin C

Vitamin C (also called ascorbic acid) is a water-soluble antioxidant that plays an important role in a healthy immune system and the formation of collagen—a main component of tissue throughout the body. Though rare today in the United States, the most serious result of an extended deficiency in vitamin C is scurvy, which occurs when the soft tissues of the body start to break down. The first symptoms of scurvy are typically tender and bleeding gums. With time, though, the condition can advance to more serious types of bleeding.

As with the other antioxidant vitamins, a great deal of research has assessed the link between vitamin C and a number of chronic diseases, including cardiovascular disease, cancer, and cataracts. For coronary heart disease and cancer, there is little evidence that getting extra vitamin C has any benefit. For stroke, the data are more supportive, and we have some preliminary results from the Nurses' Health Study that show that a high intake of vitamin C may help lower the risk of stroke. These findings are only preliminary, however, and more studies are needed before we know the exact relationship between vitamin C and the risk of stroke in women.

There is also some evidence that vitamin C supplements may lower the risk of cataracts. In a small spin-off study of the Nurses' Health Study, we found that women taking vitamin C supplements for ten or more years had a substantially lower risk of developing cloudy lenses compared to women not taking supplements. However, when looking at more severe cataracts in another assessment, we found that vitamin C was linked to only a modest decrease, if any, in risk. Other studies on this topic have had mixed results, and, again, more evidence is needed before solid recommendations can be made.

### What It All Means—Vitamin C

There is no solid evidence that getting more than the DRI for vitamin C (75 milligrams per day for nonsmoking women and 110 milligrams per day for smoking women)—from food or supplements—has any added health benefits.

## Good Food Sources of Vitamin C

Oranges

Grapefruit

Lemons

Limes

Green and red peppers

Collard greens

Broccoli

Spinach

Tomatoes

Potatoes

Strawberries

A vitamin C supplement of up to 500 milligrams per day, however, is not harmful and may possibly help lower the risk of cataracts and stroke. Very large doses of vitamin C—above 2,000 milligrams per day—may have some ill effects, such as diarrhea, nausea, and stomach cramps, and should be avoided.

### FOLATE

Folate (also called folic acid) is a B vitamin that is essential for metabolism and the production of DNA. Deficiencies in the vitamin can lead to problems with cell division and the making of protein as well as certain types of birth defects. There is also evidence that a low intake of folate may increase the risk of coronary heart disease, stroke, and colon cancer.

*Neural Tube Defects.* Neural tube defects (such as spina bifida and anencephaly) are the most common form of severe birth defects and occur when a fetus's spinal cord channel—also called the neural tube—does not close as it should. In the United States, approximately 4,000 pregnancies are affected by the condition each year. Research into the causes of neural tube defects has found that a high intake of folate before and during pregnancy can greatly lower the risk of the disease. It is estimated that half of all neural tube defects could be avoided by all women of childbearing age getting at least 400 micrograms of folate every day.

Essential to lowering the risk of neural tube defects is getting adequate folate *before* becoming pregnant, an event that is not always planned. A fetus's

> ## Vitamins at a Glance
>
> - Vitamin D is essential for strong, healthy bones and is thought to help reduce bone loss that comes with aging. Unlike other vitamins, the body can make its own vitamin D from exposure to ultraviolet light from the sun.
> - Vitamin E is helpful as an antioxidant. It also may lower the risk of coronary heart disease, but probably needs to be taken as a supplement in order to achieve beneficial levels in the body.
> - Because folate prevents certain birth defects, it is especially important for women who may become pregnant. Folate intake may also help to lower the risk of colon cancer and coronary heart disease.
> - Vitamin $B_6$ may help lower the risk of coronary heart disease and stroke.

neural tube closes around four weeks after conception, a time when most women are just realizing they may be pregnant. Therefore, it is recommended that all women of child-bearing age supplement what they eat with a daily vitamin tablet containing 400 micrograms of folate. As an added assurance, many breakfast cereals in the United States are also fortified with the vitamin. Other foods can be an excellent source of folate as well, but it can be difficult for some women to consistently get enough folate from the diet.

*Coronary Heart Disease.* A number of studies have linked a high intake of folate with a lower risk of coronary heart disease. In the Nurses' Health Study, we found that women getting an average of 400 micrograms or more a day (from food and supplements combined) had a 20 to 30 percent lower risk of the disease (see Figure 21-1). And the source of folate does not seem to matter. Folate from food or from vitamin supplements both lowered risk.

A high intake of folate—along with vitamins $B_6$ and $B_{12}$ (see below)—is thought to decrease the risk of coronary heart disease by lowering blood levels of the protein homocysteine. Many studies have shown that high levels of homocysteine in the blood can raise the risk of heart disease, possibly by increasing the risk of blood clots or injuring the walls of the coronary arteries. When looked at collectively, the evidence is fairly strong that women taking regular folate supplements will protect themselves against heart disease. However, it is not definitive. Randomized controlled trials testing the B-complex vitamins should, in the not-too-distant future, provide additional evidence.

*Stroke.* A high intake of folate may also lower the risk of stoke, though the evidence is not as strong as that for coronary heart disease. A number of stud-

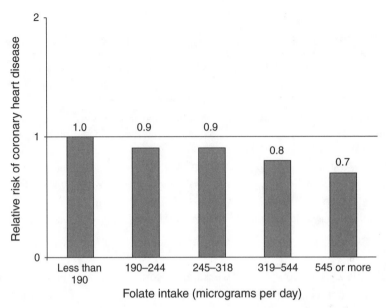

FIG. 21-1. The relative risk of heart disease drops as folate intake increases. (Source: Nurses' Health Study)

ies have linked stroke with high blood levels of homocysteine, which a low intake of folate can cause. Little evidence, though, shows directly that a high intake of folate can lower the risk of stroke.

*Colon Cancer.* Many studies suggest that a high intake of folate—either from vitamin supplements or folate-rich foods—can reduce the risk of colon cancer. Although it is not clear exactly how folate may lower risk, one possibility is that it helps protect the DNA in cells from damage that causes them to become cancerous.

The folate in foods and the folate in supplements, however, do not appear to be of equal benefit. Recent evidence suggests that a daily multivitamin with folate can lower the risk of colon cancer more than a diet rich in foods that contain folate. In the Nurses' Health Study, we found women who used multivitamins for at least fifteen years were 75 percent less likely to develop colon cancer compared to women who never took multivitamins. Notably, women whose diets were high in folate but who never took multivitamins did not have a substantial reduction in their risk of colon cancer.

Why might supplements with folate be better than the folate found naturally in food? The kind of folate contained in supplements—a synthetic version called folic acid—is absorbed more efficiently than the folate in food, which has to be broken down before it can be absorbed. As a result, a woman would have to eat about twice as much natural folate (800 micrograms) to get the amount of folic acid (400 micrograms) typically found in a multivitamin. Few women are able to consistently get that much natural folate through their diet, which would be the rough equivalent of eight servings of fruit every day.

## What It All Means—Folate

The Dietary Reference Intake for females aged 14 and over is 400 micrograms a day. For added assurance against neural tube defects, it is also recommended that all women capable of becoming pregnant get 400 micrograms of folate every day from fortified foods or supplements *in addition* to the folate they get from their diets. All other women may benefit from taking a multivitamin with folate every day as well, even though the evidence for this is not yet conclusive. Folate intake at this level is likely to protect against colon cancer and possibly cardiovascular disease.

## Good Food Sources of Folate

Wheat germ

Nuts

Green leafy vegetables

Fruit

Organ meats

Fortified breakfast cereals

Beans, such as lentils and chickpeas

## Vitamins $B_6$ and $B_{12}$

Vitamins $B_6$ and $B_{12}$, among other important functions, play vital roles in metabolism. Severe deficiency in $B_6$—which usually occurs along with a deficiency in other B vitamins—can lead to convulsions, skin problems, and anemia. Severe deficiency in $B_{12}$ can also result in anemia as well as nervous system problems. Vitamin $B_{12}$ deficiency is rare in the United States, though it becomes more common with age. Stomach acid is needed to make the $B_{12}$ in food available to be absorbed. When stomach acid levels are low—as they typically are in the elderly—$B_{12}$ from food is not readily absorbed, which can lead to deficiency even if the diet is rich in $B_{12}$. Vitamin $B_{12}$ in supplements and fortified foods, however, can be readily absorbed in the normal gastrointestinal tract, even with low levels of stomach acid.

*Coronary Heart Disease and Stroke.* A number of studies suggest that a high intake of vitamins $B_6$ and $B_{12}$ may lower the risk of coronary heart disease and stroke. As with folate, a high intake of vitamins $B_6$ and $B_{12}$ can keep levels of homocysteine in the blood low. In the Nurses' Health Study, we found that the risk of heart disease dropped as the intake of vitamin $B_6$ increased. Women getting an average of 4.6 milligrams of $B_6$ a day—more than three times the Dietary Reference Intake for adults—had a nearly 35 percent lower risk of coronary heart disease than women getting an average of 1.1 milligrams per day. When we assessed $B_{12}$ intake, we found no link with coronary heart disease, but this may be because blood levels of $B_{12}$—something we have not assessed—may be more important than the levels in food. Because most people get enough $B_{12}$ in their diet, it may only be those who have trouble absorbing $B_{12}$ that may have an increased risk of the disease.

## WHAT IT ALL MEANS—VITAMINS $B_6$ AND $B_{12}$

The Dietary Reference Intake for vitamin $B_6$ is 1.3 milligrams a day for women ages nineteen to fifty and 1.5 milligrams a day for those ages fifty-one and over. For $B_{12}$, the DRI is 2.4 micrograms a day for all adult women. To help assure

## Good Food Sources of Vitamins $B_6$ and $B_{12}$

| *Vitamin $B_6$* | *Vitamin $B_{12}$* |
|---|---|
| Chicken | Red meat |
| Fish | Chicken |
| Kidney | Fish |
| Liver | Dairy products |
| Pork | Eggs |
| Eggs | Fortified breakfast cereal |
| Oats | |
| Soybeans | |
| Walnuts | |
| Whole wheat products | |
| Fortified breakfast cereal | |

adequate intake and possibly to lower the risk of cardiovascular disease, all women may want to supplement their diets with a multivitamin containing $B_6$ and $B_{12}$. This may be especially important for women over fifty, who can have trouble absorbing enough vitamin $B_{12}$ from food.

## Minerals and Chronic Disease

Minerals perform a number of vital roles in the body, from providing structure (such as calcium in bone) to maintaining the proper amount of fluid inside and outside of cells. As with vitamins, some minerals may also help lower the risk of certain chronic diseases.

### SODIUM (SALT)

Sodium is a very important regulator of the amount of fluid in body tissues and blood. The primary source of sodium is salt (sodium chloride). Processed foods—such as canned goods, baked goods, breakfast cereals, and many snack foods—tend to be very high in salt and account for three-quarters of the sodium people consume. Fresh fruits and vegetables, on the other hand, tend to be very low in salt. Sodium deficiency is exceptionally rare in the United States, with most people consuming over 9 grams of salt per day—7 times what the body actually requires for healthy functioning.

*Hypertension.* When most people think of the consequences of a high salt diet, one condition likely comes to mind: high blood pressure (hypertension). And, while it is true that a high intake of salt can increase the risk of hypertension, it does not have as large an influence on risk as many would believe. To see a significant 3 to 6 point increase in systolic blood pressure, one large international study found that it would take a huge increase in salt intake—requiring the average American to eat more than half again as much as he or she usually does. To lower blood pressure by a similar amount, the average American would have to cut salt intake by about two-thirds, a possible yet difficult amount for most people to achieve.

For some people, though, the benefit of lowering salt intake may be greater. African Americans, people with diabetes, the obese, the elderly, and those who already have hypertension generally experience greater changes in blood pressure with changes in salt intake. One study that combined the results of numerous clinical trials found that lowering salt intake lowered blood pressure by approximately twice as much in people with hypertension as with normal blood pressure.

A more recent clinical trial sponsored by the National Heart, Lung, and

Blood Institute has further confirmed this. Called the Dietary Approaches to Stop Hypertension (DASH) trial, it found that both people with and without hypertension could significantly lower their blood pressure by lowering salt intake. People with hypertension benefited the most but even people with normal blood pressure saw improvements. When the low salt diet was combined with a diet rich in fruits, vegetables, and low fat dairy products (called the DASH diet) drops in blood pressure were even more pronounced. Compared to people eating a standard high salt diet, people with hypertension who followed the low salt DASH diet had an almost 12 mm Hg lower systolic blood pressure. Even those without hypertension had a 7 mm Hg lower systolic blood pressure.

## What It All Means—Sodium (Salt)

For the average person, salt intake is likely to have only a modest effect on the risk of hypertension. As part of an overall approach to lowering the risk of hypertension, however, keeping salt intake to a moderate level (6 grams per day—or approximately one teaspoon) is likely to be good for you. For those people who tend to have a greater response to salt intake—especially those with obesity, diabetes, or hypertension—keeping salt intake at a moderate level is even more important.

## Calcium

In addition to being a primary component of bone, calcium is also important in blood clotting as well as in the healthy functioning of muscles and the nervous system. Dairy products—milk, yogurt, and cheese—are the main sources of calcium in the United States, though leafy-green vegetables and calcium-fortified foods are also rich in the mineral.

Calcium has long been touted as the perfect agent for preventing osteoporosis. It not only helps build bone mass early in life, but also helps slow the rate of bone loss during adulthood. Despite these positive effects, however, calcium may not be as beneficial as researchers once thought. While it does lead to stronger bones, there is little solid evidence that calcium-rich diets or calcium supplements offer long-term protection against the most serious effect of osteoporosis: bone fractures.

Numerous observational studies have examined the long-term effects of calcium intake from foods, on fracture risk. To date, nearly all of these studies have shown that calcium from food has no effect on the risk of fractures. In the Nurses' Health Study, we found that women who drank two glasses of milk a day were just as likely as those who drank one glass a week to suffer a fracture of the hip or wrist. We found similar results when we looked at other foods rich in calcium.

What about calcium from supplements? A number of randomized controlled trials have shown that calcium supplements improve bone mass. However, most of these trials have not looked directly at the risk of fracture. This is because randomized controlled trials do not generally last long enough to study such long-term effects. A nine-year trial to address the issue is currently underway in the Women's Health Initiative. In that trial, researchers assigned women to take either a daily placebo or a daily supplement containing both calcium and vitamin D. At the end of the trial, researchers will determine which group has lower fracture rates: those on the placebo or those on the supplements. Two smaller trials have shown lower rates of fracture among women on supplements compared to women on placebo, but both of these studies were short in duration.

So what can women do to protect themselves against osteoporosis and bone fractures? First, there is no doubt that calcium is very important for building strong bones during childhood and adolescence. Second, although a high calcium intake has not yet been shown to provide additional protection against fractures, adult women are currently advised to get the DRI for calcium (either through diet or supplement use) as it may be an important part of a combined approach to improve bone health and lower fracture risk. That approach includes adequate vitamin D, exercise, and for some women, postmenopausal hormones.

Aside from bone health, calcium intake has shown promise as a way to lower the risk of a number of disorders, including diabetes, hypertension, stroke, and colon cancer. Calcium has also been linked to the risk of kidney stones.

*Diabetes.* Calcium has been shown in certain studies to have a beneficial effect on insulin production and blood sugar levels, which may help lower the risk of developing diabetes. When we assessed calcium intake in the Nurses' Health Study, we found that women getting the greatest amount had a 30 percent lower risk of diabetes than women getting the least.

*Hypertension.* A number of studies have found that a low calcium intake may increase the risk of hypertension, and that increasing the amount of calcium in the diet may slightly lower risk. Results from the DASH trial show that a diet rich in low fat dairy as well as fruits and vegetables can lower systolic blood pressure by 5 mm Hg compared to a standard diet. Not all studies are consistent, however, and when we assessed the topic, we found no link between calcium intake and hypertension.

*Stroke.* Although there have been a relatively small number of studies on the subject—and even fewer in women—there is some evidence that a high calcium intake may help lower the risk of stroke. In the Nurses' Health Study we found that women getting at least a modest amount of calcium (675 milligrams per day or more) had a 20 to 30 percent lower risk of stroke compared to women getting the least.

*Colon Cancer.* Cohort studies suggest that a high intake of calcium may slightly lower the risk of colon cancer. However, the evidence is not particularly consistent, and it is an issue we hope to assess in the Nurses' Health Study in the near future.

*Kidney Stones.* The few studies that have assessed the relationship between calcium and kidney stones have tended to find that a high intake of calcium increased the risk of the condition. In the Nurses' Health Study, however, we have found that the relationship may be more complicated than that. It seems that the calcium women get from dairy products and the calcium they get from supplements influences risk differently. A high intake of calcium from food seems to lower the risk of kidney stones, while a high intake of calcium from supplements actually slightly increased the risk. Dairy products, the main source of calcium in our study, may help bind and excrete the dietary oxalate that promotes the formation of kidney stones. When calcium is taken as a supplement, dietary oxalate is less likely to be excreted, which may promote stone formation.

## What It All Means—Calcium

The Dietary Reference Intake for calcium is 1,000 milligrams per day for women ages nineteen to fifty and 1,200 milligrams per day for women ages fifty-one and over, and it is currently recommended that women get this amount through diet or calcium supplements. Taking large doses of calcium much above the DRI does not seem to have any added health benefits. While dairy products are the primary source of calcium in U.S. diets, they should not be the sole source. Dairy products can be high in saturated fat and their protein content can actually cause the loss of calcium in the urine. Nuts, whole grains, and green leafy vegetables are also excellent sources of calcium.

## Good Food Sources of Calcium

Milk

Yogurt

Cheese

Nuts

Whole grains

Green leafy vegetables

Sardines and anchovies

## MAGNESIUM

Magnesium is an essential part of hundreds of chemical reactions in the body and plays a critical role in metabolism and the transmission of signals in the nervous system. Although deficiency in magnesium is very rare, if it occurs it can result in nausea, muscle weakness, irritability, and mental instability.

Many of the same chronic conditions possibly linked to calcium may also be linked with magnesium, including diabetes and hypertension.

*Diabetes.* Although studies to date have had mixed results, we found in the Nurses' Health Study that women with the highest intake of magnesium had an approximately 30 percent lower risk of diabetes than women getting the least. However, another large cohort study that included middle-aged women found no link between the two.

*Hypertension.* As with some other studies, we found in the Nurses' Health Study that magnesium intake may have small influence on blood pressure. Women in our study getting 350 milligrams or more of magnesium a day had a slightly lower blood pressure—by 1 mm Hg (millimeters of mercury) or so—than women getting less than 200 milligrams per day. We did not find, however, a direct link between low magnesium intake and blood pressure levels high enough to be called hypertension.

## WHAT IT ALL MEANS—MAGNESIUM

There is no solid evidence that getting more than the DRI for magnesium (320 milligrams per day for women over 30) has any added health benefits.

## Good Food Sources of Magnesium

Whole grains

Nuts

Seeds

Bitter chocolate (cocoa)

Leafy plants (such as spinach)

## POTASSIUM

Potassium plays a role in metabolism, muscle contractions, and the transmission of signals in the nervous system. Potassium deficiency is a rare occurrence in healthy individuals. One of the most common causes of deficiency is the use of diuretic drugs to treat hypertension, which can cause large losses of potassium in the urine. Many diuretic drugs used today, however, are designed to limit the loss of potassium. Typical symptoms of deficiency include weakness, irregular heartbeat, increased urination, and thirst.

*Hypertension.* Many studies have consistently found that a low potassium intake may increase the risk of hypertension and that increasing potassium intake may help lower blood pressure. One study that combined the result of over thirty-three randomized trials found that potassium supplements could lower systolic blood pressure by approximately 3 points and diastolic blood pressure by approximately 2 points. Our results in the Nurses' Health Study were more modest but also showed that a diet high in potassium may have a beneficial effect on blood pressure. Women in our study getting 3,200 milligrams a day or more of potassium—from both food and supplements—had blood pressure that averaged one point lower than women getting less than 2,000 milligrams a day.

*Stroke.* A relatively small number of studies have assessed the link between potassium and stroke, and even fewer have assessed the relationship in women. Many of these, however, suggest that a high potassium intake may lower the risk of stroke. One study in particular found that for every 400 milligrams (10 millimoles) of potassium consumed, the risk of stroke dropped 40 percent. In the Nurses' Health Study, our findings have been more modest. We found a weak relationship between a high potassium intake (3,500 milligrams of potassium a day) and lower risk of stroke.

*Diabetes.* Certain studies have shown that potassium may have a beneficial effect on insulin production and blood sugar levels, which may help lower the risk of developing diabetes. When we assessed this issue in the Nurses' Health Study, we found that women getting the greatest amounts of potassium—from both food and supplements—had a 40 percent lower risk of diabetes than women getting the least.

## WHAT IT ALL MEANS—POTASSIUM

There is currently no RDA set for potassium, though the lowest requirement for adults is estimated to be approximately 2,000 milligrams a day. This is a minimum requirement, however. For its potential to lower the risk of hypertension—and possibly stroke—women should strive to get at least 3,500 milligrams of potassium a day, preferably from fresh fruits and vegetables. Never take a potassium supplement without first discussing it with a health care provider, as they can cause serious problems in people with kidney conditions.

## Good Food Sources of Potassium

Whole grains

Nuts

Meats

Fruit (especially bananas, oranges, and avocados)

Vegetables (such as tomatoes, spinach, and broccoli)

## SELENIUM

Selenium is a key part of an important antioxidant enzyme and is closely tied to the functions of vitamin E. For both of these reasons, a great deal of research has been done on selenium's potential to lower the risk of cancer. While a number of small studies have had consistent, promising results, larger studies have had only mixed findings. One randomized controlled trial in men and women found that selenium supplementation could lower the risk of cancer in men but had no benefit in women. It even found a slight increase in the risk of breast cancer. In the Nurses' Health Study, we have had similar results to those of the randomized trial: a high selenium intake offered no protection against any cancer and possibly even slightly increased the risk of breast cancer. Further research is needed, however, to reveal both the risks and benefits associated with selenium intake.

## What It All Means—Selenium

There is currently not enough evidence of added health benefits to recommend more than the DRI for selenium (55 micrograms per day for adults).

### Good Food Sources of Selenium

Seafood
Kidney
Liver
Red meat
Chicken
Grains
Seeds

## Iron

Iron is a very important mineral. It is a component of the oxygen-carrying part of red blood cells (hemoglobin) and is a constituent of a number of enzymes. Long-term iron deficiency can lead to mild fatigue in early stages and advance to severe fatigue if anemia develops due to the inability of the blood to carry enough oxygen.

During the premenopausal years, women have an increased need for iron due to the loss of blood during menstruation. Even with this increased need, the majority of women in the United States get sufficient iron (18 milligrams per day) from their diets. Premenopausal women who do not get enough iron should increase their intake of healthy, iron-rich foods. Lean meat, chicken, fish, fruits, vegetables, whole grains, and fortified cereals are good sources. A multivitamin with iron may also be beneficial. After menopause, a woman's need for iron decreases, as she is no longer menstruating. If she chose to take a multivitamin with iron before menopause, she should likely stop after menopause. Exceptions include women diagnosed with iron-deficiency anemia and some women on postmenopausal hormones who still experience monthly bleeding. While it is still important to get enough iron in the diet

(8 milligrams per day for postmenopausal women), consistently consuming more than is needed can cause iron stores to increase in the body, which some studies have linked to an increased risk of coronary heart disease and cancer.

## What It All Means—Iron

It is important for all women to get the DRI for iron and to adjust their intake level as they move into the postmenopausal years. Premenopausal women should get 18 milligrams a day of iron, and may consider a multivitamin with iron to ensure they are meeting this need. Postmenopausal women only need 8 milligrams a day and should probably discontinue any iron supplement they were taking before menopause. There is currently some evidence that iron intake at the DRI levels (or above) increases the risk of coronary heart disease or cancer, although that connection is still weak at this point.

## Good Food Sources of Iron

Fortified bread
Fortified breakfast cereals
Meat
Poultry
Fish
Vegetables
Legumes
Nuts
Soy

## What It All Means—Vitamins and Minerals

Vitamins and minerals are essential for good health. In addition to playing key roles in the optimal functioning of the body, they may also help lower the risk of certain chronic diseases. However, no vitamin or mineral is a magic bullet against disease, and, while some supplements can enhance a healthy diet, they can never replace it. That said, we feel there is compelling, although still not conclusive, evidence that all women (and men) could benefit from taking a single multivitamin supplement every day.

## Minerals at a Glance

- Calcium leads to stronger bones, but there is little solid evidence to date that calcium-rich diets or calcium supplements offer long-term protection against the most serious consequence of osteoporosis: bone fractures. However, as part of a combined approach to maintaining strong, healthy bones through the years, calcium seems important for women.
- Calcium from dairy products seems to decrease the risk of kidney stones, while calcium from dietary supplements may actually increase a woman's risk of kidney stones.
- Like calcium, magnesium seems to be somewhat effective in lowering a woman's risk of diabetes and hypertension.
- High potassium intake has been linked to a decrease in the risk of hypertension in women.
- Decreasing salt intake can lower blood pressure in people with and without hypertension.

## WHAT I TELL MY PATIENTS ABOUT VITAMINS AND MINERALS

DR. NANCY RIGOTTI

When I was in medical school, we were taught that most people in the United States got all the vitamins they needed in their diet and that taking vitamin pills was unnecessary. It was a simple message, but it was probably wrong. The message I give my patients now is more complex. I tell them that:

- We now have very solid scientific evidence that a diet rich with fruits, vegetables, and whole grains is really good for you, and provides most if not all of the vitamins and minerals you need. It is a far better choice than supplementing a poor diet with vitamin and mineral supplements in pill form. Fruits and vegetables probably contain as-yet-unidentified factors besides vitamins that promote health.
- However, the typical American's diet may not contain the optimal amounts of folic acid, B vitamins, and possibly vitamins D and E.
- If you are a vegan (a vegetarian who does not eat any dairy products), your diet is probably deficient in vitamin $B_{12}$, and you need to take $B_{12}$ in a supplement such as a multivitamin. When buying a multi-

vitamin, name brand or "all natural" formulations are not necessary; a standard store-brand RDA-level multivitamin is just fine.

- If you are a woman in your childbearing years, even if you are not trying to become pregnant, you should strongly consider taking a daily multivitamin. This will provide enough folic acid (400 micrograms) to prevent your having a baby with a birth defect (neural tube defect) in case you get pregnant. A multivitamin with iron can protect you in case your daily iron intake doesn't match iron lost in your monthly flow.

- If you are a woman past your childbearing years, you should consider taking a daily multivitamin supplement to ensure you are getting enough folic acid (400 micrograms), vitamin $B_6$, vitamin $B_{12}$, and vitamin D.

- If you have risk factors for coronary heart disease, consider taking both folic acid (800 micrograms) and vitamin E (400 IU) each day. Neither of these vitamin supplements is proven to benefit you, but in these doses they do no harm, and may do some good. Because vitamin E can reduce the blood's ability to clot, women who take blood thinners should talk with their health care providers before taking a vitamin E supplement.

- If you are not meeting the Dietary Reference Intake for calcium (and most women do not unless they eat three or more servings of dairy products each day), consider taking a calcium supplement. This is one case where a supplement pill may be preferable to getting the mineral through foods.

# CHAPTER TWENTY-TWO

# Postmenopausal Hormones

## BACKGROUND

Whether or not to take postmenopausal hormones is one of the most pressing and complex health-related questions for middle-aged and older women today. There is already an overwhelming amount of information available about postmenopausal hormones, and with new evidence constantly emerging, women have an increasing number of factors to consider. Postmenopausal hormones can affect a woman's risk of the leading causes of death in the United States—cancer and heart disease—as well as a number of other conditions and diseases. Unfortunately, not all of these effects are positive, leaving most women to wonder how they can gain the benefits of postmenopausal hormones while minimizing the risks.

### The Role of Estrogen

Menopause is a complicated process in a woman's life. Although it is often defined as the cessation of menstrual periods, menopause is a gradual process that takes place over months and is often accompanied by increasingly irregular menstrual periods. This process is essentially the body's response to drastic changes in the level of the female sex hormone, estrogen.

Prior to menopause, estrogen plays an essential role not only in reproductive functions but also in the maintenance and growth of a variety of tissues and organs. Like other hormones, estrogen is produced and secreted by tissues in one part of the body—in this case, the ovaries—and then transported into the bloodstream to cells in other parts of the body. In women, estrogen affects the cells of the blood vessels, brain, skin, breast, liver, and bone, as well as the linings of the vagina and urinary tract. It stimulates these cells to release proteins that help maintain the tissues and organs.

When estrogen levels decline during menopause, the physical functioning of these tissues and organs can be altered dramatically. For example, one role of estrogen is to stimulate the tissue in the lining of the vagina. This lining is very elastic and exudes lubrication during sexual arousal. When estrogen levels decline, the vaginal lining becomes thinner, losing some of its elasticity and lubricant-producing capability. These changes result in vaginal dryness, a common menopausal symptom that can cause pain during intercourse, vaginal soreness, and annoying itching. This is one of the more noticeable results of the body's waning production of estrogen. However, it is only one of many.

## Menopausal Symptoms

More than 75 percent of women experience hot flashes, insomnia, or vaginal dryness after menopause. Characterized by sudden waves of body heat, hot flashes may be accompanied by flushing, palpitations, perspiration, and night sweats. Researchers who have studied women undergoing hot flashes have found that during these episodes, the heart beats faster and the blood vessels near the surface of the skin dilate; blood flows to the surface more quickly, releasing heat.

Experience with hot flashes varies dramatically among women who have them. Some have episodes that are fleeting, while others have flashes lasting for several minutes; some have them only occasionally, and others experience them several times an hour. Some feel only slightly warm, while others emerge wringing wet. Tolerance for these episodes also depends on the individual. Women who rarely perspire may find hot flashes extremely disconcerting, while those who are accustomed to working up a sweat, or who find it difficult to stay warm, may not mind them.

Sleep disruption is also a common symptom associated with menopause. Again, the degree of insomnia varies widely. Some women are awakened by night sweats so severe that they have to change the bedclothes, while other formerly sound sleepers find that they wake up several times during the night for no apparent reason. These sleep disruptions can cause fatigue, as well as the mood swings that are often associated with menopause.

Other symptoms that are frequently reported by postmenopausal women include achy joints, forgetfulness, headaches, and facial wrinkles. However, these may be due as much to the effects of aging as to menopause per se.

## Postmenopausal Hormone Use

By supplementing the body's waning supply of estrogen, women can alleviate the menopausal symptoms described above. This was recognized as early as the 1920s, when scientists created a synthetic estrogen that could be taken

## Postmenopausal Hormones for the Relief of Menopausal Symptoms

- Menopause is the body's response to drastic changes in the level of the female sex hormone estrogen.
- Due to the declining levels of estrogen in their bodies, more than 75 percent of women experience vaginal dryness, hot flashes, or insomnia after menopause.
- By supplementing the body's estrogen supply, postmenopausal hormones can alleviate menopausal symptoms.

orally. By the mid-1930s, however, it became clear that estrogen stimulated the growth of endometrial cells (the cells lining the uterus), thereby increasing women's risk of endometrial cancer. In the late 1970s, researchers developed a hormone regimen designed to preserve the beneficial effects of estrogen while reducing the risk of endometrial cancer. This regimen consisted of adding progestin to estrogen therapy. Progestin is a synthetic version of the natural sex hormone progesterone and curtails endometrial growth, just as natural progesterone does during the menstrual cycle. The combination of estrogen and progestin became, and still is, the treatment of choice for women who have not undergone hysterectomy and thus still have a uterus.

## LESSONS FROM THE NURSES' HEALTH STUDY AND OTHER STUDIES

Postmenopausal women first began taking estrogen for the short-term relief of menopausal symptoms. However, after years of studying women on estrogen therapy, scientists have concluded that estrogen can also have a dramatic impact on women's risk of chronic disease. Some of estrogen's effects are positive and some are negative. By knowing how estrogen might affect her overall health, a woman can begin to decide whether the benefits of estrogen outweigh the risks.

### The Benefits of Postmenopausal Hormones

RELIEF OF MENOPAUSAL SYMPTOMS

Although postmenopausal women now take estrogen for a variety of reasons, it was originally approved by the Food and Drug Administration (FDA) solely for the alleviation of menopausal symptoms. Based on evidence from randomized controlled trials, estrogen is indicated for the relief of vasomotor symptoms—hot flashes, sweats, and chills—and for the treatment of vaginal dryness. Because hot flashes and night sweats can disrupt sleep, women who take estrogen often report that it relieves insomnia. Estrogen can also alleviate the pain during sexual intercourse that often accompanies vaginal dryness. However, other claims for estrogen—that it enhances mood and concentration, relieves depression, and improves skin tone—have yet to be adequately substantiated.

## LOWER RISK OF OSTEOPOROSIS

Throughout a woman's life, her body is constantly building up and tearing down bone. Early in life, the building process dominates, but in the years immediately following menopause, bone is torn down much more rapidly than it is built up. Estrogen can prevent and even partially reverse postmenopausal bone loss by inhibiting the cells that break down bone (osteoclasts) and stimulating the cells that make new bone (osteoblasts). For this reason, estrogen has been acknowledged by the FDA to prevent and treat osteoporosis.

Women who take postmenopausal hormones tend to gain bone mass in the early years of menopause, when most women are losing it at an average of 3 percent per year. In one randomized controlled trial, postmenopausal women took estrogen and progestin daily for ten years and had a 6 percent increase in bone mass.

Estrogen's beneficial effects on the bone appear to translate into a reduced risk of hip fracture, the most serious effect of osteoporosis. Nearly a dozen epidemiologic studies have shown that women taking estrogen are about 25 percent less likely to have a hip fracture than women who have never taken estrogen (see Figures 22-1 and 22-2). Those who begin taking estrogen early in menopause and continue to do so for at least seven to ten years may attain even greater protection. Once a woman stops taking the hormones, however, the protective effect disappears, and the loss of bone mass resumes at an accelerated rate.

Though few studies have examined the effect of both estrogen and progestin on the risk of hip fracture, those that have suggest that the combined therapy is as effective as estrogen alone in preventing hip fracture.

## IMPROVED CHOLESTEROL PROFILE

High blood cholesterol is an important contributor to the development of coronary heart disease and stroke. Numerous studies have found that, when taken

Throughout this chapter, we describe how hormones might lower or raise your risk of various diseases. However, remember that some of the diseases affected by hormones are rare (like pulmonary embolism), while others are quite common (like heart disease). By knowing your chance of developing these diseases, you can better decide whether to incur the various risks and benefits associated with postmenopausal hormones. Here are the odds that a fifty-year-old woman will develop a given disease before the age of eighty.

| | |
|---|---|
| Coronary heart disease | 20 in 100 |
| Hip fracture | 15 in 100 |
| Breast cancer | 9 in 100 |
| Colon cancer | 3 in 100 |
| Ovarian cancer | 1 in 100 |
| Deep vein thrombosis/<br>    pulmonary embolism | 0.04 in 100 |

## Studying the Health Effects of Postmenopausal Hormones

Postmenopausal hormones are thought to affect women's risk of various diseases. However, some of the diseases that hormones are thought to prevent may actually be prevented by other factors. Women who use hormones tend to be different from women who do not use hormones in a variety of ways that could affect their health. For example, compared to women who do not use hormones, those who do tend to see their health care providers more regularly and may generally choose to lead healthier lives. Thus, these women might be protected in part against certain diseases not because of their hormone use, but because of their healthier lifestyles and the additional medical care they receive. Similarly, women who are ill are often not put on hormones because their providers do not want to burden them with additional medication. These women may then appear to be at higher risk of disease because they are not on hormones, when in fact they are at higher risk because of their underlying health problems.

How then can we determine that hormones affect women's health? Large studies like the Nurses' Health Study address the problem described above by collecting information on many aspects of women's lives. This allows us to better understand how different factors interact in women's lives and to be more confident in our conclusion that hormones do affect women's health.

---

*In the Nurses' Own Words . . .*

Being a member of the Nurses Health Study has been important to me in my life because I am a breast cancer survivor since age thirty-four and many topics studied and questions asked have concerned me. When they asked questions about broccoli, I ate broccoli. When they asked questions about exercise, I became an avid walker and gym bum. At age sixty-five I am alive and well and enjoy all the reports I read from your studies.

—From GK

---

orally, estrogen lowers the level of total blood cholesterol. It can also favorably affect the different types of cholesterol, lowering levels of LDL ("bad cholesterol") and raising levels of HDL ("good cholesterol").

Unfortunately, synthetic progestins may detract from the beneficial effect that estrogen has on cholesterol. Progestins tend to raise the level of LDL and lower the level of HDL. The strongest evidence of this relationship comes from a large randomized controlled trial in which the participants took either a placebo or one of three hormone regimens: estrogen alone, estrogen with natural progesterone, or estrogen with synthetic progestin. Researchers found that, over the course of the three-year study, HDL levels rose and LDL levels declined in the three groups of women on postmenopausal hormones. The extent to which the HDL levels rose differed markedly with the therapy: women taking either estrogen alone or estrogen with progesterone had a 6 percent increase in HDL levels, while women taking estrogen with progestin had only a 2 percent increase. Notably, in the women taking placebo, HDL levels *declined* by 3 percent, and LDL levels declined by much less than they did in the women on hormones. These results suggest that estrogen and progestin combined do not offer the same cholesterol benefits as estrogen alone, but that taking the combined therapy is still more beneficial than taking no therapy at all.

## IMPROVED BLOOD FLOW

When the arteries become too narrow, the flow of blood can be blocked, and this can increase the risk of cardiovascular disease. Estrogen appears to improve blood flow through a variety of mechanisms. First, it triggers the release of substances that dilate blood vessels, and this helps prevent the spasms that often contribute to heart attack and stroke. Second, by lowering the level of sub-

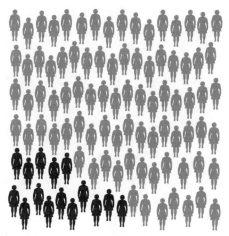

FIG 22-1. In a group of 100 women who are fifty years old and *not* taking postmenopausal hormones, 15 will suffer a hip fracture in their lifetime. (Source: Grady et al.)

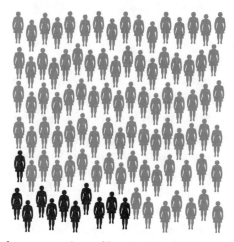

FIG. 22-2. In a group of 100 women who are fifty years old and taking postmenopausal hormones, 11 will suffer a hip fracture in their lifetime. (Source: Grady et al.)

stances that interfere with the dissolving of clots and raising the level of substances that inhibit clot formation, estrogen may help keep blood clots from blocking the arteries. Finally, estrogen lowers the level of fibrinogen, a clotting factor that at high levels can raise the risk of heart attack. In one randomized controlled trial, fibrinogen levels were 3 percent higher among women taking placebo than among women taking estrogen. This difference is not as trivial as it may sound: according to the Framingham Heart Study, a 3 percent increase in fibrinogen could increase the risk of heart disease.

## POSSIBLE LOWER RISK OF CORONARY HEART DISEASE

Postmenopausal hormones have long been recommended for the prevention of coronary heart disease. However, there is now uncertainty about this recommendation. Emerging evidence suggests that postmenopausal hormones may raise the risk of heart disease during the first one to two years that women are using them. This new evidence raises concerns about who should take the hormones and makes it doubly important for women to talk to their health care providers about this issue.

The prior recommendation that women take hormones for the prevention of heart disease is based on evidence from a large number of observational studies. Most of these studies examined the risk of heart disease among women who had never used postmenopausal hormones compared to those who had already been using them for at least five years. We combined the results of more than forty of these studies and found that while women were taking estrogen, they were about half as likely to develop heart disease as women who had never taken estrogen. This was true whether estrogen was taken alone or in combination with progestin.

Although the evidence from observational studies does suggest that hormones protect against heart disease, the relationship is not that simple. Randomized controlled trials have recently begun to examine this. In these trials, postmenopausal women take either a daily placebo or a daily dose of hormones for an extended period of time. Researchers then determine which group is less likely to develop heart disease. In the earliest trial of this nature, researchers studied the effects of estrogen on women who already *had* heart disease. During the first year of the trial, women on hormones were *more* likely to have a heart attack than women on placebo pills. As the trial progressed, however, the women on hormones became *less* likely to have a heart attack. When we looked at short-term hormone use among women with heart disease in the Nurses' Health Study, we found similar results.

Whether healthy women also experience an increase in risk during the first years of hormone use is not yet known. Preliminary results from the ongoing Women's Health Initiative suggest that they do. In that trial, researchers are studying the effects of hormones on healthy women—that is, women with no prior history of heart disease. During the first one to two years of the trial, women on hormones were slightly more likely than women on placebo pills to experience a heart attack, stroke, or blood clot. As the trial progresses, the rate of cardiovascular events seems to be equaling out between the two groups of women, much like it did in the previous trial. Since the Women's Health Initiative is ongoing, more conclusive evidence will not be available from this trial until 2005.

In the meantime, how should postmenopausal women proceed with making decisions about the use of hormones? Unfortunately, there is no clear answer right now. The available evidence suggests an *increase* in the risk of heart disease during the first one to two years of hormone use and a *decrease* in risk during subsequent years of use. Because this is an ongoing area of research, with new evidence constantly emerging, women should periodically reassess the issue with their health care providers.

## Postmenopausal Hormones and Heart Disease: The State of the Evidence

- The relationship between hormones and heart disease is complex and is not yet fully understood.

- Available evidence suggests that there is an increase in the risk of heart disease during the first one to two years of hormone use and a decrease in risk during subsequent years of use.

- More conclusive evidence will be available when the ongoing Women's Health Initiative wraps up in 2005.

- In the meantime, women should continue to discuss this issue with their health care providers, making decisions based on the best evidence available at the time.

### PROBABLE LOWER RISK OF COLON CANCER

Estrogen therapy may reduce a woman's risk of colon cancer (or cancer of the large intestine). Although the reason for this is not yet clear, it has been suggested that estrogen can slow the production of bile acids and lower the level of an insulin-like growth factor called IGF-I. Both IGF-I and bile acids are suspected of stimulating malignant growth in the colon.

We examined the relationship between postmenopausal hormones and colon cancer by combining the results of eighteen epidemiologic studies on the topic. Most of these were conducted when estrogen alone was the predominant form of postmenopausal hormone therapy. We found that while women are taking estrogen, they have a moderate reduction in the risk of colon cancer compared to women who have never taken postmenopausal hormones. Once women discontinue the therapy, however, the protection they received diminishes and eventually disappears altogether.

To date, only three studies have examined the combined effect of estrogen and progestin on the risk of colon cancer. Of these, two demonstrated a moderate protective effect, and one found no association.

## POSSIBLE LOWER RISK OF ALZHEIMER'S DISEASE

Affecting twice as many women as men, Alzheimer's disease severely impairs a person's intellectual and social abilities. In animal studies, estrogen has important influences on the brain, in particular those parts of the brain that affect learning and memory. In humans, a growing body of evidence suggests that estrogen therapy may reduce the risk of Alzheimer's disease. However, these studies are still preliminary, and much more research needs to be done before women can consider this a benefit of hormone use.

## The Risks of Postmenopausal Hormones

### INCREASED RISK OF ENDOMETRIAL CANCER

The effect of postmenopausal hormones on endometrial cancer risk depends largely on whether women take estrogen with or without progesterone. Endometrial cancer is caused primarily by an imbalance between these two hormones or, more specifically, by too much estrogen and not enough progesterone. Consequently, women who take estrogen without progesterone have an increased risk of endometrial cancer, while those who take it with progesterone have little if any increase.

### INCREASED RISK OF BREAST CANCER

Estrogen is a key promoter of breast cancer. Rates of this disease rise rapidly during the premenopausal years, when estrogen production is high, and continue to increase more slowly through menopause, when natural estrogen levels begin to decline. Postmenopausal women with high levels of natural estrogen are at much greater risk of breast cancer than postmenopausal women with low levels of natural estrogen.

There is now abundant evidence to suggest that raising estrogen levels through postmenopausal hormones increases a woman's risk of breast cancer. In the Nurses' Health Study, we have examined many different aspects of the relationship between breast cancer and postmenopausal hormones and found that taking estrogen does increase a woman's risk of breast cancer. For each year that a woman in our study used estrogen, her risk of breast cancer went up by about 8 percent. This finding is very similar to those of numerous other reports, including a very large international analysis based on over fifty studies. We also found in the Nurses' Health Study that taking estrogen with progestin raised the risk of breast cancer more than taking estrogen alone. For each year that a woman used estrogen with progestin, her risk of breast cancer rose by about 13 percent. Two other large studies have had similiar findings.

Overall, current epidemiologic evidence suggests that taking postmenopausal hormones for a short period of time (less than five years) is likely to have little influence on the risk of breast cancer (see Figures 22-3 and 22-4). However, the longer a woman takes hormones, the more likely she is to develop the disease. In addition, the risk of breast cancer is higher if a woman takes estrogen and progestin than if she takes estrogen alone.

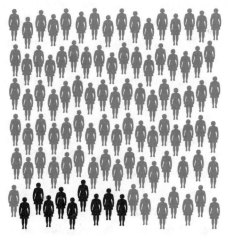

FIG. 22-3. In a group of 100 women who are fifty years old and who have not been taking postmenopausal hormones for five or more years, 9 will develop breast cancer before they reach the age of eighty. (Source: National Cancer Institute)

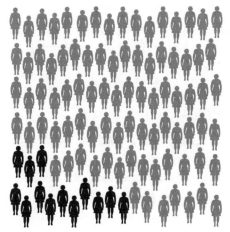

FIG. 22-4. In a group of 100 women who are fifty years old and who have been taking post-menopausal hormones for at least five years, 13 will develop breast cancer before they reach the age of eighty. (Source: Nurses' Health Study)

## Postmenopausal Hormones and Breast Cancer: The State of the Evidence

- For each year that a woman takes estrogen, her risk of breast cancer goes up slightly. If she takes estrogen with progestin, it goes up even more.
- After five years of hormone use, women are at moderately increased risk of breast cancer.

### INCREASED RISK OF GALLBLADDER DISEASE

The gallbladder is a storage site for bile produced by the liver. When bile contains too much cholesterol or pigment, small crystals form and fall to the bottom of the gallbladder. These crystals fuse together to form gallstones. By raising the level of cholesterol in the bile and decreasing bile acid concentration, estrogen promotes the growth of gallstones.

In the Nurses' Health Study, we examined whether postmenopausal estrogen use increased women's risk of having their gallbladder surgically removed. More than 500,000 Americans undergo this procedure (called a cholecystectomy) each year simply because of gallstones. We found that estrogen, with or without progestin, substantially increased the risk of cholecystectomy. The longer a woman used estrogen, and the higher the dose, the more likely she was to have her gallbladder removed. This detrimental effect of estrogen lingered after women discontinued therapy. Five years after the cessation of use, women still had a slightly higher risk of cholecystectomy than women who had never used estrogen.

## INCREASED RISK OF DEEP VEIN THROMBOSIS AND PULMONARY EMBOLISM

Deep vein thrombosis occurs when a blood clot forms in one of the deep veins, such as those in the leg or pelvis. If a clot dislodges or a fragment of it breaks away (called an embolus), it may travel through the bloodstream to the lungs. There it can become lodged in a pulmonary blood vessel, cutting off circulation to a portion of the lung. This blockage, called a pulmonary embolism, occurs suddenly and can be fatal if not treated promptly.

A growing body of evidence has established that current estrogen use, alone or with progestin, more than doubles a woman's risk of deep vein thrombosis and pulmonary embolism. However, these conditions are rare, affecting only 4 in 10,000 postmenopausal women each year. Thus, even among postmenopausal women using hormone therapy, the rate of these conditions is still less than 10 per 10,000 women per year.

## PROBABLE INCREASED RISK OF OVARIAN CANCER

Several studies have suggested that postmenopausal hormones may also increase the risk of ovarian cancer. In the only large cohort study to examine this relationship to date (the American Cancer Society Cancer Prevention Study II), researchers found a small increase in the risk of fatal ovarian cancer among women who had ever used postmenopausal hormones. The risk increased with duration of use and was greatest among those who were currently on hormones and had been for at least ten years. These women had a twofold increase in risk compared to women who had never used postmenopausal hormones. Smaller studies have corroborated these findings but have not been entirely consistent. Taken collectively, the current evidence suggests that the long-term use of postmenopausal hormones has at least a moderate effect on the risk of ovarian cancer.

## POSSIBLE INCREASED RISK OF ASTHMA

Several observations have led researchers to speculate that hormones might play a role in the development of asthma. First, the rate of asthma becomes higher among girls than boys with the onset of puberty and remains higher throughout the reproductive years. Second, women tend to be hospitalized with asthma for longer periods than men, suggesting that asthma may be more severe among women. Finally, the severity of asthma symptoms appears to vary with the menstrual cycle. Several studies have reported that nearly a third of all women with asthma have exacerbated symptoms before and/or during menstruation.

Although there is little direct evidence to support a relationship between hormones and asthma, our findings in the Nurses' Health Study are consistent with the idea that higher levels of estrogen are linked with higher rates of asthma. We found that premenopausal women had higher rates of asthma than postmenopausal women. However, among postmenopausal women, the rate of asthma was elevated among those taking estrogen. Women who were currently using estrogen, as well as those who had used it in the past, were 50 percent more likely to develop asthma than women who had never used estrogen. The longer women used the hormone, and the higher the dose, the more likely they were to develop the condition.

## POSSIBLE INCREASED RISK OF SYSTEMIC LUPUS ERYTHEMATOSUS

Systemic lupus erythematosis is a rare autoimmune disease that causes inflammation in various parts of the body, including the skin, joints, blood, and kidneys. Lupus is more common among women than men at all ages, though the difference between women and men varies markedly with age-related changes in women's estrogen levels.

The relationship between postmenopausal hormone use and the risk of lupus has not been well studied. In the Nurses' Health Study, we found that women taking estrogen were about twice as likely to develop lupus as women who had never used estrogen. The longer a woman used estrogen, the more likely she was to develop the disease. Because lupus is a relatively rare disease, additional research to confirm this relationship will require large-scale studies.

## How Postmenopausal Hormones Affect Length of Life

Using postmenopausal hormones tends to lower women's risk of premature death. However, the longer a woman is on hormones, the less benefit she gets from them in terms of mortality—and once she stops taking the hormones, the benefits disappear completely.

In the observational Nurses' Health Study, we followed postmenopausal women for an eight-year period and examined which group had lower rates of death: those who had never been on hormones, those who had previously been on hormones, and those who were currently on hormones. We found that the women who were currently on hormones had about a 40 percent lower risk of dying prematurely than either the women who had never used hormones or the women who had used them only in the past. Among those who were currently on hormones, the mortality benefit began to diminish for those who had been on them for more than ten years (see Figure 22-5).

If hormones are beneficial in terms of mortality, why isn't more better? It likely has to do with the opposing effects that hormones have on the risk of heart disease and breast cancer. In the Nurses' Health Study, women who were on hormones had stable reductions in the risk of dying from heart disease, but their risk of dying from breast cancer increased steadily with each year that they continued their hormone use. This suggests that after long periods of hormone use, estrogen's potential cardiovascular benefits may be offset in part by an increased risk of dying from breast cancer.

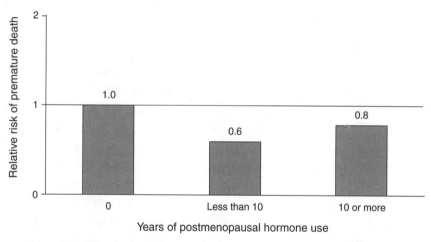

FIG. 22-5. Using postmenopausal hormones for less than ten years lowers the risk of premature death. Using them longer also lowers risk but to a lesser extent. (Source: Nurses' Health Study)

## WHAT IT ALL MEANS

To say that women have a lot to consider when deciding whether to use post-menopausal hormones is a vast understatement. Estrogen therapy has a wide range of effects on women's health, and those effects appear to vary substantially with duration of use. While women are taking estrogen, they are protected against osteoporosis and, likely, colon cancer and heart disease.

However, they are also at increased risk of breast cancer, blood clots in deep veins, gallbladder disease, and, if they are taking estrogen alone, endometrial cancer. When women stop taking estrogen, they lose many of its beneficial effects, but they also avoid some of the risks.

Since women only recently began taking estrogen with progestin, many of the effects of this combined therapy are not yet well established. Women on estrogen and progestin are known to have a much lower risk of endometrial cancer than women on estrogen alone. However, they also appear to have a higher risk of breast cancer. More conclusive evidence on this will be available in the future from ongoing observational studies, including the Nurses' Health Study, and from randomized controlled trials, like the Women's Health Initiative. As evidence continues to emerge from these studies, women should periodically discuss the use of postmenopausal hormones with their health care providers.

## Strategies for Postmenopausal Hormone Use

### TYPES OF ESTROGEN

There are several different types of estrogen (see the table on page 454). Each behaves slightly differently in the body and may be used in different regimens. Nonetheless, all fulfill certain conditions necessary for hormones to be effective. They can be absorbed, metabolized, and released into the bloodstream. And they can survive in the blood long enough and at levels high enough to reach the target tissues before the body eliminates them.

The most widely used estrogen in the United States is Premarin. Taken in the form of a pill, Premarin was designed to be easily absorbed from the digestive tract. It consists primarily of mixed estrogens derived from the urine of pregnant mares (thus the trade name). Although higher doses may be necessary for symptom relief, the standard dose is 0.625 milligram a day. Because so many of the major studies of postmenopausal hormones have been conducted with Premarin, more is known about its effects than about any other commercially available estrogen. As a result, the risks and benefits of postmenopausal hormones, discussed earlier, were determined primarily by studying women who have used Premarin.

Consisting of a plant-derived combination of estrogens similar to Premarin, Estratab is also available as a pill. Because it is thought to have similar potency to Premarin, the standard dose is the same: 0.625 milligram. Recent evidence from a two-year study suggests that lower doses are also effective in increasing bone mass. Thus, a daily dose of 0.3 milligram has also been approved for osteoporosis prevention.

Other commonly used forms of estrogen that are available as pills include Estrace, Ogen, and Ortho-est. Estrace contains a form of estradiol (the predominant form of estrogen in premenopausal women) that can easily be absorbed and converted to estrone (the predominant form of estrogen in postmenopausal women). The standard daily dose of Estrace is 1 to 2 milligrams to relieve menopausal symptoms and 0.5 milligram to prevent osteoporosis. Ogen and Ortho-est both contain estrone and are usually taken in doses of 0.625 milligram. However, because they are less potent than Premarin, higher doses may be necessary.

Although estrogen is most commonly taken in the form of pills, it can also be delivered transdermally (through the skin) by an adhesive patch worn on the skin. Dosage is controlled by a gel layer inside the patch. Alora, Climara, Estraderm, Fempatch, and Vivelle are common brands of transdermal estrogen and contain estradiol. Estradiol passes through the skin almost unaltered and enters the blood rapidly, reaching target tissues in high levels. As a result, much lower daily doses of transdermal estrogen are required to produce the same effect as standard doses of oral estrogen. Because it initially bypasses the digestive system, transdermal estrogen has somewhat different effects on the body than oral estrogen. It may not improve blood cholesterol to the same extent, but it is less likely to increase the risk of gallstones.

Estrogens are also available in creams, which are used to relieve vaginal dryness. Although hormone creams are often promoted for the treatment of menopausal symptoms and the preservation of bone mass, they are absorbed into the body in widely varying amounts, depending on the thickness of the vaginal wall. Thus their systemic effects are unknown.

An alternative way to supplement the body's estrogen supply, without actually raising the level of estrogen in the blood, is Estring. Estring is a soft ring that is inserted, like a diaphragm, into the vagina. Like an estrogen cream, it helps relieve vaginal dryness. Because it does not affect blood estrogen levels, it is often recommended for the relief of vaginal symptoms in women who have had breast cancer.

## TYPES OF PROGESTOGENS

Progestogens are chemical compounds that are available in both a natural form (progesterone) and a synthetic form (progestin) (see table on page 457).

Natural progesterone is an exact chemical duplicate of the progesterone that is normally produced by the ovaries. Progestin mimics the action of natural progesterone. However, because it has a different chemical structure than progesterone, the body does not respond to it in the same way. Progestin use can be associated with bloating, mood swings, headaches, and other PMS-like side effects. Natural progesterone appears to produce fewer side effects than progestin and tends to preserve more of estrogen's beneficial effects on cholesterol.

Progestins are more widely used than natural progesterones, with medroxyprogesterone acetate (MPA) and norethindrone acetate being the most commonly used compounds. Provera and Cycrin are popular brands of MPA and are taken orally in doses ranging from 2.5 to 10 milligrams. Aygestin and Micronor are common brands of norethindrone acetate, with a standard dose of 2.5 milligrams. Natural progesterone is available in the form of a pill (Prometrium) and a vaginal gel (Crinone).

## REGIMENS FOR POSTMENOPAUSAL HORMONE USE

As the options for postmenopausal hormone use grow, so do the ways in which the hormones can be taken and/or combined. The sole purpose of taking estrogen with progestin is to curtail the endometrial growth stimulated by estrogen alone. While some women with an intact uterus may choose to take estrogen alone, this regimen is not recommended by the American College of Obstetricians and Gynecologists and is intended only for women who have had a hysterectomy. Most women with an intact uterus now take a combination of estrogen and progestin. There are basically two ways to do this: cyclic therapy and continuous therapy (see the table on page 458).

Cyclic therapy involves taking estrogen alone for part of each month and then taking estrogen and progestin together for the rest of the month. Physicians may prescribe estrogen and progestin pills separately for cyclic therapy, so that women take one pill during the first half of the month and two pills during the second half. However, the most widely used cyclic regimen in the United States is Premphase, an FDA-approved one-tablet therapy that is available in calendar packs marked with each day of the week.

Cyclic therapy re-creates the menstrual cycle, with many of the attendant side effects. As many as 80 percent of women on cyclic therapy have vaginal bleeding after taking the last progestin pill each month. In addition, women who experienced unpleasant symptoms during their natural menstrual cycles—such as breast tenderness, bloating, irritability, and depression—sometimes find that cyclic therapy causes these symptoms to recur. The symptoms appear to increase in severity with the dose of progestin prescribed.

Continuous therapy was developed primarily to eliminate monthly bleeding and alleviate the side effects associated with progestin use. It involves taking both estrogen and progestin every day, but the dose of progestin is smaller (2.5 milligrams) than that taken by women on cyclic therapy (5.0 milligrams). Approved by the FDA in 1995, Prempro is the most commonly used continuous regimen in the United States. Women on this type of therapy may experience some irregular bleeding, but it usually subsides within the first year of treatment.

Some women and their clinicians have settled on a third option for combining estrogen and progestin: they add progestin to their estrogen therapy once every three months. Women on this type of therapy still experience heavy bleeding and PMS-like symptoms when they are taking the progestin, but they endure these side effects much less frequently than women on other combined regimens. The major disadvantage of this approach is that it may not adequately prevent endometrial hyperplasia (abnormally excessive cell growth) and thus may lead to a higher risk of endometrial cancer.

Although most women on postmenopausal hormones take a combination of estrogen and progestin, some women may choose to take a combination of estrogen and testosterone, like Estratest. Testosterone is a male-like hormone that is made naturally in the body. However, at menopause, levels of this hormone drop dramatically, and this can contribute to menopausal symptoms.

## Taking Estrogen Alone

Although it is known to be associated with an increased risk of endometrial cancer and is not recommended by the American College of Obstetricians and Gynecologists, some women with an intact uterus still choose to take estrogen alone. These women should have an annual endometrial biopsy or transvaginal ultrasound to evaluate whether there is any abnormal cell growth.

Lower doses of estrogen are currently being studied to determine if they raise the risk of endometrial cancer to the same extent as higher doses. In preapproval studies of a 0.3-milligram dose of Estratab, the rate of endometrial hyperplasia was no higher among women taking the low dose for two years than among women taking a placebo. However, this is a fairly short follow-up period, and additional research is needed to determine the safety of taking low dose estrogen alone.

Women whose menopausal symptoms are not relieved by estrogen with pro-gestin may consider taking estrogen with testosterone. However, in terms of its effect on the uterus, this combination is comparable to taking estrogen alone. Because it does not contain a progestogen, the combination of estrogen and testosterone substantially raises the risk of endometrial cancer.

## ALTERNATIVES TO POSTMENOPAUSAL HORMONE USE

Some women may choose to forgo postmenopausal hormones completely, opt-ing for more natural ways of alleviating menopausal symptoms. Commonly used alternatives include herbs and edible plants, vitamin E, and relaxation and biofeedback techniques. There is a varying degree of scientific evidence for the effectiveness of each of these strategies.

The growing interest in herbs and other edible plants as treatments for menopausal symptoms has been prompted in part by reports that menopausal symptoms are rare among women in Asian countries whose diets are rich in soy. Soy contains phytoestrogens, plant-derived compounds similar to estro-gen. Laboratory studies on soy protein suggest that it acts on the blood vessels of postmenopausal women in a manner similar to that of estrogen. In at least one controlled trial, hot flashes were reduced among women who drank an 8-ounce soy beverage daily containing 40 milligrams of the phytoestrogen genistein. However, no standard dose has been established yet for soy, or for any of the other popular herbal remedies like ginseng, black cohosh, licorice root, or dong quai.

Daily doses of vitamin E (400 to 1,200 IU) are often recommended for the relief of hot flashes, although there is little evidence of its effectiveness. In a randomized controlled trial, women who took vitamin E were no less likely to experience hot flashes than women who took a daily placebo.

The concept of alleviating hot flashes with relaxation and biofeedback tech-niques has some foundation in physiology, since both techniques work on the autonomic nervous system. This system is responsible for regulating essential functions like breathing and heart rate. Because hot flashes increase in num-ber and severity when women are under pressure, techniques that effectively reduce stress are likely to reduce hot flashes as well.

Vaginal moisturizers like Astroglide and Replens are remarkably similar to natural vaginal lubricants and have become another popular alternative. Re-plens in particular is often recommended because it does not contain estrogen and its moisturizing effects last longer than water-based lubricants like As-troglide. Some women have also been relieved by progesterone creams that are available from mail-order pharmacies. However, effective doses and potential side effects have not yet been established for these creams.

## "Designer Drugs"

In an ideal world, postmenopausal women would take a drug that gave them the benefits of estrogen without the risks. Such a drug would mimic estrogen by positively stimulating bone and cardiovascular cells, but would block estrogen from stimulating breast and endometrial cells. Such drugs are currently being developed to do just that. Referred to as designer drugs, they are designed to act in specific ways at each of the tissue sites that estrogen usually affects.

Unlike the postmenopausal hormones discussed above, designer drugs are not taken for the short-term alleviation of menopausal symptoms. Instead, they are taken specifically for the long-term prevention of chronic disease, such as osteoporosis and breast cancer. Thus, they are not always alternatives to postmenopausal hormone use. Women might take estrogen early in menopause for symptom relief and then switch to designer drugs for long-term chronic disease protection.

Under the trade name Evista, raloxifene was the first designer drug to be approved by the FDA for protection against osteoporosis. Evista appears to have a somewhat weaker effect than estrogen on most types of tissues. It increases bone mass in postmenopausal women by 1 to 2 percent compared to 3 percent for estrogen. And although it lowers total cholesterol and LDL cholesterol, it does not raise HDL cholesterol like estrogen does. In addition, it increases, rather than reduces, hot flashes.

Evista's biggest advantage lies in its ability to block estrogen's stimulation of breast and endometrial tissue. In the studies required for FDA approval, women taking Evista were 50 to 75 percent less likely to develop breast cancer than women taking a placebo. While promising, these few studies were relatively small, and overall, data remain limited.

Under the trade name Nolvadex, tamoxifen was recently approved by the FDA for protection against breast cancer in women who are at high risk of the disease. This drug offers substantial protection, reducing the risk of breast cancer by 40 to 50 percent. In addition, Nolvadex appears to increase bone mass, which is important for reducing the risk of osteoporosis. However, it does not appear to have the same beneficial cardiovascular effects as estrogen—and it does have some of estrogen's negative effects. In the studies required for FDA approval, rates of cardiovascular events (like heart attacks) were the same among women taking Nolvadex as among women taking a placebo. However, rates of both endometrial cancer and stroke were higher among women on Nolvadex. Overall, the risks and benefits of this drug remain uncertain and are under study.

# WHAT I TELL MY PATIENTS ABOUT POSTMENOPAUSAL HORMONES

DR. CELESTE ROBB-NICHOLSON

Few choices cause as much concern for my patients as the decision about whether to use postmenopausal hormones. There is no one-size-fits-all approach to this issue. Instead, each woman has to weigh the benefits and risks of postmenopausal hormones in light of her own unique medical history and values. And research is rapidly bringing us new evidence about hormones, which slightly tips the risk-benefit ratio for every woman.

Once she decides to take postmenopausal hormones, a woman is faced with additional choices. She needs to decide what form of therapy to take (pills, patches, rings, or creams), and what type to take (estrogen alone or estrogen combined with a progestogen). Once she has taken hormones for a while, she will also face the decision of how long to continue them. The health benefits and risks of hormones last while a woman is taking them. So depending on her reasons for taking hormones, a woman can choose her own duration of therapy.

If you are overwhelmed by the decision, you are not alone. The best approach is to carefully consider both your own medical history and your personal values, and to weigh the risks and benefits of hormones one by one. Then step back and consider the whole picture before making a decision. You will probably want to discuss it with your health care provider. And remember: estrogen is not a panacea for menopause. It is an adjunct to tried and true lifestyle factors that help to promote health and prevent disease. For every condition that estrogen is meant to help, there are other medical therapies and lifestyle approaches that can be used to reap a similar benefit. In the end, the decision is a highly personal one, and one that can be altered if you change your mind along the way.

## Medical Factors to Consider

*BREAST CANCER.* If you have a family or personal history of breast cancer or are concerned about developing this disease, you may not want to take postmenopausal hormones or you may want to take them only temporarily. Studies show that women who take estrogen are more likely to develop breast cancer than women who are not on the hormone. And there is recent evidence that progestin further increases this risk. However, the increased risk of breast cancer exists only while you are taking the hormone therapy, and studies indicate that the risk disappears once you stop, at least if you take it for less than ten years. For this reason, some women decide to take postmenopausal hormones only temporarily to cope with symptoms of menopause, but then stop to ensure they do not permanently increase their risk of breast cancer. Another option is to take estrogen early in menopause and then switch to one of the designer estrogens, such as tamoxifen, to further reduce the risk of breast cancer.

*CHOLESTEROL.* If you have a high cholesterol level already, you may want to consider taking postmenopausal hormones. Taking estrogen alone lowers total blood cholesterol and tends to raise the level of HDL ("good cholesterol") while decreasing the level of LDL ("bad cholesterol"). When progestin and estrogen are taken together, the picture grows murkier. Progestin tends to counter the beneficial effects of estrogen somewhat. Nevertheless, any type of hormone therapy appears to lower blood cholesterol.

*COLON CANCER.* If you have a family or personal history of colon cancer or are concerned about this disease, you may want to consider taking postmenopausal hormones. Estrogen may reduce the risk of developing colon cancer by about 35 percent for as long as you take the hormone. This protective effect disappears once you stop.

*GALLBLADDER DISEASE.* If you are concerned about developing gallstones, then you may *not* want to take postmenopausal hormones. Estrogen use increases the chance that you will develop gallstones and have to have your gallbladder removed.

*HEART DISEASE.* This issue has become complicated in the past few years. Many studies of healthy women indicated that postmenopausal hormones may reduce the risk of coronary heart disease—the leading cause of death among women—by as much as 50 percent, as long as you take them. However, several recent studies of women with heart disease have indicated that hormones may not be beneficial and may even be harmful. I used to encourage my patients who had risk factors for heart disease to take postmenopausal hormones. Now, like many other health care providers I know, I don't push as hard. We need to wait for the results of the Women's Health Initiative and other ongoing studies before deciding.

*MENOPAUSAL SYMPTOMS.* Although each woman is different, typical symptoms of menopause include hot flashes, vaginal dryness, and insomnia. In fact, three out of four women will experience these symptoms, although their severity and duration vary greatly. If you are experiencing such symptoms and are not comfortable or satisfied with alternative therapies such as herbs, relaxation, and biofeedback, then you may want to consider taking postmenopausal hormones. Some women decide to take hormones only temporarily, to help them ease through the transition. Others opt for remaining on the therapy.

*OSTEOPOROSIS.* If you are concerned about developing osteoporosis, you may want to consider taking postmenopausal hormones. Studies have shown that estrogen can prevent bone loss while you are taking the hormone, and that you may even gain bone mass. This is significant because it could also reduce your chance of suffering a hip fracture later on in life, which can be disabling or even lead to premature death. Women taking estrogen are 25 percent less likely to suffer a hip fracture. However, these benefits stop once you stop taking estrogen. If you decide not to take estrogen because of other risks, consider raloxifene, another designer estrogen that reduces the risk of osteoporosis without increasing breast cancer risk.

## Other Factors to Consider

*YOUR OWN COMFORT WITH RISK.* Much of what makes the decision about whether to take postmenopausal hormones so hard is that while it is possible to predict *general* risks and benefits, it is impossible to determine *exactly* what your particular set of risks and benefits will be. For example, I tell my patients that most studies indicate that taking postmenopausal hormones increases the risk of getting breast cancer, but that I cannot tell them what their personal risk is. No one knows that.

There are also other risks to consider. In addition to the medical conditions described in detail in the preceding pages, postmenopausal hormones double the risk of blood clots that can lead to pulmonary embolism (which is rare, but can occur suddenly and be fatal if not treated right away). And although the research is less clear, hormones may increase the risk of asthma and systemic lupus erythematosus, an autoimmune disease.

Only you can weigh these risks and decide how comfortable you are with them.

*YOUR OWN COMFORT WITH MULTIPLE CHOICES.* If you decide to try postmenopausal hormones, you face a dizzying array of choices. One decision—whether to take estrogen alone or estrogen combined with progestin—will depend largely on whether you have had a hysterectomy or not. Others are not as straightforward. If you take both hormones, do you take progestin every day of the month or for only part of the month? Do you take hormones in pill form, or try a patch, ring, or cream? And how long will you take them? The section "Strategies for Postmenopausal Hormone Use" (page 443) will help you narrow your choices, but you will still need to talk to your health care provider about which approach is best for you.

*YOUR PERSONAL VALUES AND PREFERENCES.* Some of your decision-making about postmenopausal hormones will depend on your personal view of which risks are more acceptable than others. Some women fear breast cancer so much that even a temporary increase in developing this disease is too much. Others are more worried about the chance of disability down the road because of a hip fracture.

These decisions may also depend on your view of the whole process of menopause and of how Western medicine deals with this transition. Some women have little tolerance for symptoms like hot flashes, vaginal dryness, and insomnia, or find that they interfere with life at work and home, and so want to take something to alleviate them. Others view menopause as a natural transition, not a disease that must be treated, and they prefer not to take hormones at all.

If you are one of them, you have other options for dealing with the symptoms of menopause. These include topical applications and lubricants to counter the vaginal dryness you may experience. Or you might try relaxation and biofeedback techniques to reduce stress that only exacerbates symptoms. The jury is still out on vitamin E and soy drinks, so talk with your health care provider before trying these.

You can also manage many of the diseases that hormone therapy is meant to forestall by making changes in your lifestyle. Exercise and diets that are high in fiber and low in saturated fat are cornerstones of managing high cholesterol and reducing risk for heart disease. The statins are cholesterol-lowering drugs that reduce heart disease risk and treat high cholesterol. Weight-bearing exercise and high calcium intake are basic ingredients of osteoporosis prevention. If you are at more than usual risk for osteoporosis, there are excellent new drugs (raloxifene and Fosamax) that prevent osteoporosis, as well as treat the disease. Estrogen was never meant to substitute for a healthy lifestyle.

And no decision is final. No matter what you decide, you can always modify your approach to menopause if you find your initial strategy isn't working.

## Types of Estrogen—Pills

| Trade Name | Generic Name | Usual Daily Dose | Benefits | Possible Side Effects and Risks |
|---|---|---|---|---|
| Premarin | Conjugated estrogen | 0.3 to 1.25 mg | • Relieves menopausal symptoms<br>• Increases bone mass by 3 to 5%<br>• Raises HDL cholesterol and lowers LDL cholesterol<br>• May lower the risk of heart disease, colon cancer, and Alzheimer's disease | • Increases the risk of endometrial cancer when taken without a progestogen<br>• May increase the risk of breast cancer, gallbladder disease, and deep vein blood clots |
| Estratab and Menest | Esterified estrogens | 0.3 to 1.25 mg | • 0.625 mg dose has about the same benefits as Premarin<br>• 0.3 mg dose has less effect on bone and cholesterol, but may not increase endometrial cancer risk | • Thought to be similar to Premarin, but less widely studied |
| Estrace | Estradiol | 0.5 to 2 mg | • Thought to be similar to Premarin, but less widely studied | • Thought to be similar to Premarin, but less widely studied |
| Ogen and Ortho-est | Estropipate | 0.625 to 5.0 mg | • Thought to be similar to Premarin, but less widely studied | • Thought to be similar to Premarin, but less widely studied |

## Types of Estrogen—Patches

| TRADE NAME | GENERIC NAME | USUAL DAILY DOSE | BENEFITS | POSSIBLE SIDE EFFECTS AND RISKS |
|---|---|---|---|---|
| Alora | Estradiol | 0.0375 to 0.1 mg | • Alleviates vaginal dryness and hot flashes<br>• Lowers the risk of osteoporosis<br>• Associated with beneficial changes in blood cholesterol, but not as dramatic as with oral estrogen use<br>• Associated with a lower risk of liver disease and gallstones than oral estrogen | • Irritates the skin<br>• Associated with an increased risk of breast cancer and deep vein blood clots<br>• Associated with an increased risk of endometrial cancer when taken without a progestogen |
| Climara | Estradiol | 0.025 to 0.1 mg | • Similar to Alora | • Similar to Alora |
| Esclim | Estradiol | 0.025 to 0.1 mg | • Similar to Alora | • Similar to Alora |
| Estraderm | Estradiol | 0.0375 to 0.1 mg | • Similar to Alora | • Similar to Alora |
| FemPatch | Estradiol | 0.025 mg | • Similar to Alora | • Similar to Alora |
| Vivelle | Estradiol | 0.0375 to 0.1 mg | • Similar to Alora | • Similar to Alora |
| CombiPatch | Estradiol and norethindrone acetate | 0.05 mg estradiol with 0.14 or 0.25 mg norethindrone acetate | • Similar to Alora | • Similar to Alora, but does not increase the risk of endometrial cancer |

455

## Types of Estrogen—Creams and Rings

| TRADE NAME | GENERIC NAME | USUAL DAILY DOSE | BENEFITS | POSSIBLE SIDE EFFECTS AND RISKS |
|---|---|---|---|---|
| *Creams* | | | | |
| Ortho Dienestrol cream | Dienestrol (synthetic estrogen) | Amount necessary to control symptoms | • Alleviates vaginal dryness<br>• May help prevent urinary tract infections | • The degree to which it is absorbed systemically is not yet known<br>• May increase the risk of endometrial cancer |
| Premarin cream | Conjugated estrogen | 2 to 4 gm cream (1.25–2.5 mg conjugated estrogen) according to symptoms | • Similar to Ortho Dienestrol cream | • Similar to Ortho Dienestrol cream |
| *Vaginal ring* | | | | |
| Estring | Estradiol | 0.0075 mg | • Alleviates vaginal dryness<br>• May help prevent urinary tract infections | • May be expelled when straining to have a bowel movement |

# Types of Progestogen

| Trade Name | Generic Name | Usual Daily Dose | Benefits | Possible Side Effects and Risks |
|---|---|---|---|---|
| *Pills* | | | | |
| Provera and Cyrin | Medroxyprogesterone acetate (MPA) | 2.5 to 10 mg | • Lowers the risk of endometrial cancer<br>• Slightly reduces estrogen's effects on blood cholesterol | • Cyclic regimen produces menstrual-like bleeding<br>• Daily administration should eventually eliminate bleeding<br>• Produces PMS-like side effects |
| Aygestin and Micronor | Norethindrone acetate | 2.5 mg | • Lowers the risk of endometrial cancer | • Produces more severe side effects than Provera<br>• May lower HDL cholesterol |
| Prometrium | Natural progesterone | 200 mg | • Lowers the risk of endometrial cancer<br>• Has a less adverse effect on HDL cholesterol than Provera | • Appears to have fewer side effects than Provera |
| *Vaginal gels* | | | | |
| Crinone | Natural progesterone | 4% and 8% concentrations | • Lowers the risk of endometrial cancer | • Few systemic side effects |

## Types of Combination Therapies

| Trade Name | Generic Name | Usual Daily Dose | Benefits | Possible Side Effects and Risks |
|---|---|---|---|---|
| Premphase | Conjugated estrogens and MPA (cyclic regimen) | 0.625 mg Premarin with 5.0 mg MPA for 12 days; 0.625 mg Premarin alone for 16 days | • Same as for Premarin and MPA individually | • Bleeding continues cyclically |
| Prempro | Conjugated estrogens and MPA (continuous regimen) | 0.625 mg Premarin with 2.5 or 5 mg MPA | • Same as for Premarin and MPA individually | • Eliminates bleeding eventually |
| Estratest | Esterified estrogens and methyltestosterone | 0.625 to 2.5 mg estrogen with 1.25 to 5.0 mg testosterone | • Same as for Estratab<br>• May improve libido | • May reduce beneficial effects on lipids<br>• Long-term effects unknown |

# CHAPTER TWENTY-THREE

# Birth Control

## BACKGROUND

What is the safest, most convenient, and most effective method of birth control available? If you ask that question of ten different women, you will most likely get ten different answers. Birth control is a very personal decision. What one woman considers to be convenient, another may find to be a hassle. By being aware of your many options for birth control, and clearly understanding the advantages and disadvantages of each, you can find the method right for you.

### Shifting Priorities

If you are like most women, you will probably use different forms of contraception at different points of your life. This is partly because your contraceptive priorities will most likely shift throughout life. For example, prior to your first pregnancy or between planned pregnancies, your major contraceptive concern is probably that your birth control not be permanent or affect your fertility in any way. Because sexually transmitted diseases can influence your fertility, you would want to choose a form of contraception that protects you from infection. If you have decided not to have children or never want to become pregnant again, your main contraceptive priority is probably to have long-term, continuous, reliable protection against pregnancy.

Another reason that your contraceptive choices may shift throughout life is that the health-related risks and benefits of contraception change with age. For example, taking birth control pills can temporarily raise your risk of breast cancer and cardiovascular disease. Thus, you might want to use the pill only while you are younger and still have a very low age-related risk of these diseases. When you reach your forties, you would want to reevaluate your use of the pill (particularly if you have high blood pressure, diabetes, or other risk factors for cardiovascular disease) and consider a form of contraception that has fewer associated risks.

### Effective Birth Control

Although your contraceptive priorities and age-related risks may shift throughout life, one priority will most likely remain constant: you want your contraceptive to keep you from getting pregnant. At the age when you will typically use birth control (that is, prior to menopause), your risk of getting pregnant is much greater than your risk of getting most chronic diseases. Thus, while it is important to consider how different contraceptives affect your overall health, your main concern will most likely be that you avoid pregnancy.

Although no method of birth control is foolproof (other than abstinence), the effectiveness of any method depends on the consistency with which you use it. For some methods—hormone implants, injections, and IUDs—consistent use is pretty much guaranteed, because the contraceptive is inserted into your body. Tubal ligation is similar, because the surgery permanently blocks the fertilization of eggs. As a result, these are among the most effective forms of birth control available.

Other methods, such as birth control pills and barrier methods, have the potential to be highly effective, but only if you use them consistently and correctly. For example, in the case of condoms, they must be used correctly with every act of sexual intercourse. For these methods, the reliability depends largely on the user, and so two rates of effectiveness are often given. The first is for perfect use, in which the method is always used as directed. The second is for typical use, in which the method may be used incorrectly or less consistently than recommended.

## BIRTH CONTROL PILLS

Birth control pills are one of the most effective and popular forms of reversible contraception in the United States. Approved by the Food and Drug Administration (FDA) in 1960, birth control pills quickly became a popular form of contraception. Within five years, more than 5 million American women were taking what is commonly referred to as "the pill." By the late 1960s, however, it became clear that taking the pill posed serious health threats for some women in the form of blood clots, heart attack, and stroke. These effects were due to the high doses of synthetic hormones that were originally contained in the pill: 100 to 150 micrograms of estrogen and 10 milligrams of progestin.

In the past thirty years, high dose pills have been removed from the market and replaced with lower dose pills that contain as little as 30 micrograms of estrogen and 0.5 milligram of progestin. The lower doses have made the pill considerably safer without compromising its effectiveness in preventing pregnancy. In the first year that women take low dose birth control pills, they have less than a 1 in 100 chance of getting pregnant, assuming they take them as directed. If their use of the pill is less than perfect (that is, they miss pills occasionally or do not use backup contraception when they are on antibiotics), their chance of getting pregnant goes up to 5 in 100. When a woman goes off the pill, her fertility may continue to be affected for several months. After this short period, however, her fertility will return to normal.

The pill prevents pregnancy primarily by overriding the hormonal changes that cause a woman to ovulate. It also thickens the mucus in the cervix, which blocks the passage of sperm, and alters the lining of the uterus, making it difficult for a fertilized egg to implant itself and grow.

In addition to preventing pregnancy, the two hormones contained in birth control pills can have a variety of other effects on a woman's body. The most common involve changes in the menstrual cycle and usually occur only within the first three months of pill use. During this time, women often experience lighter menstrual flow, changes in the length of their cycle (generally shorter), and bleeding between periods (or spotting). Some women may skip periods occasionally or, less commonly, stop having them altogether. Other side effects that are common, particularly during the first few months of pill use, include abdominal cramping or bloating, acne, tenderness or swelling of the breasts, nausea or vomiting, dizziness, and fatigue. Though not as common, some women on the pill also experience headaches, changes in weight, elevations in blood pressure, vaginal yeast infections, and changes in libido.

## The Benefits and Risks of Birth Control Pills

The birth control pill is among the most extensively studied drugs in medical history. In fact, it was the introduction of the pill—and the lack of information on its long-term effects—that led to the inception of the Nurses' Health Study in 1976. Since this study began, scientists have concluded that the two hormones in birth control pills can have a dramatic impact on the risk of chronic disease. Some of the pill's effects are positive, while others are negative. Some are temporary, and others long-lasting. By knowing how the pill might affect your overall health, your can begin to decide whether the benefits of the pill outweigh the risks.

*Lower Risk of Ovarian Cancer.* Ovarian cancer is a relatively rare disease.

However, because it is difficult to detect early and claims the lives of most of the women it affects, scientists have placed great emphasis on identifying factors that might help prevent it. Birth control pills are one such factor.

The pill may reduce the risk of ovarian cancer in at least two ways. First, it suppresses ovulation, and the number of times that a woman experiences ovulation may affect her risk of ovarian cancer. In addition, the pill lowers the level of hormones that may stimulate cell growth in the ovaries.

We examined the relationship between birth control pills and ovarian cancer by combining the results of more than twenty epidemiologic studies on the topic. We found that the pill substantially lowers the risk of ovarian cancer, particularly if used for at least five years (see Figure 23-1). This reduction in risk has been observed in almost all of the studies that have assessed the relationship. We also found that after women stop taking the pill, they remain protected against ovarian cancer for at least another decade if not longer. Although this evidence pertains to older high dose pills, recent study findings suggest that the modern low dose pills probably offer a similar pattern of protection against ovarian cancer.

*Lower Risk of Endometrial Cancer.* Although it is a relatively rare disease, endometrial cancer (cancer of the uterine lining) is the most common gynecologic cancer in American women. More than a dozen epidemiologic studies have confirmed that birth control pills provide long-term protection against this disease, with the most conclusive results coming from a large study conducted by the U.S. Centers for Disease Control. In that study, women who used

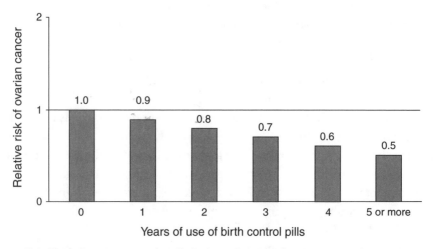

FIG 23-1. The longer women use the pill, the lower their risk of ovarian cancer. (Source: Nurses' Health Study)

the pill for one year received moderate protection against endometrial cancer, while those who used it for at least two years received substantial protection (see Figure 23-2). After women stopped taking the pill, they remained at reduced risk of endometrial cancer for at least another fifteen years. When we examined this relationship in the Nurses' Health Study, we found similar results.

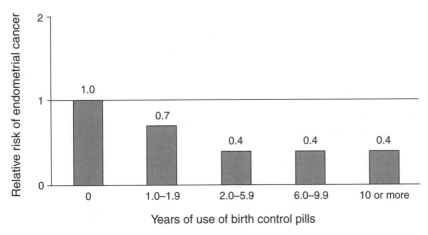

FIG. 23-2. The risk of endometrial cancer is largely reduced among women who take birth control pills for at least two years. (Source: Centers for Disease Control and Prevention)

Researchers are not yet sure why this long-term protective effect exists, but suspect that the short-term benefits are due to the fact that birth control pills contain both estrogen and progestin. In the absence of natural progesterone or synthetic progestin, estrogen stimulates the growth of endometrial cells. Since birth control pills contain both hormones, they may reduce the amount of time that a woman's endometrium is exposed to estrogen alone.

*Probable Lower Risk of Colon Cancer.* Taking birth control pills may reduce a woman's risk of colon cancer. Although the reason for this is not yet clear, it has been suggested that estrogen can slow the body's production of bile acids and lower the level of an insulin-like growth factor called IGF-I. Both IGF-I and bile acids are known to stimulate malignant growth in the colon.

Many studies have shown that birth control pills reduce the risk of colon cancer, but the results have not been strong enough to be considered a definitive relationship. This may be because most studies evaluated the effects of short-term use. The pill may need to be used for an extended period of time before it affects a woman's risk of colon cancer. In the Nurses' Health Study, we found that women had to take the higher dose pill for at least eight years before receiving even moderate protection against this disease.

To date, there is little evidence on the relationship between low dose pills and colon cancer. Since women have only taken low dose pills in recent years, and long-term use seems necessary to confer protection, it may be some time before this relationship is fully elucidated.

*Increased Risk of Breast Cancer.* Numerous epidemiologic studies have examined the relationship between birth control pills and breast cancer. Although results have been somewhat inconsistent, overall, they are reassuring. The pill seems to have only a modest—and temporary—effect on a woman's risk of breast cancer.

Some studies have suggested an increased risk of breast cancer among women who used the pill for a long time before they had any children. However, data from the Nurses' Health Study do not support this. In our study, women who had used the pill in the past were not at increased risk of breast cancer—even if they had previously used the pill for an extended period of time. Only women who were currently on the pill were at increased risk; these women were about 50 percent more likely to develop breast cancer than those who had never been on the pill.

A very large analysis that combined fifty-four international studies corroborated these findings. In that study, researchers found a small elevation in breast cancer risk among women who were currently on the pill. This excess risk gradually disappeared within ten years after women stopped taking the pill (see Figure 23-3).

Since most women are young and premenopausal while they are on the pill, the elevated risk of breast cancer should not be of great concern. Young women have a very low age-related risk of this disease, and so even if they have a moderately increased risk while they are on the pill, they are still very unlikely to develop breast cancer.

*Increased Risk of Deep Vein Thrombosis and Pulmonary Embolism.* Deep vein thrombosis occurs when a blood clot forms in one of the deep veins, such as those in the leg or pelvis. If a clot dislodges or a fragment of it breaks away (called an embolus), it may travel through the bloodstream to the lungs, where it can become lodged in a pulmonary blood vessel. This blockage is called a pulmonary embolism.

Women who are currently on the pill have a much greater risk of deep vein

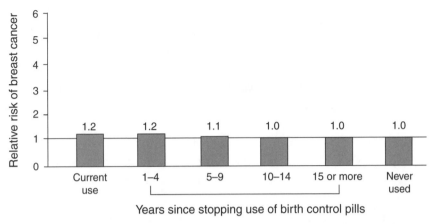

FIG. 23-3. Women have a slightly increased risk of breast cancer while taking the pill. Once they stop, their risk begins to decrease to that of women who never used the pill. (Source: Collaborative Group)

thrombosis and pulmonary embolism than women who have never used the pill. However, this increase in risk should not be of great concern. Young women have a very low age-related risk of deep vein thrombosis and pulmonary embolism. Thus even if they are at substantially elevated risk, women on the pill will most likely not develop either of these conditions.

*Probable Increased Risk of Malignant Melanoma.* Of the three types of skin cancer, malignant melanoma is the least common and most deadly. It arises in the cells that give skin its color (melanocytes) and can spread rapidly to other parts of the body.

Researchers have long suspected that the estrogen in birth control pills might influence a woman's risk of melanoma. Estrogen is known to stimulate the growth of melanocytes and to increase the amount of melanin (or pigment) in the cells. In addition, women taking birth control pills sometimes notice that their skin darkens, which is direct evidence of estrogen's effect on the melanocytes.

Although not all studies have been consistent, birth control pills do appear to increase a woman's risk of melanoma, but only while she is taking them. In the Nurses' Health Study, we found that women who were on the higher dose pill were twice as likely to develop melanoma as women who had never used the pill. Once women stopped taking the pill, however, their risk returned to that of women who never used the pill. Data from the Nurses' Health Study II suggest that the modern low dose pill might also increase the risk of melanoma, but to a lesser extent.

*Probable Increased Risk of Heart Attack.* The extent to which the pill affects a woman's risk of heart attack depends largely on whether she smokes. This is because smoking, in combination with using the pill, can greatly increase the risk of blood clots that lead to heart attack.

Taking the pill appears to have little effect if any on a nonsmoker's risk of heart attack. However, women who use the pill and smoke cigarettes have a substantially elevated risk of heart attack, especially if they are over the age of thirty-five or have hypertension or diabetes. In two separate studies, researchers showed that women who smoke twenty-five cigarettes a day and use the pill are at least 30 times more likely to have a heart attack than women who do neither.

Fortunately, any increase in risk that a woman experiences while she is on the pill disappears shortly after she discontinues it. In the Nurses' Health Study, women who used the pill in the past were no more likely to have a heart attack than women who never used the pill. This was true regardless of whether the women had smoked or used the pill for an extended duration.

Heart attacks are very rare among young women. Thus, even if women have an increased risk of cardiovascular disease while they are on the pill, they are still unlikely to have a heart attack.

*Possible Increased Risk of Stroke.* Characterized by the blockage of blood flow to the brain, stroke is a leading cause of death and permanent disability. High dose birth control pills may increase the risk of stroke by promoting the formation of blood clots.

Many studies have shown that high dose pills increase the risk of stroke, especially among smokers and those over the age of thirty-five. Even with these high dose pills, however, the risk of stroke is elevated only in women who are currently using the pill. We found in the Nurses' Health Study that after women stop taking the pill, their risk of stroke slowly drops to that of women who never used the pill.

Because most of the women in our study took the higher dose pills (if they took birth control pills at all), we do not have information on the risk of stroke among women on the lower dose pills. However, this issue is being studied by other researchers. Available evidence suggests that there is only a small to moderate increase in risk while women are on the pill. As with the high dose pill, any risk linked to the low dose pill would likely disappear after a woman stops taking the pill.

Again, since most women are young while they are on the pill, the elevated risk of stroke should not be of great concern. Young women have a very low age-related risk of this condition, and so even if they have a moderately increased risk while they are on the pill, they are still unlikely to have a stroke.

## How Birth Control Pills Affect Length of Life

Taking birth control pills can increase a woman's risk of dying from some diseases, but it can also lower her risk of dying from other diseases. In the Nurses' Health Study, we found that these risks and benefits balance each other out. For example, while a woman is on the pill, she has an increased risk of dying from breast cancer and a decreased risk of dying from ovarian cancer. Once she goes off the pill, her risk of breast cancer diminishes to that of a woman who never used the pill, while her risk of ovarian cancer remains lower than that of someone who never used the pill. Her overall risk of dying from cancer, then, is no greater than that of a woman who never used the pill—and may even be lower.

A similar balance of risks and benefits can be seen among women who used the pill for at least ten years in the past. Compared to women who never used the pill, these women have an increased risk of dying from cardiovascular disease and a decreased risk of dying from cancer. Their overall risk of mortality, then, is about the same as that of women who never used the pill.

## Birth Control Pills: What It All Means

Most of what scientists currently know about birth control pills pertains to the high dose pill used in the 1960s and '70s. Although evidence on the modern,

---

### Birth Control Pills

- Birth control pills are a highly reliable form of contraception.
- The health-related benefits include long-lasting protection against ovarian cancer, endometrial cancer, and probably colon cancer.
- On the negative side, the pill increases a woman's risk of breast cancer, deep vein thrombosis, heart attack, stroke, and malignant melanoma. Fortunately, these risks disappear shortly after a woman stops taking the pill.
- Overall, women who take the pill (and women who took it in the past) tend to live just as long as women who never used the pill.

low dose pill is not as abundant, scientists have definitively established that the low dose pill is a safe and reliable means of contraception. Overall, the available evidence on birth control pills should be reassuring if you used to take high dose pills—or now take low dose pills.

While you are on the pill—high dose or low dose—you have a slightly elevated risk of both breast cancer and cardiovascular disease. This may sound frightening, but it is important to remember that at the time in your life when you are taking birth control pills, you are most likely young, premenopausal, and consequently at extremely low risk of developing breast cancer and cardiovascular disease. In a group of a thousand women who are thirty years old, about four will develop breast cancer, and less than one will develop cardiovascular disease, before they reach the age of forty. Thus it is highly unlikely that you will develop either of these diseases while you are on the pill, even if you are at slightly elevated risk.

It is also unlikely that you will develop these diseases later in life as a result of your past pill use. The detrimental effects of the pill appear to wear off shortly after you stop using it. Thus, by the time your age-related risk of breast cancer and cardiovascular disease has substantially increased, your risk has returned to that of a woman the same age who never used the pill.

Fortunately, the benefits of the pill, namely protection against ovarian cancer and endometrial cancer, linger much longer than the risks, and extend well into the age range when the rates of these cancers are beginning to rise. If you discontinue your pill use at age thirty-five, you will still have a reduced risk of endometrial and ovarian cancer at age fifty and perhaps even longer.

Overall, birth control pills provide a safe and reliable means of contraception for most women, while offering long-term protection against cancers of the ovary and endometrium. However, they do slightly raise the risk of breast cancer and cardiovascular disease and so are not recommended for women who are already at high risk of these diseases, including:

- Women who smoke and are over age thirty-five.
- Women who have a personal history of diabetes, blood clots, or high blood pressure (hypertension).
- Women who have a personal history of breast cancer or endometrial cancer. (Even though the pill protects against endometrial cancer, once a woman has had this cancer, the estrogen in the pill may increase the chance of it recurring.)

## The Mini-Pill

Unlike most birth control pills, the mini-pill contains no estrogen and only a small dose of progestin. Though it has received less study than other birth control pills, researchers suspect that the mini-pill offers protection against ovarian cancer and endometrial cancer without raising the risk of breast cancer or affecting the risk of heart disease. Thus it is the pill of choice among women who smoke, women who are breastfeeding, and women who have a history of diabetes, blood clots, hypertension, or other diseases that estrogen can complicate.

The mini-pill prevents pregnancy primarily by suppressing ovulation and thickening the cervical mucus. It also interferes with the growth of the endometrium. Though slightly less effective than most birth control pills, the mini-pill is still very reliable. As with birth control pills, the most common side effect is a change in menstrual cycles. Less common effects include headaches, breast tenderness, nausea, and dizziness.

In addition, women with a family history of breast cancer or blood clots should be sure to discuss this with their health care provider.

## HORMONAL IMPLANTS AND INJECTIONS

Just as female hormones can be taken in the form of a pill, they can also be injected into your muscle or implanted under your skin. Once in the body, the hormones prevent pregnancy the same way they do when they are ingested, by suppressing ovulation and thickening cervical mucus. The advantage of these hormonal implants and injections is that they allow you to have long-term reliable protection without having to take a pill every day.

### DEPO-PROVERA

The injection most commonly used for contraception in the United States is Depo-Provera. Administered by a health care provider every three months, Depo-Provera contains a high dose of progestin only. This causes most women to stop having menstrual periods while they are on it. More than half will stop menstruating within a year of the first injection, and nearly three-quarters will stop within two years. In addition, some women on this contraceptive experience headaches, nervousness, decreased libido, breast discomfort, and depression.

Because its effectiveness does not depend on regular or proper usage, Depo-Provera is one of the most effective forms of contraception available:

fewer than 1 in 100 women experience an unintended pregnancy in the first year of use. Notably, Depo-Provera can have short lingering effects on a woman's fertility. After a woman gets her last injection, her fertility may be affected for six to twelve months. After that time, however, her fertility will return to normal.

*The Benefits and Risks of Depo-Provera.* Although hormonal injections have not been studied as extensively as birth control pills, they are simply different delivery systems for progestin, a hormone with fairly well-known risks and benefits. In the absence of estrogen, progestin most likely offers the same protection against ovarian cancer and endometrial cancer as birth control pills, without raising the risk of breast cancer or affecting the risk of heart disease.

## NORPLANT

The most commonly used set of hormonal implants in the United States is Norplant. These implants are soft match-like capsules that are inserted by a health care provider just under the skin of the upper arm. They release an extremely small dose of progestin every day for five years. Like Depo-Provera, Norplant is extremely effective: fewer than 1 in 100 women experience an unintended pregnancy in the first year of use.

Women who take Norplant may experience a wide range of menstrual irregularities, but usually only during the first two years of use. Overall, about 80 percent of women on Norplant experience heavier menstrual flow, changes in the length of their cycle, spotting, or cessation of periods. Often women on Norplant are given a few cycles of birth control pills to alleviate some of these menstrual disturbances. Other possible side effects include headaches, breast tenderness, nervousness, and weight gain.

*The Benefits and Risks of Norplant.* Although the long-term risks and benefits of Norplant are thought to be similar to other progestin-only contraceptives, there is very little research to confirm this. A large study currently being conducted by the World Health Organization will provide additional information about Norplant in the future.

## IUDs (INTRAUTERINE DEVICES)

In the early 1970s, the IUD was an extremely popular means of reversible birth control in the United States. Touted for its convenience and high level of effectiveness, this small plastic device could be inserted into the uterus by a health care provider and left in place to provide long-term continuous protection against pregnancy. By 1973, however, researchers began to question the safety of one particular type of IUD, the Dalkon Shield. Dalkon Shield users seemed to be more likely than other IUD users to experience excessive bleeding from miscarriages and to develop pelvic inflammatory disease, an infection that can lead to infertility and ectopic pregnancy. Because of these perceived health risks, the Dalkon Shield was removed from the market, and many women turned to other forms of birth control.

There are two types of IUDs now available in the United States, and both are known to be safe and effective in preventing pregnancy. The most commonly used is the copper IUD (called copper T 380A or ParaGard), which can remain in the uterus and provide continuous protection for up to ten years. Although researchers are not exactly sure how this IUD prevents pregnancy, the copper may evoke an inflammatory response that either immobilizes the sperm before it can reach the fallopian tube or prompts the egg to move through the fallopian tube too quickly to be fertilized. Women who use the copper IUD have less than 1 in 100 chance of getting pregnant in the first year of use.

The other IUD available in the United States is somewhat less popular, probably because it has to be replaced annually. This IUD, called Progestastert, contains and gradually releases progesterone. This hormone causes a thickening of mucus in the cervix, which blocks the passage of sperm into the uterus. It also disrupts ovulation and can alter the surface of the endometrium. Progestastert is not as effective as the copper IUD but still provides ample protection against pregnancy: women who use it have a 2 in 100 chance of getting pregnant in their first year of use.

The side effects associated with IUDs are related to changes in the menstrual cycle. Copper IUDs may cause spotting, heavier menstrual flow, and increased menstrual cramping. Though Progestastert may also cause spotting, it is often associated with lighter menstrual flow and a decrease in painful periods.

## THE BENEFITS AND RISKS OF IUDS

*Increased Risk of Pelvic Inflammatory Disease.* Since the Dalkon Shield incident, modern IUDs have been studied extensively, particularly in terms of their association with pelvic inflammatory disease. Researchers have found that IUDs do increase the risk of this disease, but only in two very specific circumstances. First, if an IUD is not inserted under sterile conditions, it can introduce bacteria into the uterus, thereby raising a woman's risk of pelvic inflammatory disease for about three weeks after insertion. Second, if a woman is using an IUD and is exposed to a sexually transmitted infection, she is more likely to contract the infection and to subsequently develop pelvic inflammatory disease than a woman who uses another form of contraception. Although the reason for this is not yet clear, it may be that the IUD lowers a woman's resistance to viruses and bacteria. Overall, these findings suggest that IUDs are much safer than researchers once thought, particularly for women who are not at risk of being exposed to sexually transmitted infections.

## BARRIER METHODS

Condoms, cervical caps, and diaphragms are often referred to collectively as barrier methods of contraception because they physically block the passage of sperm into the uterus, thereby preventing pregnancy. There are very few side effects associated with these types of contraception. Condoms and diaphragms can trigger latex allergies, and diaphragms can irritate the urethra.

*Male Condoms.* The male condom is a latex or polyurethane sheath that covers the erect penis during sexual activity and prevents semen (and the sperm in semen) from being released into the vagina. When male condoms are consistently and properly used without spermicide, a woman has about a 3 in 100 chance of getting pregnant. If condoms are used with spermicide, the likelihood of pregnancy is even lower. If, however, condoms are not used during every act of sexual intercourse or are not used properly, a woman's chance of getting pregnant goes up significantly—to about 14 in 100.

*Female Condoms.* Approved by the FDA in 1993, the female condom is a relatively new form of contraception. It is a polyurethane sheath that lines the inside of the vagina during sexual activity and prevents semen from entering the vagina. Like the male condom, the female condom must be worn during every act of sexual intercourse and must be inserted before there is any genital contact. Even with proper and consistent usage, however, it is slightly less effective than the male condom: women who use the female condom as directed have about a 5 in 100 chance of getting pregnant in the first year of use. Women who are less consistent in their condom use have a much higher chance of getting pregnant: 21 in 100.

*Cervical Caps.* The cervical cap is a thimble-shaped rubber cup that a woman fills with spermicide, inserts into her vagina, and pushes up until it fits snugly over her cervix. Once in place, the cap provides continuous protection against pregnancy for forty-eight hours, regardless of the number of times intercourse occurs. It does this primarily by holding spermicide in place over the cervix so that sperm are killed before they can enter the uterus. The effectiveness of the cervical cap depends not only on how consistently and correctly it is used, but also on whether or nor the user has had children. Women who use the cap as directed have a 9 in 100 chance of getting pregnant if they have not already had children and a 26 in 100 chance if they have. Women who use the cap less than perfectly have a 20 in 100 chance of getting pregnant if they have not already had children and a 40 in 100 chance if they have.

*Diaphragms.* The diaphragm is a shallow, dome-shaped cup that fits in the vagina and over the cervix. Like the cervical cap, it cannot block the passage of sperm into the uterus unless accompanied by a spermicide. Women who use a diaphragm as directed with spermicide have a 6 in 100 chance of getting pregnant in the first year of use. If the diaphragm is used with spermicide inconsistently or incorrectly, the chances of pregnancy go up to 20 in 100.

## THE RISKS AND BENEFITS OF BARRIER METHODS

*Lower Risk of Sexually Transmitted Infections.* By minimizing genital contact during sexual activity and preventing the exchange of bodily fluids, male condoms can protect women against a variety of sexually transmitted infections, including HIV. Ten cohort studies have evaluated the relationship between male condom use and HIV infection among heterosexual couples. In all of these studies, the risk of HIV infection was substantially reduced among those who used condoms consistently.

Because female condoms are relatively new to the contraceptive market, there are fewer studies of their effectiveness in preventing sexually transmitted infections. However, they are believed to be as effective as male condoms in preventing infections, since they are made of polyurethane and line the vagina completely.

Diaphragms with spermicide may also offer protection against sexually transmitted infections, but probably not to the same extent that male condoms do. Some studies have shown that diaphragms offer substantial protection, but most evidence suggests that the protection is only modest.

*Lower Risk of Cervical Cancer.* Cervical cancer is caused primarily by infection with a sexually transmitted virus called the human papilloma virus (HPV). This virus is usually passed by direct skin-to-skin contact during sexual activity, though recent scientific evidence suggests that it may also be transmitted through the exchange of bodily fluids. It can survive undetected in the body for many years and can eventually cause cells on the surface of the cervix to transform into cancer cells.

Male condoms and diaphragms are the only barrier methods for which there is solid evidence to support a protective effect against HPV. Numerous studies have shown that male condoms protect against this viral infection and thereby reduce a woman's risk of cervical cancer by as much as 80 percent. Diaphragms have also been shown to protect against HPV, though researchers are not sure why, since they do not prevent skin-to-skin contact. It has been suggested that the spermicides used with diaphragms have antiviral properties.

Although there is no evidence to support it yet, scientists believe that female condoms are probably as effective as male condoms in preventing cervical cancer. Cervical caps, on the other hand, do not appear to offer any protection against HPV and cervical cancer. The reason for this is not yet clear.

## TUBAL LIGATION

Tubal ligation is a surgical procedure that is often referred to as "having your tubes tied." Although there are some ways of doing this procedure that are potentially reversible, tubal ligation is considered a permanent form of contraception and is usually chosen only by women who have completed their families or are certain they never want to have children. It is almost 100 percent effective; fewer than 1 in 100 women get pregnant after having this procedure.

During tubal ligation, a woman's fallopian tubes are cut, tied, or clamped. The fallopian tubes serve as a passageway for the egg to travel between the ovary and the uterus and as a meeting place for the egg and sperm (see Figure 23-4). When a woman's tubes are tied or sealed, ovulation still occurs, but the pathway for the egg to be fertilized is blocked.

### THE RISKS AND BENEFITS OF TUBAL LIGATION

*Lower Risk of Ovarian Cancer.* A growing body of evidence suggests that having a tubal ligation reduces the risk of ovarian cancer. In the Nurses' Health Study, we found that women who had a tubal ligation were about 65 percent less likely to develop ovarian cancer than women who had not had this procedure (see Figure 23-5).

Researchers have proposed several explanations for this. First, high levels of circulating hormones in the blood may increase the risk of ovarian cancer. After a tubal ligation, there may be less blood flowing to the ovaries and thus less exposure to circulating hormones. Second, having a tubal ligation may alter the length of a woman's ovulatory cycle, so that she experiences ovulation less frequently. The fewer times a woman experiences ovulation during her lifetime, the less likely she is to develop ovarian cancer. Finally, researchers have speculated that some ovarian cancers might be caused by direct exposure to carcinogens that have been introduced into the vagina and then traveled to

**FRONT VIEW**

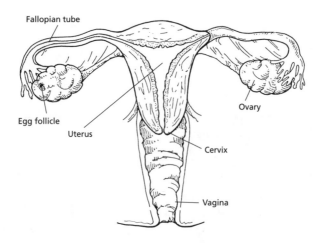

**SIDE VIEW**

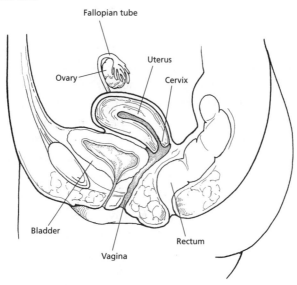

FIG. 23-4. Internal Female Reproductive System. The female reproductive system consists of two ovaries (where eggs are stored), two fallopian tubes, the uterus, cervix, vagina, and outer genitals. Each month during menstruation, an egg is released from the ovaries. If fertilized by a sperm cell, the egg begins its journey to the uterus for implantation.

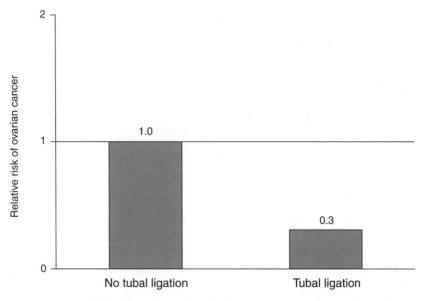

FIG. 23-5 Having a tubal ligation can lower the risk of ovarian cancer. (Source: Nurses' Health Study)

the ovaries via the uterus and fallopian tubes. After a tubal ligation, the pathway between the fallopian tubes and ovaries is blocked, preventing the passage of carcinogens from the genital tract to the ovaries.

*Increased Risk of Ectopic Pregnancy.* Though rare, fertilization can occur after tubal ligation. In a normal pregnancy, the fertilized egg travels through the fallopian tubes to the uterus, where it attaches itself to the uterine wall and begins to grow. In an ectopic pregnancy, the fertilized egg attaches to an organ other than the uterus (usually the fallopian tubes) and is unable to develop normally. If the embryo continues to grow and the organ is stretched beyond its capacity, the organ wall can burst, causing heavy internal bleeding.

Although ectopic pregnancies are extremely rare, they seem to occur more frequently among women who become pregnant after a tubal ligation. However, since very few pregnancies occur in women who have had this procedure, the overall risk of ectopic pregnancy is still extremely low. In one study, the rate of ectopic pregnancy was only 0.4 percent (or less than 1 in 100) among women who had a tubal ligation.

## Vasectomy

A vasectomy is a simple operation designed to make a man sterile. Like tubal ligation, it is highly effective and should be considered a permanent means of contraception. It is chosen only by those who have completed their families or are certain they never want to have children. We have examined the risks and benefits of vasectomy by studying the husbands of the women in the Nurses' Health Study. We found that this procedure does *not* increase a man's risk of coronary heart disease, as was once thought. However, it may still have serious health consequences in the form of prostate cancer. We found that men who had a vasectomy were 50 percent more likely to develop prostate cancer than men who had not had a vasectomy. Although not entirely consistent, other studies have had similar results, and couples should consider these findings when making contraceptive decisions.

## NATURAL METHODS

Natural family planning methods are the least reliable means of preventing pregnancy. Their effectiveness depends largely on a couple's willingness to avoid sexual intercourse completely for at least ten days per month—about a week before ovulation and several days afterward. This method of birth control requires scrupulous attention to the signs of ovulation that occur throughout a woman's menstrual cycle.

How can women tell when ovulation (or the release of an egg) is likely to occur? There are several methods. In the cervical mucus method, women chart the consistency of their vaginal mucus, which is secreted by the cervix. The days surrounding ovulation are identified by the consistency of the mucus. During a woman's most fertile time, the mucus is slick, clear, and stretchy and feels like raw egg white. The mucus becomes cloudy and thick during safer times after ovulation. Some women cannot reliably use this method because they do not secrete enough mucus to evaluate.

In the body temperature method, a woman takes her temperature every day (before she gets out of bed) with a special highly sensitive thermometer and charts each day's temperature on a monthly graph. Since temperature rises slightly at the time of ovulation, women can avoid intercourse during that time. However, they also need to be able to anticipate ovulation so that they can avoid intercourse in the days leading up to it. Women who have regular periods can do this based on their patterns of previous ovulatory cycles. They then avoid having unprotected intercourse for several days (ideally, a week) before

> ## Beyond the Pill
>
> - Hormonal injections offer long-term reliable protection against pregnancy. They are thought to have the same health-related benefits as birth control pills, but do not carry the same risks.
> - The modern IUD is a safe and effective form of long-term contraception. It has little effect on a woman's overall health.
> - Barrier methods include condoms, diaphragms, and cervical caps. They are not as reliable as other forms of contraception, but they do protect against sexually transmitted diseases.
> - The only permanent forms of contraception are tubal ligation and vasectomy. Tubal ligation offers women protection against ovarian cancer, while vasectomy may increase men's risk of prostate cancer.

the expected day of ovulation—and for at least seventy-two hours after the temperature rise indicates that they have ovulated.

Women who follow their cycles and are strict in avoiding intercourse around the time of ovulation have a 2 in 100 chance of getting pregnant with natural methods. Those who use natural methods less optimally have a 20 in 100 chance of getting pregnant.

## STRATEGIES FOR BIRTH CONTROL USE

There are many effective forms of birth control available to women, and while the choice is certainly empowering, it can also be overwhelming. It is important to make your decision about birth control carefully and to reassess this decision periodically. As you review your contraceptive options, both now and in the future, ask yourself the following questions:

### IS THE METHOD EASY TO USE AND CONVENIENT?

Contraception is effective only if it is used consistently. Ask yourself if you will remember to take a birth control pill every day or if you will be diligent about inserting a diaphragm or condom every time you have intercourse. Forgetting even one time can lead to pregnancy.

- If you prefer not to think about taking a pill every day but want long-term continuous contraception, you may want to consider IUDs, hormone implants, or injections.

- If you have sex infrequently, you may find it more convenient to use a condom or diaphragm with spermicide than to take a pill every day.
- Some couples choose to abstain from intercourse for about ten days per month (the week before ovulation and a few days afterward). This method requires not only discipline but also scrupulous attention to the signs of ovulation that occur throughout a woman's menstrual cycle.

## Is the Method Reliable?

The most reliable means of birth control are those that provide continuous long-term protection (hormone implants, injections, and IUDs) or permanent contraception (tubal ligation and vastectomy). Other forms vary in their reliability and depend largely on your using them properly and consistently.

The table on page 480 shows the pregnancy rate for various methods of birth control. This number is calculated by determining what percentage of women had an unintended pregnancy during the first year that they were using a particular form of contraception. Two rates are given in the table for each contraceptive. The first is the chance that a woman will get pregnant if she always uses the method exactly as directed (perfect use). The second is the chance that she will get pregnant if she uses the method incorrectly or less consistently than recommended (typical use). As demonstrated in the table, there can be sizable differences in the reliability of a method, depending on how well you use it.

Usually, the longer a woman uses a particular form of birth control, the more consistently and correctly she uses it. Thus the pregnancy rates for most forms of birth control improve (get lower) after the first year of use.

Finally, remember that any method, even the least reliable, is better than no method. A sexually active woman who does not use birth control for a year has an 85 in 100 chance of getting pregnant during that year. The chances of getting pregnant for women who use the least effective method inconsistently (a female condom without spermicide) are a quarter of that: 21 in 100. This means that if you are in a situation where your ideal contraceptive is not available, use an alternative method; it is bound to offer you at least some protection against pregnancy.

## Does the Method Protect Against
## Sexually Transmitted Infections?

The only contraceptive methods that offer protection against sexually transmitted infections are male condoms. Female condoms are probably also effec-

| Method | Pregnancy Rate with Perfect Use* | Pregnancy Rate with Typical Use** |
|---|---|---|
| No method | 85 | 85 |
| Birth control pills | 0.1 | 5 |
| Mini-pills | 0.5 | 5 |
| Depo-Provera | 0.3 | 0.3 |
| Norplant | 0.05 | 0.05 |
| IUD (intrauterine device) | | |
|   Progesterone IUD | 1.5 | 2 |
|   Copper IUD | 0.6 | 0.8 |
| Condoms without spermicide | | |
|   Male condom | 3 | 14 |
|   Female condom | 5 | 21 |
| Cervical cap with spermicide† | 9 | 20 |
| Diaphragm with spermicide | 6 | 20 |
| Tubal ligation | 0.5 | 0.5 |
| Vasectomy†† | 0.10 | 0.15 |
| Natural methods | 2 | 20 |

\* In a group of 100 women who always use the method exactly as directed, this is the number who will get pregnant in the first year using the method.

\*\* In a group of 100 women who *do not* always use the method exactly as directed, this is the number who will get pregnant in the first year using the method.

† Pregnancy rates among women who use this method and have not yet had children.

†† Vasectomy does not immediately clear the reproductive tract of sperm. During the first few weeks after the procedure, unprotected intercourse is not recommended and can result in pregnancy.

Source: Hatcher, R. A., et al., *Contraceptive Technology*, 17th rev. ed. (New York: Ardent Media, 1998).

tive, but there is little direct evidence to support this. Unless you are certain that you and your partner are both free of infection, use a latex or polyurethane condom every time you engage in sexual activity.

## What Are the Health Benefits and Risks of the Method?

Some forms of contraception (such as birth control pills, implants, and injections) alter your hormone levels and thus impact your risk of hormone-related diseases. For example, birth control pills offer long-term protection against ovarian cancer and endometrial cancer. Other methods (such as IUDs, condoms, and diaphragms) may influence your risk of infection, which in turn can affect your fertility and risk of cervical cancer. You will also need to consider how different methods of contraception affect your partner's health. For example, your partner's having a vasectomy may increase his risk of prostate cancer.

## WHAT ARE THE SIDE EFFECTS OF THE METHOD?

Most forms of reversible birth control can have one or more side effects. These are summarized in the table below and should be considered carefully when selecting a form of birth control. Most of the hormonal contraceptives cause irregular menstrual cycles. Some, like the pill, cause irregularities only in the first few months of use, while others, like Depo-Provera, cause the cessation of periods throughout use.

| METHOD | MOST COMMON SIDE EFFECTS | LESS COMMON SIDE EFFECTS |
| --- | --- | --- |
| Birth control pills | *Only within the first 3 months of use:* | Headaches |
| | Lighter menstrual flow | Gains or losses in weight |
| | Changes in menstrual cycle length | Elevations in blood pressure |
| | Spotting | Vaginal infections |
| | Irregular intervals between periods | Changes in libido |
| | Cessation of periods | |
| | Abdominal cramping or bloating | |
| | Changes in acne levels | |
| | Breast tenderness or swelling | |
| | Nausea or vomiting | |
| | Dizziness | |
| | Fatigue | |
| Mini-pills | Lighter menstrual flow | Headaches |
| | Spotting | Breast tenderness |
| | Irregular intervals between periods | Nausea |
| | Decrease in menstrual cramping | Dizziness |
| | Cessation of periods | |

| Method | Most Common Side Effects | Less Common Side Effects |
|---|---|---|
| Hormone injections (Depo-Provera) | *Throughout use:* Cessation of periods | Headaches Nervousness Decreased libido Breast tenderness Depression |
| Hormone implants (Norplant) | *Within the first two years of use:* Heavier menstrual flow Changes in menstrual cycle length Spotting Cessation of periods | Headaches Breast tenderness Nervousness Weight gain |
| Copper IUDs (ParaGard) | Spotting Heavier menstrual flow Increased menstrual cramping | |
| Progesterone IUDs (Progestastert) | Spotting Lighter menstrual flow Decrease in painful periods | |
| Male and female condoms | Latex allergies | |
| Diaphragm | Irritation of the urethra Latex allergies | |

## How Expensive Is the Method?

Birth control pills, IUDs, and hormonal implants may be more expensive initially, but over time they can be less expensive than other methods.

## WHAT METHOD BEST SUITS YOUR MEDICAL HISTORY?

Ask your health care provider which form of contraception he or she would recommend, based on your overall medical history. For example, if someone in your family has had cancer of the ovary or endometrium, the birth control pill may be recommended because it has been shown to reduce the risk of those cancers.

If you smoke and are over the age of thirty-five, you may be advised against birth control pills because of the increased risk of blood clots. Mini-pills, hormone injections, and hormone implants might be recommended. Tubal ligation might also be an option if you never want to become pregnant. If you have had infections of the reproductive tract, or are at increased risk of infection, your health care provider may discourage you from considering an IUD, because it can increase your chances of infection. Overall, your health care provider can help you make the best choice.

## WHAT I TELL MY PATIENTS ABOUT BIRTH CONTROL

DR. CAROL BATES

Few decisions are as personal as which form of birth control to use. Most women will use several different methods through their reproductive lives as their circumstances change. Many factors should be considered, including contraceptive effectiveness, personal and family medical history, sexual practices, convenience, and preference. After all, the whole point of birth control is to use it—and you won't use a method that makes you feel uncomfortable.

Before going into the specific options, I review the following questions with my patients. You may want to answer them yourself, to articulate your own priorities and preferences before you decide which birth control method is right for you.

### Reproductive History

1. What is your past experience with contraceptives? What did you like and dislike about prior methods?
2. Have you had any unintended pregnancies? Were you using any contraceptive method at that time?
3. Are you planning to have children? Do you know when you would like to conceive?

4. Are you approaching menopause?

5. Have you ever had a sexually transmitted infection?

6. Do you currently have more than one sexual partner?

7. Do you believe that your partner is monogamous?

## Medical History

1. How old are you?

2. Do you smoke?

3. Do you have (or have you ever had) cancer (what type), heart disease, stroke, blood clots, or diabetes?

4. Is there any family history of blood clots or ovarian cancer?

## Preferences

1. Can you remember to take a pill every day at the same time of day?

2. Barrier methods require insertion or application each time you have intercourse. Do you think you will do this faithfully?

3. Do you have any objection to taking pills, inserting something into your vagina, or having injections?

Once you've answered the questions above, you and your doctor will be better able to weigh the relative risks and benefits of a given method. You may also decide to combine birth control methods. For instance, if you are sexually active and have multiple partners, you may ask that your partner use a male condom so that you will be protected against sexually transmitted diseases. But you might also take a birth control pill, which is a more reliable form of birth control. Or you might use spermicide with the condom, which also increases this method's reliability.

As always, have frank and open discussions with your health care provider so you can make an informed decision that is right for you.

# CHAPTER TWENTY-FOUR

# Aspirin and Other Nonsteroidal Anti-inflammatory Drugs (NSAIDs)

## BACKGROUND

Aspirin is the most commonly used medicine in the world. Americans alone consume approximately 29 billion tablets each year. And while you have likely taken aspirin to relieve a variety of aches and pains, you may not be aware of its other potential health benefits, such as preventing heart attack, stroke, and possibly even cancer of the colon and rectum. But aspirin has a complex effect on health, not only lowering the risk of some conditions but also increasing the risk of others. Because aspirin is so widely used—in part due to its availability over the counter—and its health effects are so extensively studied, we feel the topic deserves an in-depth discussion in this book.

### How Aspirin Works

Although some of its benefits are just coming to light, aspirin has a very long history. As early as the fifth century B.C., Hippocrates noted that a bitter willow bark extract was effective at relieving pain. This extract contained salicin, a chemical closely related to the ingredient in today's aspirin (acetylsalicylic acid) that makes it effective not only at relieving pain but also at reducing inflammation, fever, blood clotting, and possibly the uncontrolled cell growth related to certain cancers.

#### INFLAMMATION

Inflammation—swelling caused by the response of the body's immune system to an infection or injury—is the major cause of pain and disability in a large number of health problems, from rheumatoid arthritis and lupus to simple injuries such as sprains and bruises. Aspirin combats inflammation by stopping the production of chemicals called prostaglandins, which make blood vessels and tissue more likely to swell when the body responds to an injury or infection.

## FEVER

Aspirin is also effective at lowering fever, most likely by blocking prostaglandin production in the hypothalamus—the part of the brain that regulates body temperature—and relaxing blood vessels throughout the body, which helps the body release heat.

## BLOOD CLOTS

The ability to relieve pain and reduce inflammation has long been recognized as an important benefit of aspirin. Not until the 1970s, though, was one of its most important properties discovered: the potent ability to prevent blood clots. In addition to blocking prostaglandins, aspirin also blocks production of a chemical in platelets that promotes clotting. Platelets are small particles in the blood that play a key role in the formation of blood clots. When levels of this chemical are reduced, blood clots take longer to form. While this increases the time it takes to stop a cut or scrape from bleeding, it can also make it less likely that dangerous blood clots will form in the arteries that can cause a heart attack or stroke.

## UNCONTROLLED CELL GROWTH

Finally—although it is not understood exactly how—aspirin may protect against uncontrolled cell growth that can lead to cancer in certain tissues.

### Nonsteroidal Anti-inflammatory Drugs (NSAIDs)

Aspirin is part of this larger group of drugs. NSAIDs get their name because they are not steroids and their primary function is to reduce inflammation. Although certain types of steroids (such as prednisone or hydrocortisone) are very powerful anti-inflammatories, they can also have a number of serious side effects, especially if used for extended periods. NSAIDs, on the other hand, can very effectively fight inflammation but generally have a lower frequency of serious side effects.

In addition to aspirin, other common NSAIDs that are available without a prescription include ibuprofen (also sold under the names Advil, Motrin, and Nuprin) and naproxen (also sold under the name Aleve). Examples of NSAIDs requiring a prescription include diclofenac, indomethacin, ketoprofen, nabumetone, oxaprozin, and sulindac. Most NSAIDs work in a manner similar to aspirin, blocking the production of certain chemicals, primarily prostaglandins. Therefore, like aspirin, in addition to fighting inflammation, most other NSAIDs also reduce fever and may help stop uncontrolled cell growth in certain tissues. Most NSAIDs also increase the time it takes blood to clot, though none is as effective at this as aspirin. Aspirin hampers a platelet's ability to form a clot for the life of the platelet (several days), whereas the effect of other NSAIDs on platelets is less prolonged.

## LESSONS FROM THE NURSES' HEALTH STUDY AND OTHER STUDIES

### Benefits of Aspirin and Other NSAIDs

Most women take aspirin and other NSAIDs to lower a fever or to treat the inflammation and pain associated with a variety of conditions, from rheumatoid arthritis and menstrual cramps to headaches and ankle sprains. In addition to these common uses, however, research shows that NSAIDs have other important benefits as well, lowering the risk of heart attack and stroke in certain groups and possibly even lowering the risk of some cancers.

Women who take aspirin and other NSAIDs to treat serious inflammatory conditions, such as rheumatoid arthritis, tend to take relatively high doses of the medicine. It is not uncommon for women suffering from rheumatoid arthritis to take an average of eight standard aspirin tablets (325 mg) a day, which totals approximately 2,800 milligrams. Much smaller amounts, however, seem to be needed to lower the risk of heart attack and stroke.

### LOWER RISK OF CORONARY HEART DISEASE

Coronary heart disease occurs when the arteries that feed the heart narrow. If severe enough, the narrowing can reduce blood flow and cause chest pain (angina). When blood flow becomes completely blocked, which often occurs when a blood clot forms at the site of a buildup, part of the heart muscle may die, which is called a heart attack (myocardial infarction). A number of studies have found that aspirin can help prevent a heart attack in women who already have heart disease, limit the damage of a heart attack in progress, and possibly even lower the risk of women initially developing coronary heart disease. Aspirin helps prevent or limit the damage of a heart attack primarily by hampering the formation of blood clots that can completely block the flow of blood in an artery, though it may also help fight inflammation in an artery.

*Heart Attack in Those with Coronary Heart Disease.* A great deal of evidence shows that both men and women with coronary heart disease—those who have angina or have had a previous heart attack—who take aspirin regularly can significantly lower their risk of having a subsequent heart attack. A large study that combined the results of over 170 randomized controlled trials assessing the effect of aspirin on cardiovascular disease found that both women and men with coronary heart disease who regularly took aspirin had about a 30 percent lower risk of having a second heart attack compared to those who did not take aspirin.

Doses of aspirin from 75 to 325 milligrams per day seem equally effective at reducing the risk of a heart attack in women with coronary heart disease. This equals about a quarter to one full aspirin a day, and while it is unclear what the best daily amount of aspirin is within this range, taking much larger amounts does not appear to further reduce the risk of a heart attack. In fact, some studies have shown that in addition to increasing the chances of side effects, very large amounts of aspirin may not be as effective as lower amounts at decreasing the risk of blood clots.

Because women who have angina or who have had a previous heart attack have a large risk of having subsequent heart attacks throughout their lives, it is generally recommended that they take aspirin regularly and indefinitely—but not without first checking with their health care provider.

*Heart Attack in Progress.* Aspirin is also very effective at limiting the damage of a heart attack in progress. A randomized trial of over 17,000 men and women who were thought to be having a heart attack found that those who took 162.5 milligrams of aspirin (half of a standard tablet) during and for each of the thirty days after a heart attack had a 25 percent lower risk of death compared to those who did not take aspirin. Aspirin's potent ability to decrease blood clotting, as well as to relax blood vessels, can help keep blood flowing during a heart attack and keep clots from forming again in the month after. Aspirin is now commonly given to the large majority of the 1.2 million men and women in the United States admitted each year to hospitals for heart attacks. A half to a full 325-milligram tablet is generally recommended for the first twenty-four hours after a heart attack is suspected. After that, a half tablet (162.5 mg) is recommended for each of the next thirty days.

*Initial Coronary Heart Disease Development.* Aspirin has clear benefits for people who already have coronary heart disease or who are in the process of having a heart attack. Its ability to help prevent the initial development of coronary heart disease, however, is a bit less well established, especially in women. While a large randomized controlled trial of U.S. male physicians found clear benefits from taking a 325-milligram aspirin every other day—lowering the risk of a first heart attack by nearly 45 percent—a smaller study of male British physicians found no benefit from taking aspirin regularly. These contrasting results, however, may simply reflect the difference in size between the two studies. The larger U.S. study, which had four times as many participants, may have been better able to detect a link between aspirin and a lower risk of heart disease.

Only a few observational studies in women have assessed the aspirin/heart disease issue, and these have had mixed results. In the Nurses' Health Study, we found that women who took one to six 325-milligram aspirins a week had an approximately 25 percent lower risk of coronary heart disease than women who did not take any aspirin. Women over fifty years of age seemed to benefit the most, showing a slightly greater drop in risk than younger women. Taking more than six aspirins a week did not seem to provide any additional benefit. While our results suggest that aspirin may help lower women's risk of initially developing coronary heart disease, more studies are needed before clear recommendations can be made. One study that may help clarify this issue is the ongoing Women's Health Study, a randomized controlled trial of 40,000 American women who are taking either aspirin (100 mg) or an inactive placebo every other day. Results from this study should be available in one to two years.

### Other NSAIDs

While NSAIDs other than aspirin can hamper the ability of blood to clot, none does so as effectively or at such low doses as aspirin. To date, no studies support NSAIDs other than aspirin as an effective way to prevent heart attack in those with heart disease or to limit the damage of a heart attack that is in progress.

## LOWER RISK OF ISCHEMIC STROKE

Nearly 100,000 women die each year from stroke. There are two main types of stroke, ischemic and hemorrhagic. A hemorrhagic stroke occurs when there is bleeding (hemorrhaging) in a blood vessel in the brain. An ischemic stroke, like a heart attack, occurs when an artery that supplies blood to the brain becomes totally blocked, causing the brain tissue fed by that artery to die. Blood clots are the most frequent cause of an ischemic stroke. Clots either form at the site of an atherosclerotic buildup in an artery in the neck or brain or develop elsewhere in the body and travel through the bloodstream and get lodged in an artery. Strokes are often preceded, from days to months, by events called transient ischemic attacks. Often referred to as ministrokes or precursors to stroke, transient ischemic attacks occur when blood flow to a small portion of the brain is blocked by tiny blood clots that dissolve fairly quickly, before any permanent damage can be done.

As with coronary heart disease, a great deal of evidence shows that aspirin can reduce the risk of ischemic stroke in people who experience transient ischemic attacks or have had a previous stroke. The large study of aspirin and cardiovascular disease that combined the results of over 170 trials found that men and women with a history of stroke or transient ischemic attacks who regularly took aspirin had an approximately 25 percent lower risk of stroke compared to those not taking aspirin. Similar to reducing the risk of a second heart attack, the best aspirin dosage for preventing a stroke in this population likely falls somewhere between a fourth to a full aspirin a day.

The evidence for regular aspirin use lowering the risk of a *first* stroke is much less solid. In the Nurses' Health Study, we have had positive results, finding that women who took one to six aspirins a week had a small reduction—approximately 15 percent—in the risk of a first stroke compared to women who took no aspirin at all. Many other studies on this topic, however, have found no link between regular aspirin use and a lower risk of a first stroke. As with aspirin and a first heart attack, the large Women's Health Study trial should help clarify whether or not regular aspirin use can lower the risk of a first stroke in women.

### Other NSAIDs

No NSAIDs other than aspirin have been found to be effective at lowering the risk of stroke in either men or women.

## PROBABLE LOWER RISK OF COLORECTAL CANCER

An increasing amount of evidence suggests that aspirin and other NSAIDs may lower the risk of cancer of the colon and rectum (colorectal cancer). Although it is not yet known exactly how aspirin and other NSAIDs lower this risk, it may be that they block the production of certain chemicals that indirectly inhibit the growth of tumors in the colon and rectum.

Early studies assessing the affect of aspirin on the risk of colorectal cancer generally found no relationship between the two, but they tended to assess only short-term aspirin use (five years or less). For example, a large randomized con-

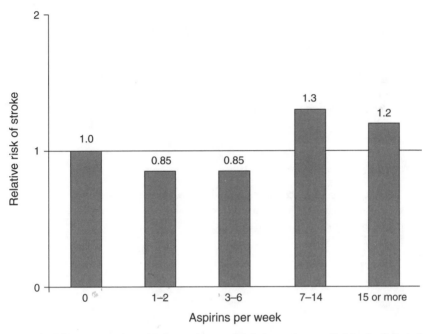

FIG. 24-1. Taking one to six aspirins a week may slightly lower the overall risk of a first stroke (ischemic and hemorrhagic combined) in women. Taking more than six aspirins per week slightly increases risk. (Source: Nurses' Health Study)

## Stroke Risk and Other Antiplatelet Agents

For those people unable to take aspirin—either because of side effects or allergic reactions—other drugs (such as Persantine and Ticlid) are occasionally prescribed to try to lower the risk of stroke. Like aspirin, these drugs are antiplatelet agents that hamper the ability of platelets to form blood clots. Compared to aspirin, though, these other drugs either are not as effective at lowering the risk of stroke or often cause side effects, sometimes very severe—such as life-threatening blood disorders. When appropriate, aspirin is usually preferred to these other antiplatelet drugs, although some studies suggest a combination of the two may be better than aspirin alone for certain patients.

trolled trial of male physicians found no benefit from taking a 325-milligram aspirin every other day for five years.

More recent studies, however, suggest that it may take at least ten years of regular aspirin use before women receive any protection against the disease. In

## Aspirin Use and Cardiovascular Disease— The Evidence for Benefit Depends on Disease History

When it comes to the cardiovascular benefits of aspirin, it is very important to distinguish between aspirin's effect on the risk of a heart attack or stroke in people with prior cardiovascular disease, and its potential effect in those *without prior* cardiovascular disease.

### PEOPLE WITH CARDIOVASCULAR DISEASE

There is strong evidence that both men and women with cardiovascular disease—such as those who have had a previous heart attack or stroke—can significantly benefit from taking aspirin regularly. In this group, regular aspirin use can lower the risk of:

- Stroke by 25 percent
- Heart attack by 30 percent
- Death from a heart attack in progress by 25 percent

### PEOPLE WITHOUT CARDIOVASCULAR DISEASE

There is much less evidence (especially for women) of the cardiovascular benefits of regular aspirin use in those people without known cardiovascular disease. While there is strong evidence that regular aspirin use can lower the risk of a first heart attack in men, the data are much less solid for women. There may be a benefit, but it is still not completely clear. As for protecting against a first stroke, studies to date have found no benefit of regular aspirin use in healthy men. In women, it is still not clear whether or not aspirin has any benefit. The result from a large, ongoing randomized trial in women looking at the cardiovascular effects of regular aspirin use should help clarify these issues.

one study, researchers found a very large reduction in risk among people who took aspirin regularly for at least ten years but no benefit among those who took it for less time. In the Nurses' Health Study, we found that the longer women took aspirin, the lower their risk of colorectal cancer. Women who took at least two 325-milligram tablets a week for ten years had a 30 percent lower risk of colorectal cancer compared to women who did not take aspirin. Women taking aspirin for twenty or more years had an even lower risk: 45 percent lower compared to women who did not take aspirin.

## Selective Cox-2 Inhibitors

A new group of nonsteroidal anti-inflammatory drugs called selective Cox-2 in-hibitors are currently being studied and approved for use to treat a number of conditions, from arthritis to severe menstrual pain. As with other NSAIDs, these new drugs can effectively combat inflammation, fever, and pain. What makes the selective Cox-2 inhibitors unique is that they seem to cause fewer problems with ulcers and bleeding in the stomach and intestine. The drugs work by blocking an enzyme (Cox-2) that plays an important role in inflamma-tion, but—unlike most other NSAIDs—they do not block an enzyme (Cox-1) that seems to be important to blood clotting and the health of the stomach and intestines.

Because they do not hamper blood clotting, the selective Cox-2 inhibitors most likely provide few, if any, cardiovascular benefits.

As with heart attack and stroke, fairly low doses of aspirin seem to protect against colorectal cancer. We found that two or more 325-milligram tablets a week offered protection against the disease, but that four to six tablets a week may offer even greater benefit. However, it is still unclear exactly what the op-timal amount of aspirin is to lower the risk of colorectal cancer and for how long a time a person has to take it to receive benefit.

### Other NSAIDs

A number of studies have found that NSAIDs other than aspirin may also lower the risk of colorectal cancer. One large cohort study found that female arthritis sufferers, who tend to take a variety of NSAIDs regularly to treat their condition, had a 40 percent lower risk of colon cancer compared to women without arthritis. Other, smaller studies specifically assessing the link between nonaspirin NSAIDs and colorectal cancer have also found that regular users have a moderate to large decrease in the risk of the disease compared to nonusers. One specific nonaspirin NSAID, sulindac, has also been found in some studies to reduce the number of colon polyps—noncancerous growths that can turn into cancer—in certain groups of people.

It is not clear if any one NSAID is better than the others at lowering the risk of colorectal cancer. Nor is it clear what dose or length of use of nonaspirin NSAIDs is optimal for lowering the risk of the disease. Future research, how-ever, should help clarify these issues.

## Unproven Benefits of Aspirin and Other NSAIDs

There are a number of other disorders where aspirin has been proposed to influence risk, but the evidence to date is either inconsistent or very limited. Three such disorders are breast cancer, cataracts, and dementia.

### BREAST CANCER

Because an increasing number of studies have linked NSAIDs with a decreased risk of colorectal cancer, there has been a great deal of interest in examining whether aspirin can lower the risk of other cancers as well. Although results have been inconsistent, a few studies have found that taking aspirin regularly can reduce the risk of breast cancer. One large study based on a sample of the U.S. population found that women who regularly used aspirin had a 30 percent lower risk of breast cancer than women who did not. Other studies, however, have shown no benefit to aspirin use. In the Nurses' Health Study, we found that regular aspirin use, even for twenty or more years, did not affect the risk of breast cancer. Overall, current data do not support a link between aspirin and breast cancer.

### CATARACTS

While a few studies have suggested that aspirin use can lower the risk of cataracts, most others have not. In the Nurses' Health Study, we found no link between aspirin use and a lower risk of cataracts, even in women who took one or more tablets a week for ten or more years.

### DEMENTIA

Some research suggests that regular aspirin use may lower the risk or delay the onset of dementia, including Alzheimer's. Although it is not completely clear how aspirin use might lower risk, one likely possibility is that it helps prevent multiple small strokes that together can result in a drop in mental ability. Although we have not assessed this topic directly in the Nurses' Health Study, a fairly large cohort study of the elderly has. With over 60 percent of its participants women, the study followed approximately 4,000 elderly over six years and found no link between aspirin and mental ability.

## Risks of Aspirin and Other NSAIDs

Although aspirin and other NSAIDs have a number of important benefits, they are not without their risks as well. In general, the risk of problems associated with NSAID use increases with the amount taken. A woman who takes 2,000 milligrams of an NSAID every day to treat her arthritis is more likely to experience a problem than a woman who takes one 325-milligram aspirin tablet every third day. Serious risks associated with NSAIDs include:

## ULCERS AND BLEEDING IN THE STOMACH AND INTESTINES

NSAIDs can injure the lining of the stomach and intestine, causing a painful ulcer. In some instances, the ulcer can begin to bleed, possibly seriously. At aspirin doses that appear to lower the risk of heart attack and stroke, the risk of ulcers and bleeding appears small. A study that reviewed the results of numerous antiplatelet drug trials (including those of aspirin) found that antiplatelet drugs cause about three extra cases of severe bleeding for every thousand people taking them regularly, and the randomized trial of U.S. male physicians found that one 325-milligram aspirin taken every other day only slightly increased the risk of ulcer. A similar trial in women, the ongoing Women's Health Study, should help clarify how long-term low-dose aspirin use specifically affects the risk of ulcers and bleeding in women.

## HEMORRHAGIC STROKE

NSAIDs, particularly aspirin, can increase the risk of hemorrhagic stroke—bleeding from a blood vessel in the brain. In the Nurses' Health Study, we found that women who took fifteen or more aspirins a week had double the risk of hemorrhagic stroke compared to women who did not take any (see Figure 24-2). Though this increase in risk may seem large, when compared to the possible benefits of aspirin in lowering the risk of heart attack, the risk of hemorrhagic stroke linked to aspirin use is relatively small because this type of stroke occurs much less frequently. A large study that combined the results of sixteen randomized trials on aspirin and cardiovascular disease—largely containing high-risk men—found that while aspirin use was linked to 137 fewer cases of heart attack for every 10,000 people, it was linked to only 12 extra cases of hemorrhagic stroke. Unfortunately, the study did not present separate findings for the women included in the trials.

## OTHER POTENTIAL RISKS

Ulcers and hemorrhagic stroke are two of the most common, serious risks associated with NSAID use. However, other risks also exist. These include kidney damage (most common in the elderly), dizziness, tinnitus (ringing in the ears), and hearing loss.

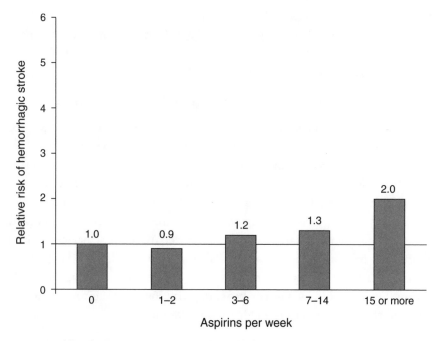

FIG. 24-2. Although one to six aspirins a week may slightly lower the overall risk of a first stroke (ischemic and hemorrhagic combined) in women, we found that women regularly taking fifteen or more aspirins a week had double the risk of subarachnoid hemorrhage, a type of hemorrhagic stroke. (Source: Nurses' Health Study)

## WHAT IT ALL MEANS

In addition to their effectiveness at treating inflammation, pain and fever, aspirin and other NSAIDs are also proving effective at lowering the risk of numerous serious disorders, including heart attack, ischemic stroke, and potentially colorectal cancer. However, taking NSAIDs is not without risk. Serious conditions, such as intestinal bleeding and hemorrhagic stroke, are linked with the use of aspirin and other NSAIDs. Therefore, except for relieving minor aches and pains, you should never begin regular aspirin (or other NSAID) use without first talking with your health care provider. Together, you can discuss the risks and benefits associated with regular NSAID use and decide if it is appropriate for you.

# WHAT I TELL MY PATIENTS ABOUT THE PROPER AND SAFE USE OF ASPIRIN AND OTHER NSAIDS

DR. CAROL BATES

Aspirin and many other NSAIDs can be purchased over the counter and so strike many of my patients as innocuous. Why should such familiar pills cause any concern? The answer is that any medication can cause side effects, and the risk increases with the dosage.

Aspirin and other NSAIDs can effectively treat many types of pain and inflammation, including that of menstrual cramps, headaches and arthritis. They also reduce your risk of developing coronary heart disease, stroke, and colon cancer. But especially when taken in large quantities, for a prolonged period, they can cause ulcers and bleeding in the stomach and intestines, as well as increase your risk of a brain hemorrhage.

Fortunately, you should be able to take aspirin and other NSAIDs safely as long as you take the following precautions.

## Medication Strategies

• **Don't overdo it.** More is not always better when it comes to pain relief or prevention of serious disease. To get the benefits of aspirin or other NSAID use while reducing your risk of complication, exercise some precautions when it comes to how much you take.

If you are at high risk of coronary heart disease or ischemic stroke, take one to six tablets of aspirin a week (75 mg–325 mg per day). This appears to be the safest effective dose range until a large-scale study currently underway tells us more. I generally suggest that my patients take 75 milligrams a day, as daily therapy may be easier to remember.

If you have arthritis or some other type of condition that causes severe pain, then you may need to take higher doses of aspirin or other NSAIDs— perhaps as many as eight aspirin (2,800 mg) per day. At this level, your risk of side effects increases significantly.

Talk with your health care provider about the safe dose of whatever medication he or she prescribes. Take as low a dose as possible. If the NSAID is not adequate to treat your pain, talk it over with him or her, rather than increase the dose on your own. No matter why you are taking aspirin or another NSAID, the best way to reduce the dosage is to supplement the medication with another pain-reducing strategy or medication.

- **If you experience stomach upset or bleeding, call your health care provider immediately.** Your provider may suggest that you stop your NSAID and substitute acetaminophen (Tylenol) or another pain reliever less likely to cause stomach upset. He or she may also prescribe omeprazole (Prilosec) or related medications known as proton pump inhibitors (PPIs) that suppress acid production. You may be able to tolerate NSAID therapy if you take it along with a PPI or misoprostol (Cytotec); this reduces your risk of developing an ulcer.

- **If you have had previous problems with NSAIDs,** talk with your health care provider about whether you should take a medication to prevent stomach problems, or at least to minimize them should they occur. You may be able to tolerate NSAID therapy if you take it along with a PPI or misoprostol (Cytotec); this reduces your risk of developing an ulcer. Alternatively, consider taking one of the Cox-2 inhibitor medicines. Cox-2 inhibitors provide effective relief from pain and inflammation, with a lower risk of causing stomach ulcers and bleeding. Two Cox-2 inhibitors have been approved by the FDA: celecoxib (marketed under the name Celebrex) and rofecoxib (Vioxx). The Cox-2 inhibitor medicines are no more effective in relieving pain than the older NSAIDs. You should consider using them if the older NSAIDs have caused stomach ulcers, gastritis or bleeding in the past.

## NSAIDs: Benefits and Side Effects

### Benefits

WELL-ESTABLISHED

*Aspirin lowers the risk of:*

- **Heart attack in men and women with coronary heart disease.** The optimal dose is likely between 75 mg (1/4 tablet) and 325 mg (1 tablet) per day and should probably be continued indefinitely.
- **Death in men and women who are having a heart attack**. The optimal dose is likely 325 mg (1 tablet) when the heart attack starts and 162.5 mg (1/2 tablet) once per day for at least the next 30 days.
- **Ischemic stroke in men and women with transient ischemic attacks or who have had a previous stroke**. The optimal dose is likely between 75 mg (1/4 tablet) and 325 mg (1 tablet) and should probably be continued indefinitely.

- **A first heart attack in men.** A large randomized trial of U.S. male physicians found that regular aspirin use could lower the risk of a first heart attack. The optimal dose is likely 162.5 mg (1/2 tablet) once per day or 325 mg (1 tablet) every other day and should probably be continued indefinitely.

PROBABLE

*Aspirin and other NSAIDs may lower the risk of:*

- **Colorectal cancer in women.** Aspirin and other NSAIDs have been linked in many studies to a lower risk of colorectal cancer. However, it is still unclear exactly what doses and duration of use are needed to lower the risk of the disease.

POSSIBLE

*Aspirin may lower the risk of:*

- **A first heart attack or stroke in women.** Although our Nurses' Health Study data suggest that regular aspirin use may help lower the risk of a first heart attack and stroke in women, more information from randomized trials in women is needed before it is known whether the benefits of regular aspirin use outweigh the potential risks.

## Potential Side Effects

*Aspirin may increase the risk of*

MOST COMMON

- Ulcers and bleeding in the stomach and intestine
- Dizziness
- Tinnitus (ringing in the ears)

RARE

- Hemorrhagic stroke

# Types of Epidemiologic Studies

THERE ARE THREE BASIC TYPES of epidemiologic studies: descriptive studies, observational studies, and randomized controlled trials. In descriptive studies, researchers are simply trying to describe the basic pattern of a disease. They do not speculate beforehand whether a certain factor is causing the disease, but instead try to get a sense of the bigger picture. Although the findings of descriptive studies are never definitive, they often demonstrate the need for additional research, which is then conducted in the form of an observational study or randomized controlled trial.

In both observational studies and randomized controlled trials, the research is grounded in the scientific method. That is, researchers start with a hypothesis about a relationship between a factor (such as exercise) and a disease (such as heart disease) and then perform a study to test their hypothesis. They record and analyze the results of their study, forming a conclusion about whether the factor and disease are related. Although they are similar conceptually, observational studies and randomized controlled trials differ in the way that they are conducted and in the strength of the conclusions they reach.

## Descriptive Studies

There are several different ways that descriptive studies can be conducted. In the first, researchers either compare populations to see which has a higher rate of disease or look at the rate of disease in the same population on two different occasions. For example, we might look at the rate of heart disease among adult women in the United States in 1960 and again in 2000 to see whether there have been changes in the rate of the disease. If we did see a change, we could speculate on what caused it, but we could not arrive at any firm conclusions.

In the second type of descriptive study, health care providers simply describe what happened to their patients. For example, a physician might note that several of her patients developed a rash while they were on a particular medication. While she cannot conclude that the rash is linked to the medication, her observation might lead to additional research on the side effects of that particular treatment.

In the final type of descriptive study, researchers ask participants at one point in time about both their lifestyle factors and their health status. Because people are reporting this information simultaneously, researchers cannot determine whether the factor occurred prior to the disease. For example, a nationwide survey might show that people with heart disease are less active than people without heart disease. However, it is not clear from this finding whether people developed the disease in part because they were sedentary or whether they are now sedentary because they are too ill to be active. An observational study or randomized controlled trial would be needed to answer this question, since these types of studies allow researchers to clearly follow the progression from factor to disease.

## Observational Studies

In observational studies, the study participants live their daily lives as they choose: they exercise when they want, eat what they like, and take the medications their physicians prescribe. They then report their activities to researchers, who use this information to understand how lifestyle choices affect health.

There are two types of observational studies: cohort studies and case-control studies. A cohort study follows a group of people over time—some who have a particular characteristic and some who do not—to see who develops the disease being studied. For example, to do a cohort study on exercise and heart disease, researchers would choose a large group of women, only some of whom exercise regularly. They would assess each woman's exercise habits, usually with a questionnaire or interview, and then follow the women to see who is more likely to develop heart disease: those who exercised regularly or those who were sedentary. The Nurses' Health Study is an example of a cohort study.

To study this same relationship, a case-control study would take a very different approach. Researchers would identify two groups—one group with people who already have heart disease, the cases, and one with people who do not, the controls. They would ask both groups about their lifestyles in the past and then compare the groups to see if any characteristic (such as level of exercise) was more common in the history of one group compared to the other.

Cohort and case-control studies each have their own advantages and limitations. A cohort study is generally considered to provide stronger evidence than a case-control study because information about lifestyle factors is collected from participants before they have been diagnosed with the disease being studied. In a case-control study, the information is collected after some of the participants (the cases) have already been diagnosed with the disease, and this has the potential to bias the study results.

Despite their limitations, case-control studies also have inherent strengths. They are often the most efficient way to identify factors related to less common diseases. In a cohort study, researchers start with healthy participants and then follow them over time, essentially waiting to study a given disease until a large group of participants has developed it. For some of the less common diseases, like ovarian cancer or melanoma, researchers may need to wait decades before having enough participants with the disease. In contrast, all of the cases in a case-control study already have the disease when they enter the study, and so researchers can begin studying the disease immediately.

## Randomized Controlled Trials

Sometimes, in contrast to observational studies, researchers intervene and change the participants' behavior or provide a particular therapy to see how it affects their health. These studies are called randomized controlled trials because the participants are randomly assigned (as if by coin toss) to a particular behavior or treatment. For example, to do a randomized controlled trial on exercise and heart disease, researchers might randomly assign half of the participants to walk ten minutes a day and half to walk two hours a day. They would then follow the participants over time to see who was more likely to develop heart disease.

Randomized controlled trials, if done well, are considered a definitive source of epidemiologic information, because they provide stronger evidence of cause-and-effect relationships than observational studies do. It is the controlled conditions of these trials that allow for this. Often, certain behaviors are naturally linked to others, and only a randomized controlled trial can disentangle the effects of one behavior from the effects of another. For example, if researchers were conducting an observational study on the health effects of multivitamins, they would need to consider that people who take multivitamins might also be likely to exercise regularly. If they did not take this into account, and their observational study showed a health benefit from multivitamins, it would not be clear whether the benefit was due to the multivitamin—or to the exercise. In a randomized controlled trial, behaviors do not cluster together like they do in the real world. Since researchers would randomly assign some women to take a multivitamin and some a placebo, there would be similar numbers of women who exercise and women who do not in each assigned group. This would allow researchers to determine the specific health effects of multivitamins.

Despite their strengths, randomized controlled trials do have several limitations that are not found in observational studies. First, they are often stopped when it becomes clear that one behavior or medication is better than the other (so that participants are not knowingly deprived of a healthful agent or assigned to a harmful one) or when no relationship has been observed over the short term and continued conduct of the study is considered too expensive. As a result, randomized controlled trials generally cannot determine long-term health effects, either beneficial or harmful. These effects must be examined through observational studies. Second, randomized controlled trials measure the effects of specific behaviors, but in the real world, most behaviors occur on a spectrum. For example, researchers could assign women to take 325 milligrams of aspirin a day versus a placebo. While this would provide useful information about the effects of that particular dose of aspirin, it would yield no information on the effects of 81 milligrams (baby aspirin) or 500 milligrams (extra-strength). In situations like this, observational studies are much more useful because they allow researchers to observe the full spectrum of behavior that people actually engage in. Finally, many behaviors, like smoking, cannot be tested experimentally, because participants can't be assigned to a behavior that is known to be harmful. Instead, researchers learn about the effects of smoking through observational studies, where they compare those who choose to smoke with those who do not.

## Summary

Each type of epidemiologic study has its own set of advantages and limitations. Descriptive studies are useful for demonstrating patterns of disease and generating hypotheses (and tend to be inexpensive to conduct), but they do not yield conclusive findings. Observational studies and randomized controlled trials, on the other hand, can demonstrate that certain factors are linked to the risk of a given disease. However, they too have their limitations. It is only when the evidence from a number of studies is compiled and seen to be consistent that one can reach firm conclusions about a given epidemiologic relationship.

# Being an Informed Consumer of Health Information

TODAY WE HAVE UNPRECEDENTED ACCESS to health information. In addition to the "classic" sources of television, radio, and print, the meteoric rise of information technology now provides nearly instant access to health-related publications from governments, health organizations, universities, businesses, and individuals the world over. Gone are the days when we relied solely on our primary care providers for advice about health. More likely, we now go to our regular checkups armed with pages printed from the Internet to ask our health care providers about a new study, a new drug, or a new health recommendation.

While this can be empowering, health information should always be viewed with vigilance. It takes an informed consumer to be able to filter through the vast amount of information available today and find pertinent, reliable health information.

Here we describe two major aspects of becoming an informed consumer of health information—understanding media reports on research studies and identifying reliable sources of health information.

## Understanding Media Reports on Research Studies

*Confusing* is one word that is often applied to the way in which the mass media report on health research. Hundreds of news stories about health get reported every week; often the messages change. While the sheer volume of the information available should be helpful to the general public, it often has the opposite effect—confusing rather than informing, frustrating people rather than motivating them to make positive change to their lives.

This stems from the fact that stories often appear to contradict each other. One week you will read that physical activity can lower the risk of heart attack, and then you may read that physical activity can increase its risk. If the experts can't figure out what's going on, why should you invest any energy in making healthy choices in your life?

The problem is most often not that the experts can't agree on a particular topic, but rather that the context of an issue often gets lost in media reports on health. By necessity, health research is an active process. A particular issue—such as physical activity and the risk of heart attack—is studied repeatedly by many different researchers and in many different ways. Most studies will find that getting regular physical activity is associated with a lower risk of heart attack. Some studies may find no link between the two, and a couple may even show that physical activity is actually linked to an increased risk of heart attack. What matters most is not the results of a single study but the conclusion drawn when all of the studies are looked at as a whole, known as the weight of evidence (as we discuss in Chapter 3). For physical activity and heart attack, the weight of the evidence indicates that getting regular physical activity can significantly lower the risk of heart attack.

The media, however, usually report the results of single studies, and while they tend to do an excellent job at keeping up with the most up-to-date findings, they do a poor job describing where a finding fits in with other studies. On top of this, what often makes a study newsworthy is the fact that it contradicts the results of other studies. While one more study that shows that regular physical activity can lower the risk of heart attack is not likely to make the news, a study with the opposite result might—just because it contradicts the current weight of evidence.

Of course, not all news sources are equal. There are many that do an excellent job reporting on new research, and even if they do not state up front where a finding fits in with others, that fact will at least appear somewhere in the story. And the media are not the only ones to blame for anemic reporting on research. Their methods of reporting are, at least in part, driven by how we—the consumers—want to see the news. With our penchant in the United States for simple, brief, and dramatic reporting, it is no wonder that the nuances of health research reports often get left out. Part of the burden also falls on the researchers themselves, some of whom tout their isolated findings rather than discuss where those findings fit into the larger picture.

The good news, though, is that simply being able to distinguish between a news report on a single study and a report that discusses the entire amount of evidence on an issue can go a long way toward making sense of health-related news. The results of single studies contribute to the research process, but in general, you should not make changes in your lifestyle based on them. The entire weight of evidence on an issue—and the health recommendations based on it—should be your guide to making choices about your health. The federal government and large health organizations such as the American Cancer Society and American Heart Association tend to also be good sources of such recommendations.

## Identifying Reliable Sources of Health Information

Outside of deciphering news stories on health research, simply finding health information you can trust can be a tall order. The popularity of the Internet makes the process that much more important. In the past, it was very costly to produce and distribute health information free to a large audience, so this was a charge primarily taken up by the federal government and large nonprofit health organizations. Now, with the Internet and its ability to make health information available worldwide at very low cost, any organization or individual can, with very little time and money, produce products and websites that look as good (or even better) than those of many reputable sources.

Whether you are searching the Internet or looking at a pamphlet from the grocery store, a few sources of health information are almost always trustworthy: federal government agencies (such as the National Institutes of Health and Centers for Disease Control), well-regarded medical and public health schools, and certain large nongovernmental health organizations (such as the American Cancer Society, the American Heart Association, and the American Diabetes Association). While other reputable sources of information also exist, these types of organizations are almost always the best place to start a search. If calls to these organizations or visits to their websites (see the list on p. 508) don't produce the information you are searching for, most can provide referrals to other trustworthy sources.

While such a strategy may seem fairly drastic, it is one of the only ways to help ensure that the information you are getting is truly worth reading. The Internet, especially, is a free-for-all of health information, rife with not only useless but also potentially harmful information. Unfortunately, there is no simple way to tell whether the information on a site is reliable or not. Therefore, it is best to stick with those few organizations that have the knowledge base, motivation, and goal to provide the public with the best health information possible.

## Finding Reliable Health Information on the Internet

With the huge variability in the quality of health information available on the Internet, it is often best to begin your search at trustworthy websites. Here is a select list of these sites:

## Federal Government

National Institutes of Health
www.nih.gov

Centers for Disease Control
www.cdc.gov

Food and Drug Administration
www.fda.gov

National Library of Medicine
www.nlm.nih.gov

Healthfinder
www.healthfinder.gov

Federal Consumer Information Center
www.pueblo.gsa.gov

## Nongovernmental Health Organizations

American Heart Association
www.americanheart.org

American Cancer Society
www.cancer.org

American Lung Association
www.lungusa.org

American Diabetes Association
www.diabetes.org

## Medical Schools and Schools of Public Health

Harvard Center for Cancer Prevention
www.yourcancerrisk.harvard.edu

Harvard Medical School (Intelihealth)
www.intelihealth.com

University of Pennsylvania (OncoLink)
www.oncolink.upenn.edu

Tufts University (Nutrition Navigator)
navigator.tufts.edu

# Some Useful Tables

## Table 1. Glycemic Index of Selected Foods

Choosing more foods with a low glycemic index—those that convert more slowly to glucose—may help decrease the risk of diabetes by lowering the body's need for insulin. The lower the number, the less the food increases blood glucose levels. In this chart, glucose is the reference point, with an index of 100. (See Chapter 18 for more information.)

| HIGH (Over 65) | MEDIUM (45–65) | LOW (Under 45) |
|---|---|---|
| Glucose 100 | Raisins 65 | Grapes 43 |
| Carrots 92 | Jelly 63 | Dried beans (cooked) 42 |
| Molasses 87 | Bananas (ripe) 62 | Pear 41 |
| Pancakes 83 | Sweet corn 61 | Orange 40 |
| Cornflakes 80 | Bran muffins 60 | Apples 39 |
| Baked potato 73 | Table sugar 59 | Chocolate 36 |
| White rice 72 | Honey 58 | Wine 35 |
| Dark bread 72 | Oatmeal (cooked) 58 | Beer 35 |
| Watermelon 72 | Kiwis 58 | Milk 34 |
| Corn chips 70 | Muesli cereal 56 | Yogurt 33 |
| White bread 69 | Oatmeal cookies 55 | Ice cream (full fat) 30 |
| Bagels 69 | Orange juice 53 | Strawberries 25 |
| Pita bread 69 | Peas 52 | Barley (uncooked) 25 |
| Cornmeal 68 | Pasta 50 | Cherries 22 |
| French fries 67 | Ice cream (low fat) 50 | Peanut butter 13 |
| Brown rice 66 | Grapefruit juice 48 | Walnuts 13 |
| Pineapple 66 | Cake 47 | Broccoli 9 |
| | | Spinach (cooked) 9 |
| | | Lettuce 9 |
| | | Eggs 0 |
| | | Fish 0 |
| | | Hard cheese 0 |

Source: Nurses' Health Study Nutrient Database

## Table 2. Determining Your Body Mass Index (BMI)

To estimate your body mass index (BMI), first identify your weight (to the nearest 10 pounds) in one of the columns across the top. Then move your finger down the column until you come to the row that represents your height. Inside the square where your weight and height meet is a number that is an estimate of your BMI. For example, if you weigh 160 pounds and are 5'7", your BMI is 25.

WEIGHT

| Height | 100 | 110 | 120 | 130 | 140 | 150 | 160 | 170 | 180 | 190 | 200 | 210 | 220 | 230 | 240 | 250 |
|---|---|---|---|---|---|---|---|---|---|---|---|---|---|---|---|---|
| 5'0" | 20 | 21 | 23 | 25 | 27 | 29 | 31 | 33 | 35 | 37 | 39 | 41 | 43 | 45 | 47 | 49 |
| 5'1" | 19 | 21 | 23 | 25 | 26 | 28 | 30 | 32 | 34 | 36 | 38 | 40 | 42 | 43 | 45 | 47 |
| 5'2" | 18 | 20 | 22 | 24 | 26 | 27 | 29 | 31 | 33 | 35 | 37 | 38 | 40 | 42 | 44 | 46 |
| 5'3" | 18 | 19 | 21 | 23 | 25 | 27 | 28 | 30 | 32 | 34 | 35 | 37 | 39 | 41 | 43 | 44 |
| 5'4" | 17 | 19 | 21 | 22 | 24 | 26 | 27 | 29 | 31 | 33 | 34 | 36 | 38 | 39 | 41 | 43 |
| 5'5" | 17 | 18 | 20 | 22 | 23 | 25 | 27 | 28 | 30 | 32 | 33 | 35 | 37 | 38 | 40 | 42 |
| 5'6" | 16 | 18 | 19 | 21 | 23 | 24 | 26 | 27 | 29 | 31 | 32 | 34 | 36 | 37 | 39 | 40 |
| 5'7" | 16 | 17 | 19 | 20 | 22 | 23 | 25 | 27 | 28 | 30 | 31 | 33 | 34 | 36 | 38 | 39 |
| 5'8" | 15 | 17 | 18 | 20 | 21 | 23 | 24 | 26 | 27 | 29 | 30 | 32 | 33 | 35 | 36 | 38 |
| 5'9" | 15 | 16 | 18 | 19 | 21 | 22 | 24 | 25 | 27 | 28 | 30 | 31 | 32 | 34 | 35 | 37 |
| 5'10" | 14 | 16 | 17 | 19 | 20 | 22 | 23 | 24 | 26 | 27 | 29 | 30 | 32 | 33 | 34 | 36 |
| 5'11" | 14 | 15 | 17 | 18 | 20 | 21 | 22 | 24 | 25 | 26 | 28 | 29 | 31 | 32 | 33 | 35 |
| 6'0" | 14 | 15 | 16 | 18 | 19 | 20 | 22 | 23 | 24 | 26 | 27 | 28 | 30 | 31 | 33 | 34 |
| 6'1" | 13 | 15 | 16 | 17 | 18 | 20 | 21 | 22 | 24 | 25 | 26 | 28 | 29 | 30 | 32 | 33 |
| 6'2" | 13 | 14 | 15 | 17 | 18 | 19 | 21 | 22 | 23 | 24 | 26 | 27 | 28 | 30 | 31 | 32 |
| 6'3" | 12 | 14 | 15 | 16 | 17 | 19 | 20 | 21 | 22 | 24 | 25 | 26 | 27 | 29 | 30 | 31 |
| 6'4" | 12 | 13 | 15 | 16 | 17 | 18 | 19 | 21 | 22 | 23 | 24 | 26 | 27 | 28 | 29 | 30 |

BMI interpretation according to National Heart, Lung, and Blood Institute guidelines

| | |
|---|---|
| Underweight | under 18.5 |
| Normal | 18.5–24.9 |
| Overweight | 25–29.9 |
| Obese | 30 and over |

## Table 3. Fiber Content of Selected Foods

| FOOD | AMOUNT | TOTAL FIBER (GRAMS) |
| --- | --- | --- |
| Whole oats | 3/4 cup | 12.4 |
| Black beans | 1/2 cup | 7.5 |
| Spaghetti, whole wheat, cooked | 1 cup | 6.3 |
| Kidney beans | 1/2 cup | 5.5 |
| Bran flake cereal | 3/4 cup | 5.2 |
| Potato, baked with skin | 1 medium | 4.8 |
| Spinach, cooked | 1/2 cup | 4.3 |
| Pear, with skin | 1 medium | 4 |
| Apple, with skin | 1 medium | 3.7 |
| Brown rice, cooked | 1/2 cup | 3.5 |
| Orange | 1 medium | 3.3 |
| Oatmeal, cooked | 3/4 cup | 3.0 |
| Banana | 1 medium | 2.8 |
| Round oat cereal | 1 cup | 2.6 |
| Broccoli | 1/2 cup | 2.3 |
| Corn | 1/2 cup | 2.3 |
| Peanuts | 1 ounce | 2.3 |
| Spaghetti, cooked | 1 cup | 2.3 |
| Peanut butter, chunky | 2 tablespoons | 2.1 |
| Whole wheat bread | 1 slice | 2.0 |
| Strawberries | 1/2 cup whole | 1.6 |
| English muffin | 1 | 1.5 |
| Walnuts | 1 ounce | 1.4 |
| Popcorn | 1 cup | 1.2 |
| White bread | 1 slice | 0.6 |
| White rice, cooked | 1/2 cup | 0.6 |
| Corn flake cereal | 1 cup | 0.3 |

Source: USDA Nutrient Database for Standard Reference

# Table 4. Daily Recommended Intake of Selected Vitamins and Minerals

## Dietary Reference Intakes (DRI)

| Age | Vitamin A (mcg) | Vitamin D (mcg) | Vitamin E (mg) (a-TE) | Vitamin K (mcg) | Vitamin C (mg) | Thiamin (mg) | Riboflavin (mg) | Niacin (mg NE) | Vitamin B$_6$ (mg) | Folate (mcg) | Vitamin B$_{12}$ (mcg) | Calcium (mg) | Phosphorus (mg) | Magnesium (mg) | Iron (mg) | Zinc (mg) | Selenium (mcg) |
|---|---|---|---|---|---|---|---|---|---|---|---|---|---|---|---|---|---|
| **INFANTS** | | | | | | | | | | | | | | | | | |
| 0–6 mo | 400 | 5 | 4 | 2.0 | 40 | 0.2 | 0.3 | 2 | 0.1 | 65 | 0.4 | 210 | 100 | 30 | 0.3 | 2 | 15 |
| 7–12 mo | 500 | 5 | 6 | 2.5 | 50 | 0.3 | 0.4 | 4 | 0.3 | 80 | 0.5 | 270 | 275 | 75 | 11 | 3 | 20 |
| **CHILDREN** | | | | | | | | | | | | | | | | | |
| 1–3 years | 300 | 5 | 6 | 30 | 15 | 0.5 | 0.5 | 6 | 0.5 | 150 | 0.9 | 500 | 460 | 80 | 7 | 3 | 20 |
| 4–8 years | 400 | 5 | 7 | 55 | 25 | 0.6 | 0.6 | 8 | 0.6 | 200 | 1.2 | 800 | 500 | 130 | 10 | 5 | 30 |
| **FEMALES** | | | | | | | | | | | | | | | | | |
| 9–13 | 600 | 5 | 11 | 60 | 45 | 0.9 | 0.9 | 12 | 1.0 | 300 | 1.8 | 1300 | 1250 | 240 | 8 | 8 | 40 |
| 14–18 | 700 | 5 | 15 | 75 | 65 | 1.0 | 1.0 | 14 | 1.2 | 400 | 2.4 | 1300 | 1250 | 360 | 15 | 9 | 55 |
| 19–30 | 700 | 5 | 15 | 90 | 75 | 1.1 | 1.1 | 14 | 1.3 | 400 | 2.4 | 1000 | 700 | 310 | 18 | 8 | 55 |
| 31–50 | 700 | 5 | 15 | 90 | 75 | 1.1 | 1.1 | 14 | 1.3 | 400 | 2.4 | 1000 | 700 | 320 | 18 | 8 | 55 |
| 51–70 | 700 | 10 | 15 | 90 | 75 | 1.1 | 1.1 | 14 | 1.5 | 400 | 2.4 | 1200 | 700 | 320 | 8 | 8 | 55 |
| 71+ | 700 | 15 | 15 | 90 | 75 | 1.1 | 1.1 | 14 | 1.5 | 400 | 2.4 | 1200 | 700 | 320 | 8 | 8 | 55 |
| **PREGNANCY** | | | | | | | | | | | | | | | | | |
| under 19 | 750 | 5 | 15 | 75 | 80 | 1.4 | 1.4 | 18 | 1.9 | 600 | 2.6 | 1300 | 1250 | 400 | 27 | 13 | 60 |
| 19–30 | 770 | 5 | 15 | 90 | 85 | 1.4 | 1.4 | 18 | 1.9 | 600 | 2.6 | 1000 | 700 | 350 | 27 | 11 | 60 |
| 31–50 | 770 | 5 | 15 | 90 | 85 | 1.4 | 1.4 | 18 | 1.9 | 600 | 2.6 | 1000 | 700 | 360 | 27 | 11 | 60 |
| **LACTATION** | | | | | | | | | | | | | | | | | |
| under 19 | 1200 | 5 | 19 | 75 | 115 | 1.5 | 1.6 | 17 | 2.0 | 500 | 2.8 | 1300 | 1250 | 360 | 10 | 14 | 70 |
| 19–30 | 1300 | 5 | 19 | 90 | 120 | 1.5 | 1.6 | 17 | 2.0 | 500 | 2.8 | 1000 | 700 | 310 | 9 | 12 | 70 |
| 31–50 | 1300 | 5 | 19 | 90 | 120 | 1.5 | 1.6 | 17 | 2.0 | 500 | 2.8 | 1000 | 700 | 320 | 9 | 12 | 70 |
| **MALES** | | | | | | | | | | | | | | | | | |
| 9–13 | 600 | 5 | 11 | 60 | 45 | 0.9 | 0.9 | 12 | 1.0 | 300 | 1.8 | 1300 | 1250 | 240 | 8 | 8 | 40 |
| 14–18 | 900 | 5 | 15 | 75 | 75 | 1.2 | 1.3 | 16 | 1.3 | 400 | 2.4 | 1300 | 1250 | 410 | 11 | 11 | 55 |
| 19–30 | 900 | 5 | 15 | 120 | 90 | 1.2 | 1.3 | 16 | 1.3 | 400 | 2.4 | 1000 | 700 | 400 | 8 | 11 | 55 |
| 31–50 | 900 | 5 | 15 | 120 | 90 | 1.2 | 1.3 | 16 | 1.3 | 400 | 2.4 | 1000 | 700 | 420 | 8 | 11 | 55 |
| 51–70 | 900 | 10 | 15 | 120 | 90 | 1.2 | 1.3 | 16 | 1.7 | 400 | 2.4 | 1200 | 700 | 420 | 8 | 11 | 55 |
| 71+ | 900 | 15 | 15 | 120 | 90 | 1.2 | 1.3 | 16 | 1.7 | 400 | 2.4 | 1200 | 700 | 420 | 8 | 11 | 55 |

# Glossary

**Absolute risk:** The chance or probability that a person will develop a specific disease during a specified period of time.

**Adenomatous polyps:** Small growths on the lining of the colon that have the potential to become cancerous.

**Adult-onset diabetes (type 2):** A condition that occurs when the pancreas does not produce enough insulin or when the body does not effectively use the insulin that is produced. Also called non-insulin-dependent diabetes mellitus.

**Amenorrhea:** A disorder characterized by the absence of menstrual periods for six or more months in a woman who has not yet gone through menopause.

**Angina:** A temporary pain (burning, pressure, or aching) in the chest that usually occurs when the heart's demand for blood is more than the arteries can supply—for instance, during physical exertion. Also called angina pectoris.

**Antioxidant:** A special group of vitamins, minerals, and other compounds that counteract the damage done to cells by oxidation. Oxidation is thought to be partially responsible for the effects of aging and for certain diseases. Examples of antioxidants include vitamin C, vitamin E, and carotenoids.

**Asthma:** A persistent inflammatory disorder of the airways of the lungs. Causes seasonal or periodic episodes of wheezing and coughing that may lead to sudden and/or severe difficulty in breathing.

**Atherosclerosis:** The dangerous narrowing of a blood vessel due to the buildup of cholesterol and other debris along the vessel wall.

**Birth control pill:** A form of contraception that prevents pregnancy primarily by overriding the hormonal changes that cause a woman to ovulate. Also called oral contraceptives.

**Blood clot:** A hardened mass of blood.

**Blood pressure:** The force in the arteries created when the heart pumps blood through the body. Systolic pressure refers to the temporary increase in pressure created in the arteries when the heart pumps. Diastolic pressure refers to the temporary decrease in pressure that occurs when the heart relaxes between beats.

**Body Mass Index (BMI):** A ratio of weight to height reflecting body fat. Specifically, weight (in pounds) divided by height (in inches) squared, with this result multiplied by 704.5.

$$BMI = [(weight\ (in\ pounds)/height\ (in\ inches)^2 \times 704.5]$$

**Breast self-examination:** A method used by women to become familiar with the normal appearance and feel of their breast tissue so that if a change occurs, it can be detected early.

**Carotenoid:** A yellow to deep-red pigment found in many vegetables and some animal products. Many carotenoids are potent antioxidants.

**Cataract:** A clouding of the normally transparent lens of the eye.

**Chemoprevention:** The use of drugs to prevent disease occurrence.

**Cholesterol:** A fat-like substance produced by the liver and contained in all food from animal sources. Cholesterol is an essential component of body cells and a precursor of bile acids and certain hormones.

**Chronic obstructive pulmonary disease (COPD):** A group of respiratory diseases characterized by difficulty in breathing air out. The conditions may be totally reversible (as in asthma) or associated with chronic mucous hypersecretion (as in chronic bronchitis) and irreversible obstruction (as in emphysema). Also called chronic obstructive lung disease.

**Clinical breast examination:** A physical examination of the breasts by a trained medical professional.

**Cohort:** A large group of people. A cohort study follows a large group of people over time—some who have a particular characteristic and some who do not—to see who develops the disease being studied.

**Colon:** The longest part of the large intestine.

**Coronary heart disease:** A condition that occurs when the buildup of cholesterol and fat in the arteries causes them to become too narrow and blocks the flow of blood.

**Deep vein thrombosis:** A condition that occurs when a blood clot forms in one of the veins deep in the body, such as those in the leg or pelvis.

**Deoxyribonucleic acid (DNA):** The substance that contains the genetic code, found in the nucleus of the cell. DNA is composed of a double strand of tiny units called nucleotides. Strings of nucleotides make up genes, which are the blueprint for the structure and function of the human body.

**Diabetes:** See definitions for adult-onset diabetes (type 2) and juvenile diabetes (type 1).

**Ectopic pregnancy:** A pregnancy that develops outside of the uterus, usually in one of the fallopian tubes. Also called a tubal pregnancy.

**Embolus:** A solid material, such as a blood clot, that breaks loose from where it was formed and becomes lodged in another blood vessel.

**Endogenous estrogen:** Estrogen that is produced naturally in the body.

**Endometrium:** The lining of the uterus.

**Energy expenditure:** The amount of calories that an individual burns in a day.

**Estrogen:** A female hormone that is produced by the ovaries and adrenal glands, is important to reproduction, and may stimulate some cancers to grow.

**Exercise:** Physical activity that is planned, structured, and done specifically to improve physical fitness. Includes aerobic exercise, flexibility exercise, and strength training.

**Exogenous estrogen:** Estrogen that is produced outside the body, such as that found in birth control pills and postmenopausal hormones.

**Family history:** The occurrence of a disease or condition among family members. Assessing study participants' family history is a useful first step in identifying familial associations that may support either a genetic basis or a common environmental basis for a disease.

**Fiber:** A plant material that resists digestion by gastrointestinal enzymes. Most fiber originates from the cell walls of fruit, vegetable, and cereal grain tissues.

**Fibrinogen:** A type of protein involved in blood clotting.

**Folate:** A B vitamin that occurs in green plants, fresh fruit, liver, and yeast. Also called folic acid.

**Gallstone:** Occurs when bile in the gallbladder crystallizes, forming small stones that grow larger.

**Gene:** The basic unit of hereditary material. A gene is composed of a particular sequence of nucleic acids and found in a particular spot on a chromosome. The information in a person's genes is inherited from previous generations on both sides of a person's family.

**Gene mutation:** A mistake in or alteration of the information contained in a gene.

**Glycemic index:** A measure of how glucose levels in the blood change following the consumption of foods that contain carbohydrates.

**Hemorrhagic stroke:** A type of stroke that occurs when a blood vessel ruptures, cutting off the supply of oxygen and nutrition to part of the brain.

**High density lipoprotein (HDL) cholesterol:** A lipoprotein that protects the arteries by transporting cholesterol from body cells to the liver and other sites for elimination. Often called "good cholesterol."

**Hyperplasia:** The noncancerous growth of tissue that results in a larger but still normal appearance.

**Hypertension:** A condition in which the blood is pumped through the body at an abnormally high pressure. Also called high blood pressure.

**Hysterectomy:** The surgical removal of the uterus. Simple hysterectomy removes only the uterus. Complete hysterectomy also removes the fallopian tubes and ovaries.

**Insulin-like growth factor (IGF):** A naturally circulating hormone that is important in growth and development.

**Ischemic stroke:** A type of stroke caused by an interruption in the flow of blood to the brain, almost always due to a blood clot blocking a blood vessel.

**Juvenile diabetes (type I):** A condition that occurs when the immune system attacks the insulin-producing cells of the pancreas, usually before age thirty. Leads the pancreas to produce progressively less insulin. Also called insulin-dependent diabetes mellitus.

**Lipoprotein:** A combination of fats and proteins that, when packaged together, transport cholesterol in the blood.

**Low density lipoprotein (LDL) cholesterol:** A lipoprotein that deposits cholesterol on the walls of the arteries. Often called "bad cholesterol."

**Mammogram:** An X-ray of the breast that is designed to detect abnormal densities or masses that may require further investigation.

**Mastectomy:** The surgical removal of the breast and some surrounding tissue.

**Menarche:** The onset of menstrual periods, marking the maturation of a woman's reproductive organs and the ability to bear children.

**Menopause:** A gradual process in which menstrual periods become irregular and then stop altogether.

**Metastases:** The spread of cancer to other organs through the lymphatic and/or circulatory system.

**Monounsaturated fats:** Fatty acids that are usually liquid at room temperature. Major sources include olive, peanut, sesame, and canola oil, and in the American diet, red meat.

**Myocardial infarction:** A blockage of a blood vessel in the heart leading to the death of some of the heart tissue beyond the blockage. Also called a heart attack.

**Nutrients:** Chemical substances required by humans to maintain life and reproduce. Examples include carbohydrates, proteins, fats, vitamins, and minerals.

**Obesity:** A weight that corresponds to an amount of body fat that is linked to serious health problems.

**Observational study:** A study in which participants report their daily activities to researchers, who then use this information to understand how lifestyle choices affect health. Examples include the Nurses' Health Study and the Framingham Heart Study.

**Oligomenorrhea:** A disorder characterized by abnormally infrequent or scant menstrual flow.

**Omega-3 fatty acids:** A type of fat that is found in soybean, rapeseed, and fish oils.

**Osteoporosis:** A condition characterized by the loss of bone mass. Occurs when new bone is not created as quickly as old bone is broken down. Leads to a loss of bone tissue, brittleness, and a higher risk of fracture.

**Ovulation:** The release of an egg from the ovary, at which time it is available to be fertilized by sperm.

**Physical activity:** Any movement that substantially increases the amount of calories burned in a day. Examples include walking, gardening, and washing the car.

**Phytoestrogen:** Estrogen that is produced by plants.

**Polycystic ovary syndrome:** A condition in which many cysts develop from ovarian follicles that have failed to rupture and release eggs. Often associated with obesity, irregular menstrual cycles, and excess production of male hormone.

**Polyp:** A noncancerous growth that is found protruding from tissues. Polyps often occur in the sinuses and in the lining of the colon.

**Polyunsaturated fats:** A type of fat that is usually liquid at room temperature. Primarily from plant and fish sources. Examples include liquid vegetable oils, oil-based salad dressing, and fatty fish (such as salmon).

**Postmenopausal hormones:** Exogenous hormones that contain estrogen and sometimes a progestin. Also called hormone replacement therapy.

**Potassium:** A mineral that is involved in the electrical stimulation of nerves and muscles. Found in high concentrations in legumes, nuts, and fruits.

**Premenopausal:** Referring to women who have not yet entered menopause.

**Prevention:** The elimination of causes of disease from the population, so that the risk of disease is either reduced (as in the case of many infectious diseases today) or postponed until later in life (as in heart disease and various cancers).

**Probability:** The likelihood that a particular event will occur.

**Progesterone:** A hormone secreted by the ovaries after ovulation and/or before implantation of the fertilized egg.

**Progestin:** A synthetic version of the natural hormone progesterone.

**Progestogen:** A hormone that has the same effect in the body as progesterone; refers to both natural progesterone and progestin.

**Prophylactic mastectomy:** The surgical removal of one or both breasts to lower the risk of breast cancer. Also called preventive mastectomy.

**Pulmonary embolism:** The blockage of one or more portions of the arteries in the lungs by a blood clot that has traveled through the bloodstream.

**Randomized controlled trial:** A study in which participants are randomly assigned to a particular behavior or treatment.

**Relative risk:** The ratio of two absolute risks. The top half of the ratio is the absolute risk of disease in people who have a particular characteristic, and the bottom half is the absolute risk in people who do not have that characteristic.

$$\frac{\text{Absolute risk of disease among people with a particular characteristic}}{\text{Absolute risk of disease among people without the particular characteristic}}$$

**Rheumatoid arthritis:** An inflammatory disease that damages the tissue connecting bones and joints.

**Risk (of disease):** The probability that a disease will develop in an individual during a specified time period.

**Risk factor:** Any factor that can cause a person to be more or less likely to develop a disease. For example, smoking is a risk factor for lung cancer.

**Saturated fat:** A type of fat that is usually solid at room temperature. Found primarily in animal foods, such as red meat, poultry, butter, and whole milk.

**Screening:** A test or procedure used to detect disease in a person who does not have any symptoms of that disease.

**Trans-unsaturated fats:** A type of fat found in products such as shortening and hydrogenated oils. Hydrogenation is a process that makes oils more solid at room temperature. Hydrogenated oils give processed foods, such as margarine and crackers, a longer shelf life.

**Triglyceride:** The main chemical form of the fats that circulate in the bloodstream.

**Tubal ligation:** A form of contraception. A surgical procedure in which a woman's fallopian tubes are either cut, tied, or clamped to prevent an egg released by an ovary from moving down the fallopian tube into the uterus.

**Vitamin:** An essential substance that facilitates chemical reactions in body cells and helps process food. Each vitamin has a specific role and regulates different body processes.

# Selected Readings

## The Nurses' Health Study and Other Studies

Colditz, G.A., et al. "The Nurses' Health Study: 20-year Contribution to the Understanding of Health Among Women." *Journal of Women's Health* 6: 49–61 (1997).

Folsom, A.R., et al. "Association of Incident Carcinoma of the Endometrium with Body Weight and Fat Distribution in Older Women: Early Findings of the Iowa Women's Health Study." *Cancer Research* 49: 6828–31 (1989).

*Framingham Heart Study: 50 Years of Research Success.* National Heart, Lung, and Blood Institute, National Institutes of Health, 1998. Available from http://www.nhlbi.nih.gov/about/framingham/

Thun, M.J., et al. "Epidemiological Research at the American Cancer Society." *Cancer Epidemiology, Biomarkers & Prevention* 9: 861–68 (2000).

Women's Health Initiative Study Group. "Design of the Women's Health Initiative Clinical Trial and Observational Study." *Controlled Clinical Trials* 19: 61–109 (1998).

## Cancer

Hankinson, S.E., et al. "A Prospective Study of Reproductive Factors and Risk of Epithelial Ovarian Cancer." *Cancer* 76: 284–90 (1995).

Kelsey, J.L., et al. "Epidemiology and Prevention of Breast Cancer." *Annual Review of Public Health* 17: 47–67 (1996).

Manson, J.E., et al. "The Case for a Comprehensive National Campaign to Prevent Melanoma and Associated Mortality." *Epidemiology* 11: 728–34 (2000).

Tomeo, C.A., et al. "Harvard Report on Cancer Prevention. Volume 3: Prevention of Colon Cancer in the United States." *Cancer Causes and Control* 10: 167–80 (1999).

## Cardiovascular Disease (Heart Disease and Stroke)

Bronner, L.L., et al. "Primary Prevention of Stroke." *New England Journal of Medicine* 333: 1392–1400 (1995).

Rich-Edwards, J.W., et al. "The Primary Prevention of Coronary Heart Disease in Women." *New England Journal of Medicine* 332: 1758–66 (1995).

Stampfer, M.J., et al. "Primary Prevention of Coronary Heart Disease in Women Through Diet and Lifestyle." *New England Journal of Medicine* 343: 530–37 (2000).

## CONTRACEPTION

Hatcher, R.A., et al. *Contraceptive Technology,* 17th rev. ed. New York: Ardent Media, 1998.

## DIABETES

*Diabetes in America,* 2nd ed. National Diabetes Data Group, National Institutes of Health, National Institute of Diabetes and Digestive and Kidney Diseases. Available from http://diabetes-in-america.s-3.com/

## DIET

*Dietary Guidelines for Americans* 2000, 5th ed. U.S. Department of Agriculture. Available from http://www.usda.gov/cnpp/DietGd.pdf

Willett, W. C., editor. *Eat, Drink and Be Healthy: The Harvard Medical School Guide to Healthy Eating.* New York: Simon & Schuster, 2001.

## GENERAL HEALTH

Boston Women's Health Book Collective. *Our Bodies, Ourselves for the New Century: A Book by and for Women.* New York: Simon & Schuster, 1998.

Komaroff, A.L., editor in chief. *Harvard Medical School Family Health Guide.* New York: Simon & Schuster, 1999.

Siegal, D.L., et al. *Ourselves, Growing Older: Women Aging with Knowledge and Power.* New York: Simon & Schuster, 1994.

## OSTEOPOROSIS

Cummings, S.R., et al. "Risk Factors for Hip Fracture in White Women." *New England Journal of Medicine* 332: 767–73 (1995).

*Osteoporosis Prevention, Diagnosis, and Therapy. NIH Consensus Statement Online March 27–29, 2000.* National Institutes of Health, 2000. Available from http://odp.od.nih.gov/consensus/cons/111/111_statement.htm

## PHYSICAL ACTIVITY

*Physical Activity and Health: A Report of the Surgeon General.* U.S. Department of Health and Human Services, Public Health Service, Centers for Disease Control and Prevention, National Center for Chronic Disease Prevention and Health Promotion, 1996. Available from http://www.cdc.gov/nccdphp/sgr/contents.htm

Manson J.E., et al. "A Prospective Study of Walking as Compared with Vigorous Exercise in the Prevention of Coronary Heart Disease in Women." *New England Journal of Medicine* 341: 650–58 (1999).

Manson, J., and P. Amend. *The 30-Minute Fitness Solution: A Four-Step Plan for Women of All Ages.* Cambridge, MA: Harvard University Press, 2001.

## POSTMENOPAUSAL HORMONES

Grady, D., et al. "Hormone Therapy to Prevent Disease and Prolong Life in Postmenopausal Women." *Annals of Internal Medicine* 117: 1016–3 7 (1992).

Hulley, S., et al. "Randomized Trial of Estrogen Plus Progestin for Secondary Prevention of Coronary Heart Disease in Postmenopausal Women." *Journal of the American Medical Association* 280: 605–13 (1998).

North American Menopause Society. "A Decision Tree for the Use of Estrogen Replacement Therapy or Hormone Replacement Therapy in Postmenopausal Women: Consensus Opinion of the North American Menopause Society." *Menopause* 7: 76–86 (2000).

## SMOKING

*Smoking and Health.* Report of the Advisory Committee to the Surgeon General of the Public Health Service, 1964. U. S. Public Health Service. Available from http://www.cdc.gov/tobacco/sgr/sgr_1964/sgr64.htm

*Women and Smoking: A Report of the Surgeon General.* U.S. Public Health Service, 2001. Available from http://www.cdc.gov/tobacco/sgrpage.htm

*Treating Tobacco Use and Dependence. Quick Reference Guide for Clinicians, October 2000.* U.S. Public Health Service. Available from http://www.surgeongeneral.gov/tobacco/tobaqrg.htm

*You Can Quit Smoking. Consumer Guide, June 2000.* U.S. Public Health Service. Available from http://www.surgeongeneral.gov/tobacco/consquits.htm

WEIGHT

*Clinical Guidelines on the Identification, Evaluation, and Treatment of Overweight and Obesity in Adults.* National Heart, Lung, and Blood Institute, National Institutes of Health, 1998. Available from http://www.nhlbi.nih.gov/guidelines/obesity/prctgd_c.pdf

Manson, J.E., et al. "America's Obesity Epidemic and Women's Health." *Journal of Women's Health* 5: 329–34 (1996).

Willett, W.C., et al. "Guidelines for Healthy Weight." *New England Journal of Medicine* 341: 427–34 (1999).

# Index

adult–onset (Type 2) diabetes. *See* diabetes.

African Americans: and asthma, 255; and cancer, 72, 82, 241; and CHD, 38–39, 64; and diabetes, 38, 146, 153; and hypertension, 417; and osteoporosis, 192; and strokes, 121, 126; and weight, 38; and Women's Health Initiative, 18

age, 43, 81; and alcohol, 393, 397, 398; and aspirin/NSAIDs, 59, 489; and birth control, 459, 466, 468; and dietary fats, 356–57; at menarche, 74, 75, 89, 94, 96, 97, 100, 101, 107, 193, 215, 219; at menopause, 96, 97, 99, 100, 101, 107, 193, 215, 217–18, 219; and smoking, 99, 319, 334, 348; and vitamins and minerals, 408, 417; and weight, 51, 87–89, 297; when giving first birth, 82, 94, 95–96, 100, 107. *See also* postmenopausal women; premenopausal women; *specific disease*

alcohol, 47, 67, 90, 134, 202, 324, 325, 387, 390–99. *See also specific disease*

alpha–linolenic acid, 53, 54, 352, 354–55, 376

alternative medicine, 347, 447, 451, 452

Alzheimer's disease, 92, 267–72, 287, 437, 494

American Cancer Society: and alcohol, 396; and breast cancer, 103, 105; Cancer Prevention Study II of, 14–15, 225, 228, 396, 440; contributions to research of, 14–15; and life span, 396; and lung cancer, 116; and ovarian cancer, 225, 228, 440; and skin cancer, 251; and smoking, 347

American Indians, 18, 81, 126, 146, 153, 193

antioxidants, 266, 374–75, 403–4, 407. *See also specific antioxidant or disease*

arthritis, 201, 259–62, 271–72, 310, 485, 487, 493, 495, 497

Asian Americans, 18, 39, 81, 126–27, 146, 154

aspirin, 5, 138, 485, 486, 487–95, 496, 497; and bleeding/clotting, 5, 182, 485, 486, 487, 488, 495, 496, 497, 498, 499; and

inflammations, 485–86, 487, 496, 497; for injuries, 485, 486; medication strategies for, 497–99; and menstrual symptoms, 487, 497. *See also* nonsteroidal anti-inflammatory drugs (NSAIDs); *specific disease*

asthma, 161, 201, 254–59, 271–72, 287, 310–311, 319, 329, 335, 440–41, 452

atherosclerosis: and blood cholesterol, 133; and diabetes, 130; and diet, 54, 56, 135; and dietary fats, 140, 354; infections that may cause, 63; and nuts, 378; and other diseases, 34, 35, 36, 45, 49, 54, 56, 61, 63, 129; and physical activity, 49; and smoking, 128; and strokes, 128, 129, 130, 133, 135, 136, 140; and vitamins and minerals, 136, 401, 410

basal cell cancer, 236–37, 244, 247. *See also* skin cancer

Bates, Carol, 65–69, 143–45, 185–88, 248–53, 271–72, 483–84, 497–99

beta-carotene, 373, 374, 377, 403, 404, 405, 406, 407. *See also specific disease*

birth: age when giving first, 82, 94, 95–96, 100, 107

birth control: background/overview about, 459–60; barrier methods of, 460, 472–474, 478; benefits and risks of, 473–74, 476, 480–81; and breast-feeding, 469; expense of, 482; and fertility, 480; forms of, 459; and medical history, 468, 483–484; and menstruation, 461, 469, 470, 471, 477–78, 480; natural methods of, 477–78, 479, 480; personal preferences about, 484; and progesterone/progestin, 460–61, 463, 469, 470, 471, 480, 482; reliability of, 460, 461, 467, 478, 479, 480, 484; and sexually transmitted diseases, 272, 459, 473–74, 478, 479–480, 484; and shifting contraceptive priorities, 459, 460; and smoking, 60–61, 138, 332, 466, 468, 469, 483; strate-

# Figure Sources

Figure 3-1: Ries, L.A.G., et al. "SEER Cancer Statistics, 1973–1997." The SEER Cancer Statistics Review website (http://seer.cancer.gov/Publications/CSR 1973_1997/), 2000.

Figure 3-2: Illustration by the Channing Laboratory.

Figure 3-3: Colditz, G. A., et al. "Family History, Age, and Risk of Breast Cancer." *Journal of the American Medical Association* 270: 338–43 (1993).

Figure 4-1: Lloyd-Jones, D. M., et al. "Lifetime Risk of Developing Coronary Heart Disease." *Lancet* 353: 89–92 (1999).

Figure 4-2: Copyright © Harriet Greenfield.

Figure 4-3: Colditz, G. A., et al. "A Prospective Study of Parental History of Myocardial Infarction and Coronary Heart Disease in Women." *American Journal of Epidemiology* 123: 48–58 (1986).

Figure 4-4: Department of Health and Human Services, Office of Minority Health. "Coronary Heart Disease Death Rates" table. The Initiative to Eliminate Racial and Ethnic Disparities in Health website (http://www.raceand health.omhrc.gov/3rdpgBlue/Cardio/k12.gif), 1999.

Figure 4-5: Manolio T. A., et al. "Cholesterol and Heart Disease in Older Persons and Women. Review of an NHLBI Workshop." *Annals of Epidemiology* 2: 161–76 (1992).

Figure 4-6: National Institutes of Health; National Heart, Lung, and Blood Institute; National High Blood Pressure Education Program. *The Sixth Report of the Joint National Committee on the Prevention, Detection, Evaluation, and Treatment of High Blood Pressure*. National Heart, Lung, and Blood Institute website (http://www.nhlbi.nih.gov/guidelines/hypertension/jncintro.htm), 1997.

Figure 4-7: Manson, J. E., et al. "A Prospective Study of Walking as Compared with Vigorous Exercise in the Prevention of Coronary Heart Disease in Women." *New England Journal of Medicine* 341: 650–58 (1999).

Figure 4-8: Willett, W. C., et al. "Weight, Weight Change, and Coronary Heart Disease in Women: Risk Within the 'Normal' Weight Range." *Journal of the American Medical Association* 273: 461–65 (1995).

Figure 4-9: Rimm, E. B., et al. "Folate and Vitamin $B_6$ from Diet and Supplements in Relation to Risk of Coronary Heart Disease Among Women." *Journal of the American Medical Association* 279: 359–64 (1998).

Figure 5-1: See source for Figure 3-1.

Figure 5-2: See source for Figure 3-1.

Figure 5-3: Copyright © Harriet Greenfield.

Figure 5-4: See source for Figure 3-1.

Figure 5-5: See source for Figure 3-3.

Figure 5-6: Byrne, C., et al. "Mammographic Features and Breast Cancer Risk: Effects with Time, Age, and Menopause Status." *Journal of the National Cancer Institute* 87: 1622–29 (1995).

Figure 5-7: van den Brandt, P. A., et al. "Height, Weight, Weight Change, and Postmenopausal Breast Cancer Risk: The Netherlands Cohort Study." *Cancer Causes and Control* 8: 39–47 (1997).

Figure 5-8: Hankinson, S. E., et al. "Plasma Sex Steroid Hormone Levels and Risk of Breast Cancer in Postmenopausal Women." *Journal of the National Cancer Institute* 90: 1292–99 (1998).

Figure 5-9: Hunter, D. J., et al. "Cohort Studies of Fat Intake and the Risk of Breast Cancer—A Pooled Analysis." *New England Journal of Medicine* 334: 356–61 (1996).

Figure 5-10: Huang, Z., et al. "Dual Effects of Weight and Weight Gain on Breast Cancer Risk." *Journal of the American Medical Association* 278: 1407–11 (1997).

Figure 5-11: Willett, W. C., et al. "Moderate Alcohol Consumption and the Risk of Breast Cancer." *New England Journal of Medicine* 316: 1174–80 (1987).

Figure 5-12: Colditz, G. A., et al. "The Use of Estrogens and Progestins and the Risk of Breast Cancer in Postmenopausal Women." *New England Journal of Medicine* 332: 1589–93 (1995).

Figure 5-13: Collaborative Group on Hormonal Factors in Breast Cancer. "Breast Cancer and Hormonal Contraceptives: Collaborative Reanalysis of Individual Data on 53,297 Women with Breast Cancer and 100,239 Women without Breast Cancer from 54 Epidemiological Studies." *Lancet* 347: 1713–27 (1996).

Figure 5-14: Rosner, B., et al. "Reproductive Risk Factors in a Prospective Study of Breast Cancer: The Nurses' Health Study." *American Journal of Epidemiology* 139: 819–35 (1994).

Figure 6-1: See source for Figure 3-1.

Figure 6-2: Komaroff, A. L., editor in chief. *Harvard Medical School Family Health Guide.* New York: Simon & Schuster, 1999.

Figure 6-3: See source for Figure 3-1.

Figure 6-4: Horwitz, R. I., et al. "An Ecogenetic Hypothesis for Lung Cancer in Women." *Archives of Internal Medicine* 148: 2609–12 (1988).

Figure 6-5: Speizer, F. E., et al. "Prospective Study of Smoking, Antioxidant Intake, and Lung Cancer in Middle-Aged Women (USA)." *Cancer Causes and Control* 10: 475–82 (1999).

Figure 6-6: See source for Figure 6-5.

Figure 7-1: Grady, D., et al. "Hormone Therapy to Prevent Disease and Prolong Life in Postmenopausal Women." *Annals of Internal Medicine* 117: 1016–37 (1992).

Figure 7-2: Copyright © Harriet Greenfield.

Figure 7-3: *State-Specific Prevalence of Selected Health Behaviors, by Race and Ethnicity—Behavioral Risk Factor Surveillance System.* Centers for Disease Control and Prevention. Morbidity and Mortality Weekly Report 49(SS02): 1–60 (2000).

Figure 7-4: Rexrode, K. M., et al. "A Prospective Study of Body Mass Index, Weight Change, and Risk of Stroke in Women." *Journal of the American Medical Association* 277: 1539–45 (1997).

Figure 7-5: Hu, F. B., et al. "Physical Activity and Risk of Stroke in Women." *Journal of the American Medical Association* 283: 2961–67 (2000).

Figure 7-6: Stampfer, M. J., et al. "A Prospective Study of Moderate Alcohol Consumption and the Risk of Coronary Disease and Stroke in Women." *New England Journal of Medicine* 319: 267–73 (1988).

Figure 7-7: Joshipura, K. J., et al. "Fruit and Vegetable Intake in Relation to Risk of Ischemic Stroke." *Journal of the American Medical Association* 282: 1233–39 (1999).

Figure 7-8: Iso, H., et al. "Prospective Study of Calcium, Potassium, and Magnesium Intake and Risk of Stroke in Women." *Stroke* 30: 1772–79 (1999).

Figure 8-1: Department of Health and Human Services, et al. *Diabetes in America.* 2nd ed. Bethesda: U.S. Department of Health and Human Services; Public Health Service; National Institutes of Health; National Institute of Diabetes and Digestive and Kidney Diseases; National Diabetes Data Group, 1995.

Figure 8-2: Department of Health and Human Services, et al. See source for Figure 8-1.

Figure 8-3: National Center for Health Statistics. "Number of Selected Reported Chronic Conditions per 1,000 Persons, by Sex and Age: United States, 1995." National Center for Health Statistics website (http://www.cdc.gov/nchs/datawh/statab/pubd/ce95t58.htm), 1995.

Figure 8-4: Carey, V. J., et al. "Body Fat Distribution and Risk of Non-Insulin-Dependent Diabetes Mellitus in Women." *American Journal of Epidemiology* 145: 614–19 (1997).

Figure 8-5: See source for Figure 8-4.

Figure 8-6: Hu, F. B., et al. "Walking Compared with Vigorous Physical Activity and Risk of Type 2 Diabetes in Women: A Prospective Study." *Journal of the American Medical Association* 282: 1433–39 (1999).

Figure 8-7: Salmeron, J., et al. "Dietary Fiber, Glycemic Load, and Risk of Non-Insulin-Dependent Diabetes Mellitus in Women." *Journal of the American Medical Association* 277: 472–77 (1997).

Figure 9-1: See source for Figure 3-1.

Figure 9-2: Copyright © Harriet Greenfield.

Figure 9-3: See source for Figure 3-1.

Figure 9-4: Fuchs, C. S., et al. "A Prospective Study of Family History and the Risk of Colorectal Cancer." *New England Journal of Medicine* 331: 1669–74 (1994).

Figure 9-5: Martinez, M. E., et al. "Physical Activity, Body Size, and Colon Cancer in Women." *Journal of the National Cancer Institute* 89: 948–55 (1996).

Figure 9-6: Willett, W. C., et al. "Relation of Meat, Fat, and Fiber Intake to the Risk of Colon Cancer in a Prospective Study Among Women." *New England Journal of Medicine* 323: 1664–72 (1990).

Figure 9-7: Giovannucci, E., et al. "Multivitamin Use, Folate, and Colon Cancer in Women in the Nurses' Health Study." *Annals of Internal Medicine* 129: 517–24 (1998).

Figure 9-8: See source for Figure 9-5.

Figure 10-1: See source for Figure 7-1.

Figure 10-2: Cummings, S. R., et al. "Risk Factors for Hip Fracture in White Women." *New England Journal of Medicine* 332: 767–73 (1995).

Figure 10-3: See source for Figure 10-2.

Figure 10-4: Cornuz, J., et al. "Smoking, Smoking Cessation, and Risk of Hip Fracture in Women." *American Journal of Medicine* 106: 311–14 (1999).

Figure 11-1: See source for Figure 3-1.

Figure 11-2: See source for Figure 3-1.

Figure 11-3: Unpublished data from the Nurses' Health Study.

Figure 11-4: Centers for Disease Control and Prevention. "Combination Oral Contraceptive Use and the Risk of Endometrial Cancer. The Cancer and Steroid Hormone Study of the Centers for Disease Control and the National Institute of Child Health and Human Development." *Journal of the American Medical Association* 257: 796–800 (1987).

Figure 11-5: Unpublished data from the Nurses' Health Study.

Figure 12-1: See source for Figure 3-1.

Figure 12-2: Copyright © Harriet Greenfield.

Figure 12-3: See source for Figure 3-1.

Figure 12-4: Mink, P. J., et al. "Physical Activity, Waist-to-Hip Ratio, and Other Risk Factors for Ovarian Cancer: A Follow-up Study of Older Women." *Epidemiology* 7: 38–45 (1996). Poole, C. A., et al. "Influence of a Family History of Cancer Within and Across Multiple Sites on Patterns of Cancer Mortality for Women." *American Journal of Epidemiology* 149: 454–62 (1999).

Figure 12-5: Hankinson, S. E., et al. "A Quantitative Assessment of Oral Contraceptive Use and Risk of Ovarian Cancer." *Obstetrics and Gynecology* 80: 708–14 (1992).

Figure 12-6: Hankinson, S. E., et al. "Tubal Ligation, Hysterectomy, and Risk of Ovarian Cancer: A Prospective Study." *Journal of the American Medical Association* 270: 2813–18 (1993).

Figure 12-7: Hankinson, S. E., et al. "A Prospective Study of Reproductive Factors and Risk of Epithelial Ovarian Cancer." *Cancer* 76: 284–90 (1995).

Figure 12-8: Whittemore, A. S., et al. "Characteristics Relating to Ovarian Cancer Risk: Collaborative Analysis of 12 US Case-Control Studies. II. Invasive Epithelial Ovarian Cancers in White Women." *American Journal of Epidemiology* 136: 1184–1203 (1992).

Figure 13-1: See source for Figure 3-1.

Figure 13-2: Miller D. L., et al. "Nonmelanoma Skin Cancer in the United States: Incidence." *Journal of the American Academy of Dermatology* 30: 774–78 (1994).

Figure 13-3: See source for Figure 13-2.

Figure 13-4: See source for Figure 6-2.

Figure 13-5: See source for Figure 3-1.

Figure 13-6: D'Arcy, C., et al. "Pigmentary Traits, Ethnic Origin, Benign Nevi, and Family History as Risk Factors for Cutaneous Malignant Melanoma." *Journal of the National Cancer Institute* 72: 257–66 (1984).

Figure 13-7: Hunter, D. J., et al. "Risk Factors for Basal Cell Carcinoma in a Prospective Cohort of Women." *Annals of Epidemiology* 1: 13–23 (1991). Weinstock, M. A., et al. "Melanoma and the Sun: The Effects of Swimsuits and a 'Healthy' Tan on the Risk of Nonfamilial Malignant Melanoma in Women." *American Journal of Epidemiology* 134: 462–70 (1991). Unpublished data from the Nurses' Health Study.

Figure 13-8: Bain, C., et al. "Self-Reports of Mole Counts and Cutaneous Malignant Melanoma in Women: Methodological Issues and Risk of Disease." *American Journal of Epidemiology* 127: 703–12 (1988).

Figure 13-9: Weinstock, M. A., et al. "Nonfamilial Cutaneous Melanoma Incidence in Women Is Associated with Sun Exposure before 20 Years of Age." *Pediatrics* 84: 199–204 (1989).

Figure 14-1: Copyright © Harriet Greenfield.

Figure 14-2: Copyright © Harriet Greenfield.

Figure 14-3: Copyright © Harriet Greenfield.

Figure 15-1: Department of Health and Human Services, Public Health Service, Centers for Disease Control and Prevention, National Center for Chronic Disease Prevention and Health Promotion, Division of Nutrition and Physical Activity. *Promoting Physical Activity: A Guide for Community Action.* Champaign, IL: Human Kinetics, 1999.

Figure 15-2: See source for Figure 4-7.

Figure 15-3: See source for Figure 4-7.

Figure 15-4: See source for Figure 7-5.

Figure 15-5: See source for Figure 8-6.

Figure 15-6: See source for Figure 9-5.

Figure 15-7: Rockhill, B. J., et al. "Physical Activity and Mortality: A Sixteen-Year Prospective Study Among Women." *American Journal of Public Health* 91: 578–83 (2001).

Figure 16-1: Illustration by the Channing Laboratory.

Figure 16-2: Huang, Z., et al. "Body Weight, Weight Change, and Risk for Hypertension in Women." *Annals of Internal Medicine* 128: 81–88 (1998).

Figure 16-3: See source for Figure 16-2.

Figure 16-4: See source for Figure 8-4.

Figure 16-5: See source for Figure 8-4.

Figure 16-6: See source for Figure 4-8.

Figure 16-7: Rexrode, K. M., et al. "Abdominal Adiposity and Coronary Heart Disease in Women." *Journal of the American Medical Association* 280: 1843–48 (1998).

Figure 16-8: See source for Figure 7-4.

Figure 16-9: See source for Figure 5-10.

Figure 16-10: Unpublished data from the Nurses' Health Study.

Figure 16-11: Stampfer, M. J., et al. "Risk of Symptomatic Gallstones in Women with Severe Obesity." *American Journal of Clinical Nutrition* 55: 652–58 (1992).

Figure 16-12: Manson, J. E., et al. "Body Weight and Mortality Among Women." *New England Journal of Medicine* 333: 677–85 (1995).

Figure 17-1: Centers for Disease Control and Prevention. "Percentage of Adults Who Were Current, Former, or Never Smokers,+ Overall and by Sex, Race, Hispanic Origin, Age, and Education, National Health Interview Surveys, Selected Years—United States, 1965–1995." Centers for Disease Control and Prevention website (http://www.cdc.gov/tobacco/research_data/adults_prev/adstat1.htm), 2000.

Figure 17-2: See source for Figure 6-5.

Figure 17-3: See source for Figure 6-5.

Figure 17-4: Blot, W. J., et al. "Smoking and Drinking in Relation to Oral and Pharyngeal Cancer." *Cancer Research* 48: 3282–87 (1988).

Figure 17-5: Troisi, R. J., et al. "Cigarette Smoking and Incidence of Chronic Bronchitis and Asthma in Women." *Chest* 108: 1557–61 (1995).

Figure 17-6: Willett, W. C., et al. "Relative and Absolute Excess Risks of Coronary Heart Disease Among Women Who Smoke Cigarettes." *New England Journal of Medicine* 317: 1303–9 (1987).

Figure 17-7: Kawachi, I., et al. "Smoking Cessation and Time Course of Decreased Risk of Coronary Heart Disease in Women." *Archives of Internal Medicine* 154: 169–75 (1994).

Figure 17-8: See source for Figure 17-7.

Figure 17-9: Kawachi, I., et al. "A Prospective Study of Passive Smoking and Coronary Heart Disease." *Circulation* 95: 2374–79 (1997).

Figure 17-10: Centers for Disease Control and Prevention. "Targeting Tobacco Use: The Nation's Leading Cause of Death." Atlanta: Centers for Disease Control and Prevention, 1999.

Figure 17-11: Kawachi, I., et al. "Smoking Cessation in Relation to Total Mortality Rates in Women: A Prospective Cohort Study." *Annals of Internal Medicine* 119: 992-1000 (1993).

Figure 18-1: See source for Figure 8-7.

Figure 18-2: See source for Figure 8-7.

Figure 18-3: Liu, S., et al. "A Prospective Study of Glycemic Load, Carbohydrate Intake, and Risk of Coronary Heart Disease in US Women." *American Journal of Clinical Nutrition* 71: 1455–61 (2000).

Figure 18-4: Wolk, A., et al. "Long-term Intake of Dietary Fiber and Decreased Risk of Coronary Heart Disease Among Women." *Journal of the American Medical Association* 281: 1998–2004 (1999).

Figure 19-1: See source for Figure 7-7.

Figure 19-2: Hu, F. B., et al. "Frequent Nut Consumption and Risk of Coronary Heart Disease in Women: Prospective Cohort Study." *British Medical Journal* 317: 1341–45 (1998).

Figure 19-3: Liu, S., et al. "Whole-Grain Consumption and Risk of Coronary Heart Disease: Results from the Nurses' Health Study." *American Journal of Clinical Nutrition* 70: 412–19 (1999).

Figure 19-4: See source for Figure 9-6.

Figure 19-5: Unpublished data from the Nurses' Health Study.

Figure 20-1: See source for Figure 7-6.

Figure 20-2: See source for Figure 7-6.

Figure 20-3: See source for Figure 5-11.

Figure 20-4: See source for Figure 7-6.

Figure 21-1: See source for Figure 4-9.

Figure 22-1: See source for Figure 7-1.

Figure 22-2: See source for Figure 7-1.

Figure 22-3: See source for Figure 3-1.

Figure 22-4: Unpublished data from the Nurses' Health Study.

Figure 22-5: Grodstein, F., et al. "Postmenopausal Hormone Therapy and Mortality." *New England Journal of Medicine* 336: 1769–75 (1997).

Figure 23-1: See source for Figure 12-5.

Figure 23-2: See source for Figure 11-4.

Figure 23-3: See source for Figure 5-13.

Figure 23-4: Copyright © Harriet Greenfield.

Figure 23-5: See source for Figure 12-6.

Figure 24-1: Iso H, et al. "Prospective Study of Aspirin Use and Risk of Stroke in Women." *Stroke* 30: 1764–71 (1999).

Figure 24-2: See source for Figure 24-1.

# Senior Editors

**Susan E. Hankinson, R.N., Sc.D.** is an associate professor of medicine at Harvard Medical School, associate professor of epidemiology at the Harvard School of Public Health, and epidemiologist at Brigham and Women's Hospital. She has been an investigator with the Nurses' Health Study for the past fourteen years and has a primary interest in the relationship between hormones and cancer risk.

**Graham A. Colditz, M.D., Dr.P.H.** is a professor of medicine at Harvard Medical School, professor of epidemiology at the Harvard School of Public Health, and epidemiologist at Brigham and Women's Hospital. Dr. Colditz is the current principal investigator of the Nurses' Health Study. He has been with the Nurses' Health Study for twenty years, and his research has focused on the causes and prevention of cancer.

**JoAnn E. Manson, M.D., Dr.P.H.** is a professor of medicine at Harvard Medical School, professor of epidemiology at the Harvard School of Public Health, and chief of the Division of Preventive Medicine at Brigham and Women's Hospital. Dr. Manson has been an investigator with the Nurses' Health Study for the past seventeen years and has a primary interest in the prevention of cardiovascular disease and diabetes. She is also codirector of the Connors Center for Women's Health and Gender Biology at Brigham and Women's Hospital.

**Frank E. Speizer, M.D.** is the Edward H. Kass Professor of Medicine at Harvard Medical School, professor of environmental science at the Harvard School of Public Health, and senior physician and co-director of the Channing Laboratory at Brigham and Women's Hospital. Dr. Speizer is the founding principal investigator of the Nurses' Health Study. In recognition of the accomplishments of the Nurses' Health Study, Dr. Speizer has won many honors, including the Mott Prize, the prestigious award of the General Motors Cancer Research Foundation.

## WRITERS

**Hank Dart, M.S.** has a master's of science in health and social behavior from the Harvard School of Public Health. Currently working for the Harvard Center for Cancer Prevention, he has over ten years of health communication experience.

**Catherine Tomeo Ryan, M.P.H.** has a master's of public health in epidemiology from the Boston University School of Public Health. She has been involved in health-related research and communication for the past five years.